Veterinary Technician's Daily Reference Guide
Canine and Feline

Veterinary Technician's Daily Reference Guide

Canine and Feline

Candyce M. Jack, LVT
Sequim, Washington

Patricia M. Watson, LVT
Redmond, Washington

Mark S. Donovan, DVM
Consulting Editor
Seattle, Washington

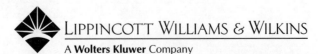

LIPPINCOTT WILLIAMS & WILKINS
A **Wolters Kluwer** Company

Philadelphia · Baltimore · New York · London
Buenos Aires · Hong Kong · Sydney · Tokyo

Editor: David Troy
Managing Editor: Rebecca Kerins
Marketing Manager: Paul Jarecha
Production Editor: Paula C. Williams
Designer: Armen Kojoyian
Compositor: Graphic World, Inc.
Printer: Data Reproductions Corp.

351 West Camden Street
Baltimore, Maryland 21201-2436 USA

530 Walnut Street
Philadelphia, Pennsylvania 19106-3621 USA

The publisher is not responsible (as a matter of product liability, negligence, or otherwise) for any injury resulting from any material contained herein. This publication contains information relating to general principles of medical care which should not be construed as specific instructions for individual patients. Manufacturers' product information and package inserts should be reviewed for current information, including contraindications, dosages, and precautions.

Printed in the United States of America

Library of Congress Cataloging-in-Publication Data
Jack, Candyce.
    Veterinary technician's daily reference guide: canine and feline / Jack Candyce, Patricia Watson.
       p. cm.
    Includes bibliographical references.
    ISBN 0-7817-3202-6
       1.Veterinary medicine—Handbooks, manuals, etc. I. Watson, Patricia. II. Title.

SF748 .J33 2002
636.089—dc21

                                                                    2002028646

The publishers have made every effort to trace the copyright holders for borrowed material. If they have inadvertently overlooked any, they will be pleased to make the necessary arrangements at the first opportunity.

To purchase additional copies of this book call our customer service department at **(800) 638-3030** or fax orders to **(301) 824-7390.** International customers should call **(301) 714-2324.**

Visit Lippincott Williams & Wilkins on the Internet: **http://www.lww.com.** Lippincott Williams & Wilkins customer service representatives are available from 8:30 am to 6:00 pm, EST, Monday through Friday, for telephone access.

02 03 04 05
1 2 3 4 5 6 7 8 9 10

This book is dedicated to all the licensed veterinary technicians doing their best for the advancement of the field and devoting themselves to providing the best care to their animal patients.

A special thanks to our medical editor, Dr. Mark Donovan, without his dedication and commitment to our goal we would not have been able to complete this book.

Patricia

To my husband, my daughter and my son, without whose patience, support and sacrifice, I would not have been able to accomplish this project.

Candyce

To JJ and Brenden—Thank you for your continuous patience, understanding and support throughout this project, without you it would not have been possible.

To my mentors:

Stu Spencer, DVM—Thank you for the constant encouragement and push to reach an even higher level of knowledge. I also thank you for helping me keep my eyes open in all aspects of veterinary medicine.

Linda Merrill, LVT—Thank you for your support and for showing me through example the high level an LVT can achieve.

Preface

The presentation of *Veterinary Technician's Daily Reference Guide: Canine and Feline* marks an exciting time for the veterinary technology profession. This manual provides a link between the formal learning environment and the daily clinical setting. Its purpose is not to present ideas for the first time, but to refresh the veterinary technician's memory about information that has already been learned and skills that have already been mastered. The goal is to increase confidence and allow veterinary technicians to provide clear client education.

This book covers all areas of the veterinary technology profession pertinent to canines and felines, from the basics of physical examinations to chemotherapy administration. We are confident that the veterinary technician will find a daily need for this invaluable resource. In the end, it is our goal that this book will facilitate improved care for patients and the owners that rely on experienced veterinary technicians.

SUMMARY OF KEY FEATURES

Comprehensive Guide. This book was written as a quick reference guide. Its purpose is to assist an already trained and licensed veterinary technician throughout the work day—providing a refresher for a seldom-taken radiograph, for example, or a pharmacology reminder to help answer a client's question. The veterinary technology student will also find this book useful as a supplement to more in-depth textbooks as they finish training and join the workforce.

Unique Chart and Table Format. The format of this book uses charts and tables for the efficient retrieval of pertinent information. As a result, very little prose text has been included. This unique format leads technicians straight to the answers they need to perform a task quickly.

Extensive Art Program. The art program, which includes more than 150 illustrations and photographs, will provide visual assistance to the technician performing laboratory tests, dentistry, client education, and much more. The color insert makes the artwork very clear and easy to use.

It is our expectation that this book will be of great assistance to the veterinary technician. Use of this book should result in enhanced performance of a veterinary technician's duties and, therefore, improved care for patients.

Candyce Jack, LVT
Patricia Watson, LVT

SUMMARY OF KEY FEATURES

Acknowledgments

We would like to express our heartfelt thanks to all the people who gave support and guidance during the forming of this book. We also appreciate the professional courtesy extended by Phoenix Laboratory, DentaLabels, the Iowa State University Press, Anne Rains, Dr. David Stansfield/ Novartis, Dr. James H. Meinkoth/ Oklahoma State University, Gary Averbeck, Dr. Robert K. Ridley/ Kansas State University, and Dr. Jay R Georgi.

Contributors

Bob Kramer	DVM, Diplomate ACVR
Brita Kraabel	DVM
Cindy Elston	DVM
Jeb Mortimer	DVM
Laura Tautz-Hair	RVT
Linda Merrill	RVT
Lisa Coyne	BS, RVT
Pat Richardson	DVM, MS
Richard Panzer	DVM, MS
Sandy Willis	DVM, MVSc, Diplomate ACVIM
Stu Spencer	DVM

x

Contents

Anatomy

For a veterinary technician to be able to accurately complete many of his or her daily tasks, a clear understanding of the anatomy of the canine and feline body is needed. The following diagrams show the basic layout of the body systems, highlighting the areas of interest that are most commonly accessed in daily medicine practices ranging from the correctly positioned radiograph to a single-stick venipuncture.

*Eye, ear, and urogenital drawings are found in Chapter 6.

OVERALL

See Figure 1-1 for overall anatomy.

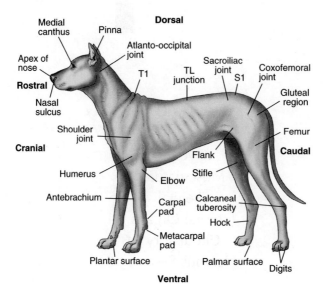

Figure 1-1 Overall.

MUSCULATURE

See Figure 1-2 for the lateral view of the musculature.

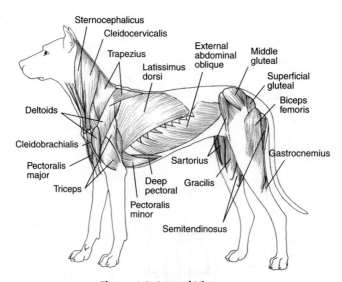

Figure 1-2 Lateral View.

SKELETAL

See Figure 1-3 for a lateral view of the skeletal system. See Figure 1-4 for a dorsal view of the skeletal system.

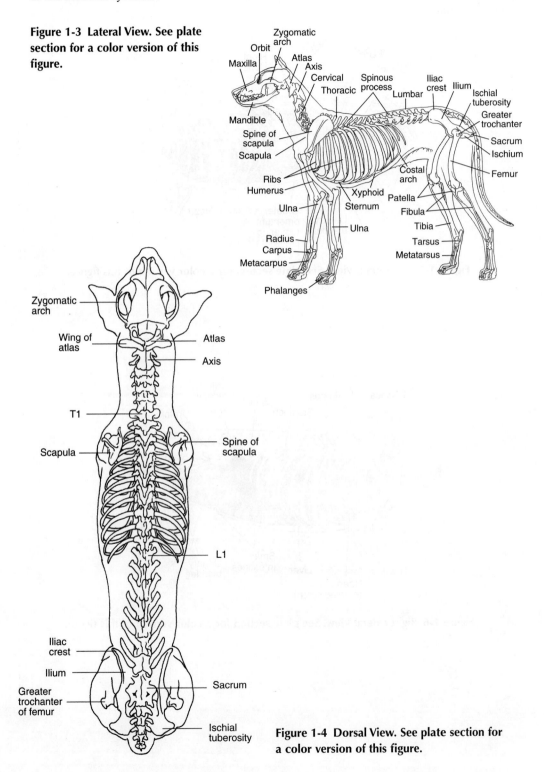

Figure 1-3 Lateral View. See plate section for a color version of this figure.

Figure 1-4 Dorsal View. See plate section for a color version of this figure.

INTERNAL ORGANS

See Figure 1-5 for the left lateral view of the internal organs. See Figure 1-6 for the right lateral view of the internal organs. See Figure 1-7 for the ventral view of the internal organs.

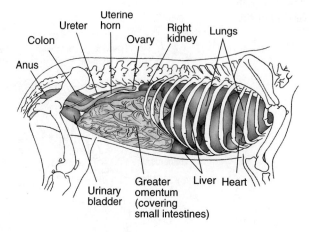

Figure 1-5 Left Lateral View. See plate section for a color version of this figure.

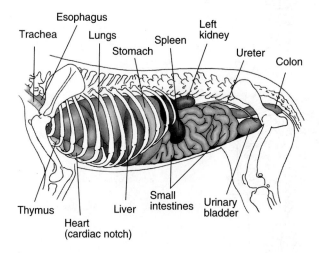

Figure 1-6 Right Lateral View. See plate section for a color version of this figure.

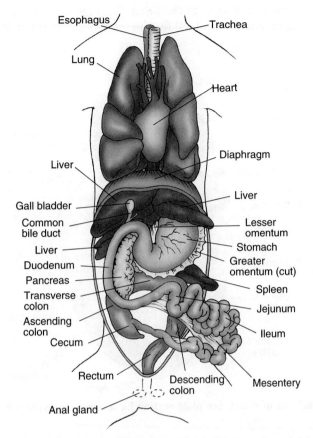

Esophagus

Trachea

Lung

Heart

Diaphragm

Liver

Liver

Gall bladder

Lesser omentum

Common bile duct

Stomach

Liver

Greater omentum (cut)

Duodenum

Pancreas

Spleen

Transverse colon

Jejunum

Ascending colon

Ileum

Cecum

Rectum

Descending colon

Mesentery

Anal gland

Figure 1-7 Ventral View. See plate section for a color version of this figure.

CIRCULATORY

See Figure 1-8 for the dorsal view of the heart. See Figure 1-9 for the lateral view of the circulatory system. See Figure 1-10 for the inside view of the heart.

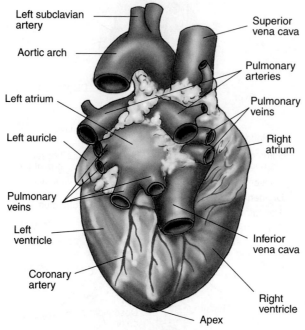

Figure 1-8 Dorsal View of Heart. See plate section for a color version of this figure.

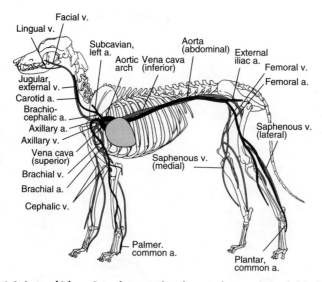

Figure 1-9 Lateral View. See plate section for a color version of this figure.

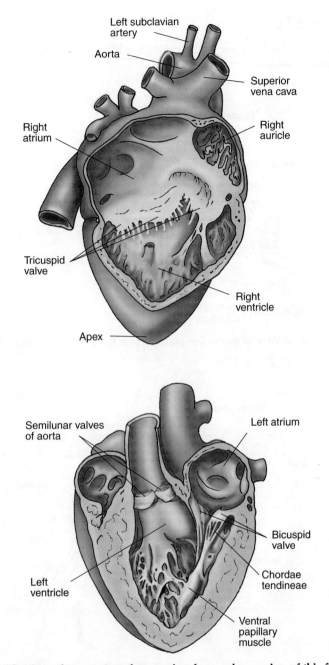

Figure 1-10 Inside View of Heart. See plate section for a color version of this figure.

NERVOUS SYSTEM

See Figure 1-11 for a lateral view of the brain. See Figure 1-12 for a lateral view of the nervous system.

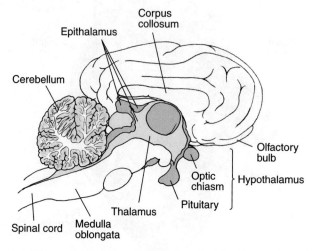

Figure 1-11 Lateral View of Brain. See plate section for a color version of this figure.

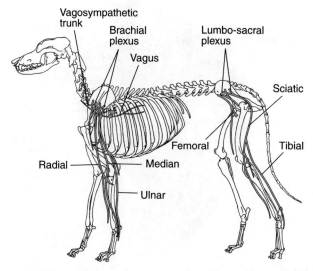

Figure 1-12 Lateral View. See plate section for a color version of this figure.

Chapter 2

Anesthesia

Anesthesia is a part of veterinary medicine often required to provide patient restraint, loss of consciousness, the elimination of pain sensation during surgical and medical procedures, and control of seizure activity. The safe and effective use of anesthetic agents is the key component in anesthesia administration. This requires a general understanding of both the pharmacologic actions of several different agents and the performance of several procedures.

Anesthesia requires a thorough preanesthetic evaluation of every patient. This evaluation aids in the formulation of an anesthesic plan based on patient characteristics, the surgical or medical procedure to be performed, drug availability, and the experience of the anesthetist. Careful monitoring is needed throughout the anesthetic period.

ANESTHETIC DRUGS
Preanesthetics

Table 2-1   Anticholinergics

Drug Class	Anticholinergics
DRUG (TRADE NAME)	• Atropine sulfate • Glycopyrrolate (Robinul-V)
MODE OF ACTION	• Works on muscarinic receptors of the parasympathetic nervous system by blocking the action of the neurotransmitter, acetylcholine • Reverses the effects of the parasympathetic nervous system
PHYSICAL EFFECTS	• ↓ Oral, pharyngeal, and respiratory tract secretions • Pupil dilation • Bronchial dilation • Prevention of bradycardia • ↓ GI motility • Blocks vagal nerve stimulation
USES	• Preanesthetic • Treatment of sinus bradycardia, sinoatrial arrest, and incomplete atrioventricular (AV) block • Treatment of bronchoconstrictive disease • Antidote of organophosphate poisoning
MONITORING	• Heart rate and rhythm • Thirst/appetite, urination/defecation correlation • Mouth; secretions and dryness
NOTES	• Glycopyrrolate has a ↓ chance of tachycardia over atropine; as well as a ↓ chance of cardiac dysrhythmias, and it suppresses salivation more thoroughly • Glycopyrrolate does not cross the blood–brain barrier or placental barriers • Can counter bradycardia that develops from laryngeal or ocular stimulation and other vagovagal stimulation

Table 2-2   Anticholinergic Drugs

Drug Class	Anticholinergics	
DRUG (TRADE NAME)	Atropine	Glycopyrrolate (Robinul-V)
DOSE/ROUTE/ DURATION	*Dose:* 0.01-0.02 mg/lb *Route:* SQ, IM, IV *Duration:* 60–90 minutes	*Dose:* 0.005 mg/lb *Route:* SQ, IM, IV *Duration:* 2–4 hours
METABOLISM	*Dog:* kidney and excreted in the urine *Cat:* liver	*Same as atropine*
PRECAUTIONS	• Mydriasis, especially in cats (can cause retinal damage if exposed to bright light for an extended period because of reduced pupillary light reflex) • Decreased tear production (eyes should be protected with an ophthalmic ointment to prevent corneal drying, especially if using ketamine) • Bronchodilation (increases the dead space and can cause thick mucous secretions, especially in cats) • Do not mix with diazepam • Increased risk of cardiac dysrhythmias and sinus tachycardia in dogs	*Same as atropine*
CONTRAINDICATIONS	• Tachycardia (dogs: >140 beats/min; cats: >160 beats/min) • Congestive heart failure • Constipation or ileus	*Same as atropine*
TOXICITY	• Dogs are more susceptible to toxicity than are cats • Drowsiness, dry mucous membranes, thirst, excitability, dilated pupils, tachycardia, and depression	*Same as atropine*

Tranquilizers and Sedatives

Table 2-3   Phenothiazines

Drug Class	Phenothiazines
DRUG (TRADE NAME)	• Acepromazine maleate (Promace)
MODE OF ACTION	• Depresses the reticular activating center of the brain
PHYSICAL EFFECTS	• Calming effect • Muscle relaxant • ↓ Motor activity • ↑ Threshold for responding to external stimuli • ↑ Analgesic effects of other drugs even though they are not personally noted for producing any analgesic qualities themselves • Antiemetic effect is very obvious at low doses during the anesthetic period, a GI upset, or motion sickness
USES	• Preanesthetic agent • Tranquilizer • Antiemetic • Antispasmodic • Antidysrhythmic effects
MONITORING	• Degree of tranquilization • Cardiac rate and rhythm • Blood pressure • Body temperature
NOTES	• Protect from light • Minimal effects on the cardiac and respiratory systems • ↓ Seizure threshold

Table 2-4 Phenothiazine Drugs

Drug Class	Phenothiazines
DRUG (TRADE NAME)	Acepromazine maleate (Promace)
DOSE/ROUTE/DURATION	*Dose: (sedation)* Dogs: 0.05-0.2 mg/lb Cats: 0.05-0.3 mg/lb *Route:* PO, SQ, IM, IV (cautiously) *Duration:* 4–8 hours
METABOLISM	Liver
PRECAUTIONS	• Lowers seizure threshold • Peripheral vasodilation (possibly leading to hypothermia or hypotension) • Excitement rather than sedation • Prolonged recovery in aged animals or those with portocaval shunts
CONTRAINDICATIONS	• Patients with epilepsy, shock, head trauma, or those undergoing procedures such as a myelogram • Geriatric, neonatal, and patients who have compromised liver may have an increased potency (cut dose by $^1/_2$) • Allergy skin testing (prevents the release of histamine therefore reducing allergic reactions)
TOXICITY	• Seizures • Hypotension • Hypothermia

Table 2-5   Benzodiazepines

Drug Class	Benzodiazepines
DRUG (TRADE NAME)	• Diazepam (Valium, Vazepam) • Midazolam HCl (Versed)
MODE OF ACTION	• Releases an inhibitory neurotransmitter in the brain, gamma-aminobutyric acid (GABA)
PHYSICAL EFFECTS	• Antianxiety and calming effect • Skeletal muscle relaxation • Anticonvulsant activity
USES	• Preanesthetic • Sedative • In animals experiencing seizures, those undergoing procedures that commonly result in seizures postoperatively (cerebrospinal fluid taps or myelograms), or with drugs that lower the seizure threshold (ketamine, opioids, and local anesthetics) • Oral diazepam may be used to curb inappropriate urination in cats • IV diazepam may be used as an appetite stimulant for cats; it is transient and dose dependent
MONITORING	• Level of sedation • Respiratory and cardiovascular function
NOTES	• Class IV controlled substance • Protect from light • Diazepam should not be stored in plastic syringes, bags, or tubing; it is readily absorbed into the plastic • Diazepam may increase the effects of digoxin • Minimal adverse effects on the cardiovascular and respiratory systems • Oral diazepam is a controlled drug that is not licensed for use in animals in the United States

Table 2-6   Benzodiazepine Drugs

Drug Class	Benzodiazepines	
DRUG (TRADE NAME)	Diazepam (Valium, Vazepam)	Midazolam (Versed)
DOSE/ROUTE/ DURATION	*Dose:* 0.1–0.2 mg/lb *Route:* IV *Duration:* 1–4 hours	*Dose:* 0.03–0.1 mg/lb *Route:* IM, IV *Duration* 2 hours (*in humans*)
METABOLISM	Liver and excreted in the urine and feces	Liver
PRECAUTIONS	• Rapid IV administration may cause bradycardia because of the propylene glycol in the formulation • Not best used as a sole anesthetic agent because it does not produce sedation • May cause significant thrombophlebitis • Crosses placenta	• Rapid IV administration may cause bradycardia because of the propylene glycol in the formulation • Not best used as a sole anesthetic agent because it does not produce sedation • May cause significant thrombophlebitis
CONTRAINDICATIONS	• Do not mix with atropine, acepromazine, barbiturates, or opioids because they will produce a precipitate • May cause either sedation or excitement in dogs • May cause behavior modification in cats; irritability or depression	• Do not mix with atropine, acepromazine, barbiturates, or opioids because they will produce a precipitate • May cause either sedation or excitement in dogs • May cause behavior modification in cats; irritability or depression
TOXICITY	• Ataxia • Central nervous system depressant • Confusion, coma, and decreased reflexes • Hypotension	• Ataxia • Central nervous system depressant • Respiratory depression • Confusion, coma, and decreased reflexes

Table 2-7 Alpha-2 Agonists

Drug Class	Alpha-2 Agonists
DRUG (TRADE NAME)	• Xylazine (Rompun, AnaSed, Gemini) • Medetomidine (Domitor)
MODE OF ACTION	• Stimulates alpha-2 receptors, causing a decrease in the level of the neurotransmitter, norepinephrine, released in the brain
PHYSICAL EFFECTS	• Calming and sedation • Muscle relaxation • Suppresses salivation, gastric secretions, and gastrointestinal motility; can trigger emesis
USES	• Preanesthetic • Sedation • Short periods of analgesia • Induce vomiting in cats after ingestion of toxins • Stimulate appetite in low doses
MONITORING	• Level of anesthesia and analgesia • Respiratory function • Cardiovascular function • Body temperature
NOTES	• Xylazine has the highest rate of anesthetic complications and death • Medetomidine is more potent than xylazine, with fewer side effects; however, it is not licensed for use in cats in the United States • Atropine is often given in conjunction with xylazine to counteract the vomiting and cardiovascular changes • Affects glucose values after drug administration; suppresses insulin release, causing increased plasma glucose concentration and glucosuria

Table 2-8   Alpha-2 Agonist Drugs

Drug Class	Alpha-2 Agonists	
DRUG (TRADE NAME)	Xylazine (Rompun, AnaSed, Gemini)	Medetomidine (Domitor)
DOSE/ROUTE/ DURATION	*Dose:* 0.2–0.5 mg/lb IV 0.05–1 mg/lb SQ, IM *Route:* SQ, IM, IV, epidurally and subarachnoidally *Duration:* 20–40 minutes	*Dose:* Dogs: 13.5–18 mg/lb IM 9–13.5 mg/lb IV Cats: 27–54.5 mg/lb IM 18–36 mg/lb IV • If using a premedication, dose can be cut by 50% *Route:* IM, IV, sublingually *Duration:* 45–90 minutes
METABOLISM	Liver and excreted in the urine	Liver and excreted in the urine
PRECAUTIONS	• Vomiting (50% of dogs and 90% of cats) usually seen within 3–5 minutes; to prevent aspiration, do not induce further anesthesia until after this time • Severe respiratory depression • Hypotension (initial increase and then subsequent decrease) • Bradyarrhythmias • Cardiac output possible decrease of 30%–50% • Depresses thermoregulatory mechanism • Can be absorbed through skin abrasions and mucous membranes (should be handled carefully)	• Mucous membranes cannot be used as a vital sign for oxygen saturation; they may appear blanched or cyanotic • Bradycardia • Respiratory depression • Depressed thermoregulatory mechanism • ↓ Blood pressure

Table 2-8 Alpha-2 Agonist Drugs (Continued)

Drug Class	Alpha-2 Agonists
CONTRAINDICATIONS	• Brachycephalic breeds (may cause stridor and dyspnea and depresses the swallowing reflex) • Patients with a history of cardiac or respiratory disease • Highly excited or nervous patients (may produce ataxia, violent reactions, or inadequate response) • Dogs prone to gastric dilatation or torsion (may cause abdominal distension) • Animals taking epinephrine	• Patients with history of cardiac disease, respiratory disorders, renal or hepatic disease • Animals in shock, severely debilitated, or stressed because of extreme heat, cold, or fatigue • Breeding or pregnant dogs • Highly excited or nervous patients should be calmed before administration and then let sit quietly for 10–15 minutes • Animals younger than 12 weeks old
TOXICITY	• Cardiac arrhythmias • Hypotension • Respiratory depression • Profound CNS depression • Seizures	• Bradycardia • Occasional AV block • Respiratory depression • Hypothermia • Vomiting • Hyperglycemia
ANTAGONIST	• Yohimbine: 0.05 mg/lb IV slowly • Tolazoline: 1–2 mg/lb IV slowly	• Atipamezole (Antisedan) give an equal volume (mL per mL) as medetomidine IM • Dose will be 5× the concentration of medetomidine • 1/2 the volume may be given IV if 45 minutes has elapsed since administration of medetomidine • May repeat 1/2 of the IM dose 10–15 minutes after atipamezole

Table 2-9   Opioids

Drug Class	Opioids
DRUG (TRADE NAME)	• Butorphanol (Torbutrol, Torbugesic) • Oxymorphone (Numorphan) • Fentanyl (Sublimaze) • Meperidine (Demerol)
MODE OF ACTION	• Acts on 3 different receptors (mu, kappa, and sigma) found within the brain • Each agent affects different receptors or combinations of receptors in different ways
PHYSICAL EFFECTS	• Central nervous system depression or excitement • Respiratory depression • Gastrointestinal function; nausea, vomiting, hypermotility, and defecation • Bradycardia • Hypotension • Cough suppression, except oxymorphone • Miosis in dogs and mydriasis in cats • Increased response to noise • Excessive salivation
USES	• Preanesthetics • Induction agents • Analgesia
MONITORING	• Respiratory and cardiovascular function
NOTES	• Rapid IV administration in dogs can cause excitement • Avoid fentanyl in cats • Meperidine usually does not cause vomiting and defecation, and fentanyl usually does not cause vomiting • Opioids can be combined with local anesthetics to provide spinal analgesia for several hours • Fentanyl is a Class II controlled substance and not approved for veterinary use

Table 2-10   Opioid Drugs

Drug Class		Opioids
DRUG (TRADE NAME)	Butorphanol tartrate (Torbugesic, Torbutrol)	Oxymorphone HCl (Numorphan)
DOSE/ROUTE/ DURATION	*Dose:* Dog: 0.05 mg/lb IV 0.2 mg/lb SQ, IM Cat: 0.05 mg/lb IV 0.2 mg/lb SQ *Route:* SQ, IM, IV *Duration:* 30 min – 2 hours	*Dose:* Dog: 0.05–0.1 mg/lb IV 0.05–0.1 mg/lb SQ, IM Cat: 0.01 mg/lb IM, IV *Route:* IV, epidurally *Duration:* 2–5 hours IV and 8 hours epidurally
METABOLISM	Liver and excreted in the urine	Liver and excreted in the urine

PRECAUTIONS	• Excitement, dysphoria
	• Apnea
	• Mild bradycardia
	• Ataxia and incoordination
	• Mild decreased blood pressure
	• Rarely causes anorexia and diarrhea
	• SQ injection absorption can be unpredictable
		• Excitement in cats when given IV
		• Respiratory depression in debilitated, neonatal, or geriatric animals
		• Bradycardia
		  ↓ Blood pressure
		  ↓ Cardiac contractility
		  ↓ Gut motility
		• Crosses placenta
		• Ataxia and incoordination in cats with high doses
		• Causes initial panting in dogs

CONTRAINDICATIONS	• Hypothyroidism • Renal and hepatic disease • Animals with Addison's • Geriatric or debilitated animals • Patients with head trauma or other CNS dysfunction	• Hypothyroidism • Renal and hepatic disease • Animals with Addison's • Geriatric or debilitated animals • Animals with diarrhea caused by toxin ingestion • Animals with head traumas or acute abdominal injuries • Animals taking monoamine oxidase (MAO) inhibitors
TOXICITY	• CNS effects • Cardiovascular changes • Respiratory depression • Seizures • Diuretic response	• Cardiovascular collapse • Hypothermia • Skeletal muscle hypotonia • Respiratory depression

ANTAGONIST	Naloxone: 0.018 mg/lb SQ, IM, IV	Naloxone: 0.018 mg/lb SQ, IM, IV
DRUG (TRADE NAME)	Fentanyl (Sublimaze)	Meperidine (Demerol)
DOSE/ROUTE/ DURATION	*Dose:* 1 mL / 6.8–13.6 lb *Route:* IM, IV *Duration:* Less than 30 minutes	*Dose:* Dog: 1.1–3 mg/lb IM, IV (very slowly) Cat: 0.5–1.8 mg/lb IM, IV *Route:* SQ, IM, IV (very slowly) *Duration:* 1–2 hours
METABOLISM	Liver and excreted in the urine	Liver and excreted in the urine
PRECAUTIONS	• Do not use in cats • Respiratory depression, may persist for several hours • Bradycardia • Ataxia • Exaggerated response to loud noises • Increases amylase and lipase levels	• Poor postoperative analgesic • Mydriasis in dogs • Nausea and vomiting → Intestinal peristalsis • Bronchoconstriction in dogs when given IV • CNS depressant • Respiratory depressant • Rapid IV administration may cause histamine release, hypotension excitement, and convulsions • Do not mix with heparin sodium, aminophylline, methylprednisolone sodium succinate, thiopental sodium, thiamylal sodium, pentobarbital sodium
CONTRAINDICATIONS	• Animals with preexisting respiratory problems • Avoid use in geriatric, very ill, or debilitated animals	• Hypothyroidism • Renal and hepatic disease • Animals with Addison's • Geriatric or debilitated animals • Animals with diarrhea caused by toxin ingestion • Animals with head traumas or acute abdominal injuries
TOXICITY	• Respiratory depression • Bradycardia • CNS depression • Cardiovascular collapse • Tremors, neck rigidity, and seizures	• Cardiovascular collapse • Hypothermia • Skeletal muscle hypotonia • Respiratory depression • Seizures • CNS excitability in cats • CNS depression
ANTAGONIST	Naloxone: 0.018 mg/lb SQ, IM, IV	Naloxone: 0.018 mg/lb SQ, IM, IV

Table 2-11 Barbiturates

Drug Class	Barbiturates
DRUG (TRADE NAME)	• Pentobarbital sodium (Nembutal, Somnotol) • Thiopental sodium (Pentothal) • Thiamylal sodium (Surital, Bio-Tal) • Methohexital (Brevital)
MODE OF ACTION	• Depresses the reticular activating center of the brain, causing a loss of consciousness
PHYSICAL EFFECTS	• High degree of respiratory depression related to dose and rate of administration • Depresses intestinal motility, have poor analgesic and muscle relaxation qualities, predispose to cardiac arrhythmias, minimally depress blood pressure • ↑ Salivary secretions, resulting in coughing, hiccoughing, sneezing, or laryngospasm • Suppresses the respiratory centers in the brain • Central nervous system (CNS) depression
USES	• Sedation • Induction agents • Sole anesthetic agents • Pentobarbital is used for seizures secondary to convulsant agents and CNS toxins
MONITORING	• Levels of consciousness • Respiratory and cardiovascular function • Seizure control • Body temperature
NOTES	• Premedication with atropine or glycopyrrolate is always recommended with barbiturate administration • Administered to effect; ⅓ given IV over 3–10 seconds, animal observed for 1 minute and then more given if needed • The effects of repeated doses are cumulative, except with methohexital • Pentobarbital can be used in the treatment of seizures associated with epilepsy and strychnine poisoning • Methohexital is the preferred barbiturate for sighthounds and brachycephalic breeds because of its rapid metabolism • Their effect ends when the drug leaves the brain and is redistributed to the muscle and adipose tissues • Avoid in pregnant animals because it may cause complete inhibition of fetal respiratory movements • All animals should be intubated and oxygen administration provided

Table 2-12   Barbiturate Drugs

Drug Class	Barbiturates		
DRUG (TRADE NAME)	*Oxybarbiturates—short-acting* • Pentobarbital sodium (Nembutal, Somnotol)	*Thiobarbiturates—ultrashort-acting* • Thiopental sodium (Pentothal) • Thiamylal sodium (Surital, Bio-tal)	*Methylated barbiturates—ultrashort-acting* • Methohexital (Brevital)
DOSE/ROUTE/ DURATION	*Dose:* 7–9 mg/lb with premedication; 10–15 mg/lb without premedication given to effect *Route:* PO, IM, IV (very slowly), IP, rectal *Duration:* 30 minutes to 2 hours	*Dose:* 6–13 mg/lb given to effect • Thiamylal is slightly more potent than Thiopental • Dose based on lean body mass *Route:* IV (SQ and IM routes may be used, but can cause tissue necrosis) *Duration:* 10-20 minutes	*Dose:* 2.3–4 mg/lb *Route:* IV *Duration:* 5–10 minutes
METABOLISM	Liver and excreted in the urine	Liver and excreted in the urine	Liver and excreted in the urine
PRECAUTIONS	• Euthanasia dose is only 2 times the anesthesia dose • Crosses the placenta • Respiratory depression • Hypothermia • Initial decrease in blood pressure • Repeated administration is cumulative and may cause excitement during recovery and an extended recovery time • Do not mix with butorphanol tartrate, glycopyrrolate, Penicillin G potassium, meperidine HCl, cimetidine, and diphenhydramine HCl • Stored at room temperature	• Doses are reduced by 80% in debilitated or sedated animals • Perivascular infiltration may cause local necrosis (infuse area with saline to decrease necrosis, and inject with 2% lidocaine to decrease pain) • Transient apnea, decreased blood pressure, and dysrhythmias may be seen with rapid induction, especially in cats • Muscle relaxation and poor analgesic • Repeated administration is cumulative • Solution is only stable for 3 days at room temperature or 7 days refrigerated; air injected into the bottle may give premature precipitation • Crosses placenta	• Because of excitement during recovery, a premedication is always recommended • Postoperative seizures are treated with diazepam • Recovery may be seen by pronounced involuntary excitement and convulsions • Crosses placenta

Table 2-12 Barbiturate Drugs (Continued)

Drug Class	Barbiturates	
CONTRAINDICATIONS	• Avoid use in sighthounds because of slow metabolism, low body fat, and being heavily muscled • Pregnant animals—almost completely inhibits fetal respiratory movements • Do not use in animals with lidocaine intoxication–induced seizures • Animals with respiratory, cardiac, or hepatic disease • Animals with signs of hypovolemic shock or anemia • Female cats are especially sensitive to respiratory depression	• Avoid use in sighthounds because of slow metabolism, low body fat, and being heavily muscled • Pregnant animals—almost completely inhibits fetal respiratory movements • Animals with cardiovascular disease, preexisting ventricular arrhythmias, shock, myasthenia gravis, asthma, or increased intracranial pressure	• Pregnant animals—almost completely inhibits fetal respiratory movements
TOXICITY	• Respiratory and cardiovascular depression • Hypothermia • Hypotension • Mimics shock	• Respiratory and cardiovascular depression • Hypothermia • Hypotension	• Respiratory depression

Table 2-13   Cyclohexamines

Drug Class	Cyclohexamines
DRUG (TRADE NAME)	• Ketamine (Ketaset, Ketalean, Vetalar) • Tiletamine (Telazol)
MODE OF ACTION	• Acts by disruption of the nervous system pathways within the cerebrum and a stimulation of the reticular activating center of the brain • Induces a state of anesthesia and amnesia by over stimulating the CNS or inducing a cataleptic state
PHYSICAL EFFECTS	• Hallucinations • Confusion, agitation, and fear • ↑ Sensitivity to sound, light, and other stimuli, especially with large doses • Excessive salivation • Respiratory depression at high doses • ↑ Heart rate and blood pressure • Normal to increased muscle tone and rigidity • ↓ Corneal reflex
USES	• Restraint • Unconsciousness • Analgesia, somatic pain • Induction agent • Sole anesthetic agent for minor procedures
MONITORING	• Level of anesthesia and analgesia • Respiratory function • Cardiovascular function • Body temperature • Monitor eyes to prevent drying or injury (lubrication recommended)
NOTES	• This agent is a dissociative anesthetic that produces catalepsy • Ocular, oral, and swallowing reflexes are only weakened • The use of a premedication such as a tranquilizer, barbiturate, or benzodiazepine is recommended to relieve increased muscle tone, decrease salivation and lacrimation, and produce visceral analgesia • Its use as an induction agent is enhanced when mixed with diazepam and given IV (especially in dogs)

Table 2-14 Cyclohexamine Drugs

Drug Class	Cyclohexamines	
DRUG (TRADE NAME)	Ketamine (Ketaset, Ketalean, Vetalar, Vetaket)	Tiletamine (Telazol- 1:1 combination of zolazepam and tiletamine)
DOSE/ROUTE/ DURATION	*Dose:* Dog: ketamine 2.5 mg/lb plus diazepam 0.15 mg/lb IV or ketamine 3–5 mg/lb plus xylazine 0.3 mg/lb IV Cat: 2–5 mg/lb IM/SQ or 0.5–1 mg/lb IV • 1–3 mg total for sick cats or those with urethral obstruction *Route:* Dog: IV Cat: SQ, IM, IV *Duration:* 10–30 minutes	*Dose:* 4.5–6 mg/lb IM *Route:* IM *Duration:* 30 minutes – 1 hour
METABOLISM	Liver and excreted in the urine	Liver and excreted in the urine
PRECAUTIONS	• Tissue irritation and pain on IM injection • Eyes remain open, central, and dilated during anesthesia; use an ophthalmic ointment to prevent corneal drying • May cause personality changes that will spontaneously resolve in a few days or weeks	• Eyes remain open, central, and dilated during anesthesia; use an ophthalmic ointment to prevent corneal drying • Produces apneustic breathing • ↑ Heart rate

- Produces apneustic breathing; can induce significant respiratory depression at high doses or if given too rapidly IV
- ↑ Heart rate, blood pressure, and nystagmus
- Recovery is hyperresponsive with ataxia
- Repeated doses can accumulate in the tissues, prolonging recovery and increasing the chance of convulsions during the recovery period

- Excessive salivation
- Initial ↑ in blood pressure, then ↓
- Coughing, swallowing, corneal, and pedal reflexes remain intact
- Hypothermia
- Possible muscle rigidity during recovery
- Crosses placenta
- Animals with renal disease have a prolonged recovery
- Can be stored in the refrigerator after reconstitution for 14 days
- Prolonged recovery, 1–5 hours
- Pain on IM injection

CONTRAINDICATIONS

- Should be avoided or used with caution with patients with hyperthyroidism, cardiomyopathy, preexisting cardiac disease, cardiac dysrhythmias
- Avoid use in animals with ingestion of strychnine, metaldehyde, marijuana, organophospahtes, or those undergoing neurologic procedures, i.e., CSF tap or myelogram, eye injury, cranial trauma, hepatic disease in dogs and renal disease in cats, or epilepsy

- Animals with pancreatic disease, severe cardiac disease, and/or pulmonary disease

TOXICITY

- Respiratory depression

- Respiratory depression leading to apnea

Table 2-15 Neuroleptanalgesics

Drug Class	Neuroleptanalgesics
DRUG (TRADE NAME)	• Innovar-Vet (the only commercial product is a combination of fentanyl and droperidol)
MODE OF ACTION	• See sections on opioids and phenothiazines
PHYSICAL EFFECTS	• Central nervous system depressant • Bradycardia • Sedation, ataxia, recumbency • Possible apnea • Stimulates defecation and flatulence • Hypotension
USES	• Analgesic • Short anesthetic procedures and cesarean sections
MONITORING	• Level of neuroleptanalgesia • Respiratory and cardiovascular function
NOTES	• Class II controlled substance • Can be used with barbiturates to increase muscle relaxation and eliminate stimulatory effects of loud noises • Protect from light

Table 2-16 Neuroleptanalgesic Drugs

Drug Class	Neuroleptanalgesics
DRUG (TRADE NAME)	Innovar-Vet (Fentanyl and Droperidol)
DOSE/ROUTE/ DURATION	*Dose:* Dog: 1 mL/40 lb IM; Cat: 1 mL/20 lb SQ. *Route:* SQ, IM, IV. *Duration:* 30 minutes – 1.5 hours
METABOLISM	Liver
PRECAUTIONS	• Respiratory depression • Bradycardia in dogs and tachycardia in cats • Ataxia • Excitement • CNS and behavioral abnormalities in some breeds • Defecation and flatulence • Panting • Nystagmus • ↑ Amylase and lipase values for 24 hours
CONTRAINDICATIONS	• Australian terriers may be resistant
TOXICITY	• Profound hypotension • Respiratory depression • Cardiovascular collapse • CNS depression • Tremors, neck rigidity, and seizures
ANTAGONIST	• Naloxone 0.018 mg/lb SQ, IM, IV

Table 2-17 Propofol

Drug Class	Propofol
DRUG (TRADE NAME)	Propofol (Diprivan, Rapinovet, PropoFlo)
MODE OF ACTION	• Induces depression by enhancing the effects of the inhibitory neurotransmitter GABA and decreasing the brain's metabolic activity • It is a short-acting hypnotic agent, unlike any other anesthetic agent
PHYSICAL EFFECTS	• Respiratory depression if given rapidly or at high doses • Hypotension • Bradycardia • ↓ Intraocular pressure • ↑ Appetite • Antiemetic properties
USES	• Sedation/short anesthesia (up to 20 min) • Induction agent • Animals with preexisting cardiac dysrhythmias
MONITORING	• Level of anesthesia • CNS effects • Respiratory depression • Cardiovascular function
NOTES	• Protect from light and shake well before using • Little to no analgesic properties • Short duration because of rapid redistribution from CNS to peripheral tissue

Table 2-18 Propofol

Drug Class	Propofol
DRUG (TRADE NAME)	Propofol (Diprivan, Rapinovet, PropoFlo)
DOSE/ROUTE/ DURATION	*Dose:* Induction: 1–3 mg/lb (Give 25% of dose every 30 seconds until intubation possible) Maintenance: 0.1–0.3 mg/lb/min *Route:* IV *Duration:* 2–5 minutes for each single bolus
METABOLISM	Liver and excreted in the urine
PRECAUTIONS	• Product must be used within 24 hours to prevent iatrogenic sepsis • Bradycardia • Respiratory depression and initial apnea • Hypotension • ↓ Intraocular pressure • ↑ Appetite • Antiemetic properties • Crosses placenta • Minimal analgesic action
CONTRAINDICATIONS	• Animals with systemic infections • Animals who have seizures • Use with caution in animals that are experiencing shock or stress or have undergone trauma • Avoid use with any premedication using acepromazine or opiates because of exacerbation of bradycardia and hypotension
TOXICITY	• Respiratory depression • Cardiovascular depression

Table 2-19   Inhalant Agents

Inhalant agents are routinely used to provide general anesthesia through muscle relaxation. Their mode of action is unknown, but two possiblities exist; 1) by inhibiting the breakdown of GABA, an inhibitory neurotransmitter or 2) by causing nerve cell membranes to lose their ability to conduct nerve impulses. Inhalant agent monitoring should include the level of anesthesia, respiratory and ventilatory function, cardiac rate and rhythm and blood pressure.

Drug Class	Inhalants			
	Nitrous oxide	Isoflurane (Aerrane, Isoflo, Florane)	Halothane (Fluothane)	Sevoflurane (Sevoflo, Ultane)
DRUG (TRADE NAME)				
ATTRIBUTES	• Can lower the levels of other inhalant agents when nitrous oxide is used • Speeds the uptake of other agents because of the "second-gas effect" • Rapid induction and recovery • Good analgesia and muscle relaxation • Little effect on respiratory, cardiovascular, hepatic, and urinary systems	• Extremely rapid induction and recovery • Great for mask and chamber induction • Recovery in 1–2 minutes after discontinuation of gas • Used for animals with cardiac disease, liver and kidney disease, and neonatal and geriatric animals • Excellent muscle relaxation	• Produces muscle relaxation and slight analgesia • Fairly rapid induction and recovery • Mask induction takes approximately 10 minutes in a tranquilized animal • Recovery takes less than 1 hour to achieve sternal recumbency	• Extremely rapid induction and recovery • Great for mask and chamber induction • Produces muscle relaxation and analgesia • Nonpungent odor
DOSE	• Maintenance concentration of 50%–66% • $N_2O:O_2 = 1:1$ or 2:1	• 5% induction • 0.5%–2.5% maintenance	• 3% induction • 0.5%–1.5% maintenance	• 5%–7% induction • 3.3%–4% maintenance
METABOLISM	• Rapid elimination through the lungs—completely in 2 minutes	• 99% eliminated unchanged by the alveoli • 0.17% metabolized by the liver	• Mostly eliminated by the lungs • 12%–40% is metabolized by the liver, and metabolites are excreted by the kidneys	• Rapid elimination through the lungs

PRECAUTIONS	• Do not use at concentrations greater than 70% • Oxygen must be kept at 30 mL/kg/min • Do not use in a closed anesthetic system, because it can displace oxygen in alveoli • Animals must be left on pure oxygen for 5–10 minutes postoperatively	• Progressive vasodilation and decreased blood pressure occur with deeper levels of anesthesia • Rapid recovery and no analgesia postoperatively can lead to pain and excitement (i.e., emergence delirium) • Respiratory depression • Slight decrease in cardiac output • Decrease in smooth muscle tone and motility • Crosses placenta • Depression of body temperature • Gastrointestinal effects; nausea, vomiting, and ileus	• Sensitizes the heart to catecholamines to give possible dysrhythmias • Decreased cardiac output • Increased vagal tone, possibly leading to bradycardia • Increased vasodilation, leading to possible hypothermia and decreased blood pressure • Depression of respiration rate and tidal volume • Depresses central nervous system • Pupils may be constricted at all stages of anesthesia • Shallow and rapid respiration • Abdominal muscles are only relaxed at deeper levels of anesthesia • Decreased intestinal tract motility, tone, and peristaltic activity	• Crosses placenta • Not stable in moist soda lime and may release carbon monoxide • Respiratory depression, hypotension, bradycardia, shivering, and nausea • Increase in concentration may cause rapid hemodynamic changes (i.e., hypotension) • The safety of this agent has not been evaluated in geriatric, debilitated, breeding, or neonate animals
CONTRA-INDICATIONS	• Preexisting pulmonary disease • Animals with intestinal obstruction, gastric torsion, pneumothorax, or diaphragmatic hernia caused by the diffusion of N_2O into air pockets	• Animals with a history of malignant hyperthermia • Use with caution in animals with increased CSF, head injury, or myasthenia gravis	• Animals with a history of malignant hyperthermia or hepatic impairment after previous halothane exposure • Hypovolemic or hypotensive animals • Animals with cardiac arrhythmias • Use with caution in animals with increased CSF, head injury, or myasthenia gravis	• Animals with a history of malignant hyperthermia

ANESTHETIC ADMINISTRATION

The administration of anesthesia allows necessary veterinary procedures to commence without difficulty. Proper administration of anesthesia ensures the comfort of the patient during administration and during and after the procedure.

Table 2-20 Local and Regional Anesthetic Administration

Types	Area and Nerves Blocked	Uses	Drug/Dose/Duration	Equipment	Method	Associated Risks
Topical	• Area directly where drug is applied • Nerve endings in peripheral tissues	• Intubation of a cat • Desensitize the cornea and conjunctiva for procedures such as conjunctival scrapings and tonometry • Urethral catheterization	*Drug:* • Butacaine • Tetracaine • Piperocaine • Proparacaine • Cetacaine • Lidocaine *Duration:* • 3–5 minutes	• Gloves	• Sprayed or brushed onto mucous membranes • Dropped into the eye • Infused into the urethra	
Infiltration Nerve Blocks	• Any nerve	• Analgesia involving superficial tissues • Skin biopsies and small skin tumors • Repair of minor lacerations	*Drug:* • Lidocaine with epinephrine (L) • Mepivacaine (M) • Tetracaine (T) • Bupivacaine (B) *Dose:* • 1–2 mL *Duration:* • L= 2 hours • M= 90–180 minutes • T= 2 hours • B= 4–6 hours	• 23- or 25-gauge needle	• Apply a surgical preparation to surgery site. Palpate the nerve to determine its location, insert syringe and then aspirate to verify placement is not in a vessel. Inject the local anesthetic in close proximity to the nerve. The drug will then diffuse through the tissues to reach the target tissues.	• Avoid injecting directly into a nerve, because temporary or permanent nerve loss can occur • Avoid IV injection, because CNS or CV effect may occur • Do not inject into inflamed areas • Cats are more sensitive to systemic effects of (L)—avoid using >1 cc/10 lb

| Line Blocks | • Tissues immediately proximal to target area
• Placed between the target area and the spinal cord | *Same as Nerve Block* | • Surgery on an area of tissue served by many nerves
• Analgesia involving superficial tissues
• Skin biopsies and small skin tumors
• Repair of minor lacerations | *Same as Nerve Block* | • Apply a surgical preparation to surgery site. Visualize a line of infiltration that is proximal to the surgery site. Insert the needle along the proposed line of infiltration and aspiration and aspirate to verify placement is not in a blood vessel. Inject small amounts of drugs as the needle is gradually withdrawn. The drug will then diffuse through the tissues to reach the target tissues. | *Same as Nerve Block* |

Table 2-20 Local and Regional Anesthetic Administration (Continued)

Types	Area and Nerves Blocked	Uses	Drug/Dose/Duration	Equipment	Method	Associated Risks
Regional						
Intra-venous	• Extremity distal to tourniquet • Nerve endings in peripheral tissues	• Biopsies • Foreign bodies from the paw	*Drug:* • 1% lidocaine *Dose:* • 2–3 mL *Duration:* • 60–90 minutes	• 22-gauge needle, 1½ inch	• Place an IV catheter in a vein distal to the tourniquet. Apply a pressure bandage to desanguinate the limb before placing the tourniquet. Remove bandage once the tourniquet is placed. Inject 2.5–5 mg/kg 1% lidocaine intravenously. Full effects are seen in 5–10 minutes. After the procedure, the tourniquet should be removed slowly over a 5-minute period to prevent overdose of local anesthetic agents (especially in cats)	• Do not use bupivacaine • Tourniquet left on for more than 90 min can lead to tourniquet-induced ischemia; 4 hours can lead to reversible shock and over 8 hours can lead to sepsis, endotoxemia, and death • Malignant hyperthermia in susceptible animals
Epidural-Anesthesia	• L5 with a drug dose of 1 mL/10 lbs • T5 with a drug dose of 1 mL/7.5 lbs	• Animals who are severely depressed, in shock, or need immediate hindquarter surgery • Aged animals, those in high risk, or those in which anesthetics agents are contraindicated • To provide analgesia after abdominal surgery or hindquarter surgery	*Drug:* • 2% lidocaine • 0.75% bupivacaine *Dose:* • 1 mL/10 lbs *Duration:* • 4–6 hours with a drug combination including epinephrine	• 2–4 inch, 18–20 g, short bevel with stylet spinal needle • 2.5-mL and 5-mL syringe • Thin-walled, 18-g, 3-inch needle for a continuous epidural	• Apply a surgical preparation to surgery site. The bevel of spinal needle should be positioned cranially. Infiltrate the area of the lumbosacral space with 2% lidocaine by inserting the spinal needle between L7 and S1. Push the needle in a slight cranial or caudal angle as needed to a needle depth of ½ to 1½. Remove the stylet and observe for blood or CSF; if none is seen, aspirate. Inject 1–2 mL air to assure correct placement. If SQ crepitus is felt, the needle is incorrectly placed; no resistance should be felt. Then inject the drug used to achieve the correct level of anesthesia.	• Improper placement of the local anesthetic into the intervertebral space • Do not use in patients with septicemia, coagulation defects, or spinal inflammation • Respiratory depression and paralysis with drug overdose; drug needs to migrate to C5 or C7 for this effect • Hypothermia • Anesthetic in vertebral sinuses: vomiting, tremors, hypotension, convulsions, and paralysis • Malignant hyperthermia for susceptible animals

Epidural-analgesic	*Same as epidural-anesthesia*	• Rear limb lacerations or fractures, abdominal surgery, perianal surgery, cesarean sections, surgical procedures of the tail, perineum, vulva, vagina, rectum, and bladder, urethrostomies, and obstetric manipulations • Intraoperative and postoperative pain • Critical care patients	*Drug:* • Morphine (M) • Oxymorphone (O) • Fentanyl (F) *Dose:* • M= 0.045 mg/lb diluted in 0.06–0.12 mL/kg 0.9% NaCl solution • O= 0.02–0.045 mg/lb diluted in 0.12 mL/lb 0.9% NaCl solution • F = 0.45–4.5 µg/lb diluted in 0.12 mL/lb 0.9% NaCl solution *Duration:* • M= 10–24 hours • O= 10–20 hours • F= 3–5 hours	*Same as epidural-anesthesia*
		Same as epidural-anesthesia		• Respiratory depression • Urinary retention • Delayed gastrointestinal motility • Vomiting • Pruritis

Skill Box 2-1 / Intramuscular Injection

- Volume: <3 mL per site
- Locations: lumbar region, semimembranous, and semitendinosus muscles
- Injections in the rear leg
  - Avoid: the sciatic nerve, femoral artery and vein, popliteal lymph node, and femur
  - Placement: chose a posterior location on the leg, on the lateral side, and caudal to the femur. Place the needle at least a thumb's width from the femur
  - Technique: inject the needle in a slightly caudal direction, aspirate for blood, and inject contents of syringe
- Injections in the lumbar region
  - Avoid: all nerves and blood vessels
  - Placement: place your thumb on the wing of the ilium and your middle finger on a vertebra of the spine. Let your index finger fall naturally; where it lands is the location for the injection
  - Technique: inject the needle straight into the muscle, aspirate for blood, and inject contents of syringe

Table 2-21 Induction to General Anesthesia

Method of Induction	Common Drugs Used	Procedure	Uses	Associated Risks	Patient Contraindications
Oral	• Ketamine • Innovar-Vet	Draw up a single dose of the drug into a syringe and squirt into the patient's mouth	• Uncooperative animals • Animals in which injections are difficult	• Aspiration • Poor administration	• Animals with gastrointestinal disease or injury
Intramuscular	• Ketamine • Innovar-Vet	Draw up a single dose of the drug into a syringe and administer intramuscularly	• Uncooperative animals • Animals in which IV injections are difficult (i.e., puppies, kittens)	• Delayed recovery • Overdose	• Old and debilitated animals that would benefit from induction to effect (i.e., lower dosing)
Intravenous	• Ketamine • Propofol • Thiopental sodium • Oxymorphone/acepromazine	Place an IV catheter or locate vein, then administer drug by either a bolus over 10–15 seconds, slow injection over 1–2 minutes, or IV fluid drip.	• Minor anesthetic procedures • Induction to general anesthesia with inhalant anesthetics • Animals in which rapid control of the airway is needed (i.e., laryngeal collapse, bracycephalics, etc.)	• Perivascular injection • Accumulation of drug with repeated dosing (i.e., Prolonged recovery)	• Obese animals in which locating a vein may not be possible • Fractious animals
Face mask	• Isoflurane • Halothane	With adequate restraint, place an anesthetic mask over the mouth and nose tightly to minimize waste gas and dead space. Run 100% oxygen at 3 liters/min for 5 minutes to allow adjustment to mask then begin anesthetic flow slowly over a few minutes to a level of 3%–4%.	• Induction to general anesthesia with inhalant anesthetics via endotracheal tube • Premedicated animals, moribund animals, or tractable dogs	• Vomiting • No control of airway • Environmental anesthetic pollution • Can be stressful to some patients	• Brachycephalic dogs • Animals with respiratory or cardiovascular disease • Animals that have not been fasted
Chamber	• Isoflurane • Halothane	Place the animal in a chamber large enough to allow laying down and extension of the neck. Run oxygen at 3–5 liters/min and the anesthetic flow at 4%–5%. Once the animal has lost its righting reflex, remove them from the chamber and place an endotracheal tube.	• Induction to general anesthesia with inhalant anesthetics • Premedicated cats and small dogs	• Inability to adequately monitor • No control of airway • Environmental anesthetic pollution	• Brachycephalic dogs • Animals with respiratory or cardiovascular disease • Animals that have not been fasted

Skill Box 2-2 / Intravenous Injection

- Volume: large volumes can be given
- Locations: Any accessible vein (e.g., external jugular vein, cephalic vein, saphenous vein, pedal veins, lingual vein during anesthesia)
- Injections of the external jugular vein
  - Avoid: Carotid artery
  - Placement: Occlude the vein in the jugular furrow at the thoracic inlet with thumb of non-syringe hand. The head should be slightly rotated toward the injection site for better visibility. The jugular vein typically lies in the cowlick of the fur running from the ramus of the mandible to the thoracic inlet.
  - Technique: Insert the needle parallel to the skin in a cranial direction, aspirate for blood, either inject contents of syringe or withdraw blood.
- Injections of peripheral veins
  - Avoid: All nerves
  - Placement: Once vein is occluded by either a tourniquet or assistant, lay thumb alongside the vein to stabilize it
  - Technique: See above

Emla cream applied to the site 20–30 minutes before venipuncture can lessen the pain

Gentle insertion of the needle typically results in much less of a reaction than thrusting

Skill Box 2-3 / Endotracheal Intubation

Technique:

1. Place small to medium patients in sternal recumbency; larger patients can be placed in lateral recumbency
2. Open patient's mouth and gently grasp tongue with a 3×3 gauze pad (prevents slipping)
3. Extend tongue for a clear view of the throat area
4. Tube should have bevel facing up and concave side facing ventrally
5. Insert tube over the epiglottis between the arytenoid cartilages into the larynx, rotating from 0° to 90° to facilitate passage
6. Tie tube in place with gauze to prevent slippage
7. Inflate cuff to ensure no leakage of gases
   - Attach a clean syringe full of air to the tubing of the cuff. Close pop-off valve and place ear next to mouth of patient to listen for escaping air while gently squeezing reservoir bag (the pressure manometer should read less than 20 cm H_2O) Depress plunger of syringe and fill cuff with air just until no air can be heard escaping around tube. Remove syringe and open pop-off valve.

To Ensure Proper Placement:

- Verify the correct tube length
  - Tube length should be the distance from the incisor teeth to the thoracic inlet
  - Use of excessively long tubes may lead to dead space and endobronchial intubation
- Palpate throat region for only one hard structure
  - Two hard tubes indicates that the tube is in the esophagus
- Check for leaking air
  - Close pop-off valve and place ear next to mouth of patient to listen for escaping air while gently squeezing reservoir bag (the pressure manometer should read less than 20 cm H_2O)
- Absence of vocalization
- Condensation of respiratory gases on the inside of the tube during exhalation

Tips:

- Always check cuff viability before use
- Wet tube with water to lessen friction
- Use lubrication on tube (e.g., KY jelly)
- Use a stylet for small floppy tubes
- Use a laryngoscope for clearer visualization of throat
- In cats, application of lidocaine (0.1 mL) to glottis will reduce spasms
- In cats, with the index finger of the hand holding the tongue, apply pressure to the trachea to elevate the larynx for better visibility of the trachea
- In cats, placement of a mouth speculum allows one-person intubation and safety from being bitten

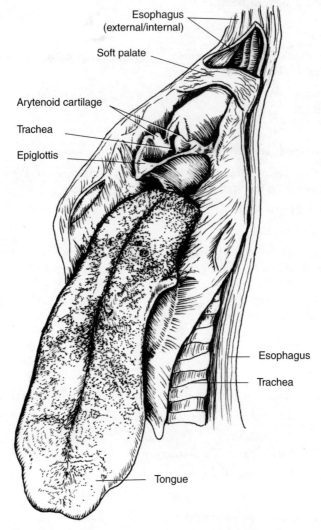

Esophagus
(external/internal)

Soft palate

Arytenoid cartilage

Trachea

Epiglottis

Esophagus

Trachea

Tongue

Figure 2-1 Endotracheal intubation

ANESTHETIC MONITORING

A variety of sophisticated and complex monitoring devices are available to monitor all situations of an anesthetic procedure. As much as these instruments are beneficial in the overall picture, nothing can take the place of an attentive and educated anesthetist. All anesthetists should be able to adequately monitor a patient under anesthesia without the use of any equipment. The equipment should be available as an assistant to monitoring, not a crutch.

Table 2-22 Stages of Anesthesia

System Affected	Characteristic Observed	Stage I	Stage II	Stage III — Plane 1 (Light)	Stage III — Plane 2 (Medium)	Stage III — Plane 3	Stage III — Plane 4 (Deep)	Stage IV
Cardiovascular	Heart rate	Normal	Increased	90–120 beats/min	Dog: 80–120 beats/min; Cat: 120–160 beats/min	Decrease	Decrease	Cardiac arrest
		Tachycardia	Tachycardia	Progressive bradycardia	Progressive bradycardia	Progressive bradycardia	Progressive bradycardia	
	Pulse	Normal	Normal	Regular and strong	Relatively strong	Weaken	Weaken	Weak or imperceptible
	Blood pressure	Normal	Hypertension	Normal	Increasing hypotension	Increasing hypotension	Increasing hypotension	Shock level
	Capillary refill time	1 second or less	1 second or less	1 second or less	Progressive delay	Progressive delay	Progressive delay	3 seconds or more
	Dysrhythmias probability	+++	+++	++	+	+	++	++++
Respiratory	Respiratory rate	Irregular or increased	Irregular or increased	12–20 breaths/min	Progressive decrease	Progressive decrease	Progressive decrease	Ceased, may gasp terminally
	Respiratory depth	Irregular or increased	Irregular or increased	Dog: 12–16 breaths/min; Cat: 20–40 breaths/min	Dog: 12–16 breaths/min; Cat: 20–40 breaths/min	Progressive decrease	Progressive decrease	Ceased
	Mucous membrane, skin color	Normal	Normal	Normal	Normal	Normal	Cyanosis	Pale to white

Table 2-22 Stages of Anesthesia (Continued)

System Affected	Characteristic Observed	Stage I	Stage II	Stage III Plane 1 Light	Plane 2 Medium	Plane 3	Plane 4 Deep	Stage IV
Respiratory (Continued)	Respiratory action	May be breath holding		Regular and smooth rhythm	Irregular rate and pattern thoracoabdominal, abdominal		Variable pattern diaphragmatic	Ceased
	Cough Reflex	+ + + +	+ + +	+	Lost			
	Laryngeal reflex	+ + +	May vocalize		Lost			
	Intubation possible		No		Yes			
Gastrointestinal	Salivation	+ + + +	+ + +	+	Diminished, absent			Absent
	Oropharyngeal reflex	+ + + +	+ + +	+		Lost		
	Vomition probability	+ + +	+ + +	+			Very slight	
	Reflux potential	None		Increases with relaxation				+ + + +
Ocular	Pupils	Constricted	Dilated	Constricted	Progressive dilation — Moderately dilated		Widely dilated	Fully dilated
	Corneal reflex	Normal	+ + +		Diminishes, lost			Absent
	Lacrimation	Normal	+ + +	+	Diminished, absent			Absent

	1	2	3	4	5	6	7
Ocular (Continued)							
Photomotor reflex	Normal	Normal	Responsive	Sluggish response	Minimal or absent response	Unresponsive	Absent
Palpebral reflex	Normal	+++	+	Diminished, absent			Absent
Eyeball position	Variable	Central	Third eyelid prolapsed		Centrally fixed		
(eyeball, cont.)			Rotated medially	Slight medial rotation			
Nystagmus	Normal	Possible nystagmus	Possible slight nystagmus		Absent		
Musculoskeletal							
Jaw tone	++++	++++		Decreased, minimal		Lost	
Limb muscle tone	++++	++++		Decreased, minimal		Lost	
Abdominal muscle tone	++++	++++	++		Decreased, minimal		Lost
Sphincters (anus, bladder)	May void			Progressive relaxation		Control lost	
Pedal reflex	++++	++++	Decreased	Absent			
Nervous							
Reaction to surgical stimulus	Increased respiratory rate and heart rate					No response	
(reaction, cont.)		Limb movement		Traction reflexes			

+ to ++++ = degree present

Table 2-23   Assessing the Depth of Anesthesia

Sign	Technique	Stage I	Stage II- Stage III, Plane 2	Stage III, Plane 3—Stage IV	Alterations With Certain Drugs
Corneal	• Touch the cornea with a sterile cotton swab, or sterile drop of water or ophthalmic ointment and observe for blinking and withdrawal of the eye into the orbital fossa	Present	Present	Absent	• Ketamine—may be retained into Stage III
Ear flick	• Gently touch the hairs on the inside of the pinna and observe for movement	Present	Maybe Present	Absent	• Ketamine—no eye rotation
Eye position	• Visual observation	Central	Ventromedial	Central	
Heart rate	• Auscultation of chest cavity • Electrocardiogram • Direct palpation	Often elevated	Variable	Often decreased	• Ketamine/atropine—increases heart rate
Laryngeal	• Touch the epiglottis and vocal cords to observe for immediate closure (i.e., endotracheal tube)	Present	May be Present	Absent	
Muscle Tone	• Open jaw to observe jaw tone • Flex and extend foreleg and observe for resistance • Observe size of anal orifice for anal tone	High	Moderate	Absent	• Diazepam/Xylazine—decreases muscle tone • Ketamine/tiletamine- increases muscle tone

Palpebral	Tap the lateral or medial canthus of the eye to observe blinking response				• Barbiturate—present • Halothane—rarely present
Pedal	Pinch or squeeze a digit or pad and observe for flexing of the leg	Maybe	None	Absent	• Pentobarbital—good sign for monitoring
Pupil size	Visual observation	Constricted	Slightly dilated	Dilated	• Atropine—may cause pupil dilation, especially in cats
Pupillary light Reflex	Shine a pen light to observe constriction of pupil	Present	Maybe	Absent	
Respiratory rate	Visual observation of movement of chest cavity Auscultation of chest cavity Pulse oximetry	Often elevated	8–30 breaths/min	Often decreased	• Almost all drugs cause some degree of respiratory change
Salivary/lacrimal secretions	Visual observation	Present	May be present	Absent	• Decreased with anticholinergics
Surgical stimuli	Visual observation of body movement, lacrimation, and salivation				
Swallowing	Sweating on foot pads Observe the ventral neck region for movement	Maybe	None	Absent	

Table 2-24   Vital Signs

Vital Sign	Significance	Normal Values	Abnormal Values	Technique Used to Evaluate Vital Sign

Heart Rate and Rhythm	• A decreased heart rate is normally seen in an anesthetized patient
	• Observance for bradycardia and cardiac rhythm
	• Cardiac function
	• Acute intraoperative blood loss can trigger compensatory tachycardia
		Dog: 70–80 beats/min
		Cat: 110–200 beats/min
			Dog: <70 beats/min
			Cat: <100 beats/min
				• *Direct palpation of chest wall or pulse*
				• *Auscultation of chest with a stethoscope*
				• *Esophageal stethoscope*
				  • A thin tube attached to a stethoscope is placed in the esophagus of the patient until an audible heartbeat is heard
				  • Allows auscultation even when patient's chest is covered during surgery
				• *Electrocardiograph (ECG)* (See Chapter 6, Cardiopulmonary)
				  • Clips are placed on the animal in a specific order to produce specific leads, typically lead II
				  • To assess the pattern and rhythm of myocardial contractions
				  • Abnormal size, duration, shape, or regularity of ECG tracing offers information on cardiac function
				• *Doppler pulse monitor*
				  • Placing a cuff on the patient to occlude a peripheral vessel and then listening to the return of blood as pressure is released
				  • Can be used to monitor heart rate indirectly

Blood pressure	• Reflects the adequacy of blood circulation throughout the body	Systolic: 110–160 mm Hg
		Diastolic: 60–100 mm Hg
			<60 mm Hg	• *Capillary refill time (CRT)*
				  • Normal is 1–2 seconds
				  • Noticeably prolonged when systolic pressure drops below 70–80 mm Hg
				• *Strength of peripheral pulse*
				  • Direct palpation of femoral, lingual, carotid, or dorsal pedal arteries
				• *Indirect monitoring*
				  • Placing a cuff on the patient to occlude a peripheral vessel and then listening to the return of blood as the pressure is released, using a stethoscope, oscillometer, or Doppler
				• *Direct monitoring*
				  • Indwelling catheter (femoral or dorsal pedal artery)
				  • See below

Parameter	Reflects/Assesses	Normal	Abnormal	Method
Central venous pressure	Allows assessment of blood return to the heart and how well the heart can receive and pump blood	<8 cm H$_2$O pressure	• Pressures over 12–15 cm H$_2$O are considered elevated • Monitor trends over time, versus a single reading	*Indwelling catheter* • A long catheter is inserted percutaneously or by cutdown into the anterior vena cava. The catheter is inserted close to the right atrium of the heart. The catheter is then connected to a water manometer to obtain a measurement. The manometer should be positioned at the approximate level of the heart
Capillary refill time	• Reflects the perfusion of the tissues with blood	1–2 seconds	>2 seconds	*Direct palpation* • Direct digital pressure is applied to the mucous membranes until blanched and then timed for blood (pink color) to return
Mucous membrane color	• Reflects blood loss, anemia, or poor perfusion	Pink	• Pale—blood loss, anemia, or poor perfusion • Purple or blue—cyanosis, shortage of oxygen	*Visual observation* • Observed at the gingiva, tongue, buccal mucous membrane, conjunctiva of the lower eyelid, mucous membrane lining the prepuce or vulva
Blood loss	• Circulation • Blood pressure	• <15% loss	• >15% loss • Packed cell volume (PCV) <20%–25%	*Visual observation* • A healthy animal can tolerate up to a 15% loss of total blood volume • 1 soaked gauze sponge equals approximately 5–6 mL blood

Table 2-24 Vital Signs (Continued)

Vital Sign	Significance	Normal Values	Abnormal Values	Technique Used to Evaluate Vital Sign
Respiration rate and depth	• Reflects proper oxygenation of body tissues	Dog: 10–30 breaths/min Cat: 25–40 breaths/min	<8 breaths/min	• *Observation of the movement of the anesthetic reservoir bag* • An anesthetized animal should be given an intermittent positive pressure ventilation (IPPV) every 5 minutes during the anesthetic procedure • The IPPV should not exceed 20 mm Hg • *Auscultation of the chest cavity* • A normal chest cavity has almost inaudible sounds • Harsh noises, whistles, and squeaks may indicate narrow or obstructed airways or the presence of fluid or secretions in the airways or alveoli • *Pulse Oximetry* • The spectrophotoelectric device is placed on a nonhaired area (i.e., tongue, between digits), and the percentage of saturated hemoglobin is displayed through light absorption • Signal is reduced by hypotension, hypothermia, and altered vascular resistance • Normal is >95% • Serious hypoxemia is <90% • Very serious hypoxemia is <75% • *Movement of the chest wall*
Blood gases	• Respiratory function • Determines acidosis and alkalosis	See Skill Box 5-2	See Skill Box 5-2	• *Blood gas analysis equipment* • Arterial blood draw • Follow manufacturer's directions
Thermoreg-ulation	• Circulation	100.5°–102.5° F	• <100° • >103° F	• *Rectal thermometer* • *Direct palpation of paws and ears* • Temperature should be monitored every 30 minutes • Hypothermia causes prolonged recovery from anesthesia because of slow rate at which the liver enzymes metabolize anesthetic drugs • Prevention of hypothermia can be done with warmed IV fluids, hot water circulating heating pads, hot water bottles, bubble packing, foil wraps, and blankets • Malignant hyperthermia can be a fatal condition and should be tended to immediately

Table 2-25   Monitored Parameters and Their Causes

Monitored Parameter	Causes
Heart rate	**Tachycardia** • Inadequate anesthetic depth (i.e., pain) • Drugs—ketamine, thiobarbiturates, and anticholinergics • Hypokalemia • Hyperthermia • Hypercarbia and hypoxemia • Anemia, hypovolemia (i.e., blood loss) • Hyperthyroidism • Anaphylaxis • Hypotension **Bradycardia** • Excessive anesthetic depth • Drugs—narcotics, xylazine, and anticholinesterases • Preexisting heart disease • Vagal reflex (i.e., eye surgery, pylorus surgery, etc.) • Terminal stages of hypoxemia • Hypothermia • Hypertension • Hyperkalemia • Elevated intracranial pressure
Respiratory rate and pattern	**Tachypnea** • Drugs—doxapram overdose • Pain/Inadequate anesthetic depth • Hypoxemia • Hyperthermia • Hypercarbia/Inadequate CO2 removal in closed system **Apnea** • Drugs—ketamine, thiobarbiturates, and propofol • Hypothermia • Recent hyperventilation under anesthesia • Musculoskeletal paralysis
Arterial blood pressure	**Hypertension** • Drugs—ketamine • Hypercarbia • Hyperthermia • Pain • Inadequate anesthetic depth • Excessive fluid administration **Hypotension** • Drugs—thiobarbiturates boluses and inhalation anesthetics • Sepsis • Shock • Blood loss • Excessive anesthetic depth • Dehydration

Table 2-26 General Concerns During Anesthetic Procedures

	Procedure	Complication	Remedy
Induction	• Inducing anesthesia	• Bodily injury when losing consciousness • Stress-induced catecholamine release with subsequent potential for harmful cardiac arrhythmias	• Support all body parts when inducing • Try to avoid Stage II anesthesia level • Reduce stress by premedication when appropriate • Induction environment should be quiet, and technique chosen according to patient sensitivity to stress
Endotracheal tube	• Intubation	• Incorrect placement, (i.e., esophagus placement) • Incorrect size • Traumatic placement into glottis (laryngitis)	• Close pop off valve and squeeze reservoir bag to listen for leaking gas • Observe for rising and falling of chest wall
	• Rolling or turning the patient	• Kinked endotracheal tube resulting in airway obstruction • Accidental dislodging	• Disconnect tube before moving
Anesthetic hoses	• Placement of anesthetic hoses	• Tracheal trauma • Removal of endotracheal tube • Kinked endotracheal tube	• Correct support of anesthetic hoses to prevent weight placed on the endotracheal tube • Correct position of anesthetic hoses to prevent a kink or bend in endotracheal tube
Surgery Table	• Tilting table	• Abdominal organs compressing the diaphragm compromising heart and lung function	• Do not tilt more than 15 degrees
	• Positioning patient	• Overextension or hyperflexion of neck and limbs causing permanent neurologic injury • Hyperflexion of the neck may occlude endotracheal tube	• Assure the patient maintains as normal a position as possible
	• Restraining devices	• Decreased peripheral blood circulation	• Avoid tight limb restraints
Drapes and Instruments	• Placement of drapes and instruments	• Compression of chest cavity of small patients	• Avoid placing heavy drapes and instruments directly on the chest of small patients

SPECIAL PATIENT CONSIDERATIONS

Each patient presented for an anesthetic procedure has many areas to consider to ensure a successful outcome. Therefore, a patient that begins an anesthetic procedure with less than optimum health needs to be properly evaluated and a specific anesthetic plan designed just for them.

Table 2-27 Special Cases

Condition	Potential Complications	Anesthetic Alterations	Special Surgical Care
Brachycephalic • English Bulldog, French Bulldog, Pug, Boston Terrier, Boxer, and Pekingese	• Dyspnea • Cyanosis • Bradycardia • Laryngeal collapse at induction with failure to intubate	• Rapid IV induction • Preoperative oxygen administration • Administration of a preanesthetic anticholinergic • Avoid deep sedation • Prepare for possible tracheostomy tube placement	• Maintain the endotracheal tube as long as possible in recovery • Possibly sedate to reduce stress during recovery period and allow tube to remain in longer • Continue oxygen administration until extubation • Closely monitor respiration for 1 hour after recovery
Cardiovascular Disease Congenital heart disease	• Bradycardia • Ventricular ectopic beats • Hypothermia	• Pediatric protocol for induction • Avoid xylazine and halothane • Preoperative oxygen administration	• Observe for overhydration
Hypotension/hypovolemia	• Cardiac arrest • Circulatory failure	• Protocol using drugs with the least hypotensive qualities • Avoid xylazine and halothane • Preoperative oxygen administration	• Animal should be stabilized with fluids and/or whole blood before anesthetic procedure • Observe for overhydration; use low-volume IV fluid rate
Impaired cardiac output	• Bradycardia • Tachycardia • Hypovolemia	• Drugs producing tachycardia should be avoided (i.e., anticholinergics, dissociative agents), except with congestive cardiomyopathy, in which increased heart rate may be beneficial • Avoid alpha-2 agonists and halothane • Perioperative oxygen administration	• Observe for overhydration

Table 2-27   Special Cases (Continued)

Condition	Potential Complications	Anesthetic Alterations	Special Surgical Care
Anemia/hypoproteinemia	• Hypoxemia • Fluid overload • Pulmonary edema • Anesthetic drug overdose	• Highly protein-bound drugs will give an increased effect, and the dose should be decreased • Avoid xylazine and halothane • Perioperative oxygen administration	• Possible blood transfusion if PCV is less than 25%–30% • Serial PCV and total proteins should be monitored during surgery and postoperatively • Conservative fluid therapy to avoid pulmonary edema caused by reduced vascular oncotic pressure (especially crystalloids)
Heartworm disease	• Cardiac dysrhythmias • Decreased cardiac output • Pulmonary dysfunction	No contraindications	
Cesarean	• Stress on the heart • Respiratory difficulty • Uterine hemorrhage • Vomiting • Hypertension • Neonatal depression from anesthetic agents	• Decrease drug dose by 40% • Perioperative oxygen administration • Opioid agents are often favored because of their reversibility with naloxone • Avoid pentobarbital because of its close to 100% mortality in neonates	• Surgical preparation should be done in an awake animal in left lateral recumbency to remove pressure from the vena cava • IV catheter and fluids should be routine • Kittens and puppies should be placed with the mother immediately after the mother's recovery from anesthesia
Endocrine Diabetes mellitus	• Hypoglycemia • Delayed recovery	• Consider drugs that can be antagonized or are rapidly metabolized	• Patient should be stabilized and regulated before an anesthetic procedure • Procedure should be scheduled in early morning after normal administration of insulin • Possibly reduce insulin dose by 50% on day of surgery • Preoperative, intraoperative, and postoperative blood glucose values should be monitored—maintaining between 150 and 250 mg/dL • IV fluid administration of 5% dextrose

Condition	Concerns	Anesthetic Considerations
Hyperthyroidism	• "Thyroid storm"—increased heart rate, hypertension, cardiac dysrhythmias, hyperthermia, and shock • Hypoxemia • Increased oxygen consumption	• Attempt to regulate thyroid level before anesthesia • Beta-blockers for severe tachycardia may be necessary
Hypoadrenocorticism	• Hypotension • Shock	• No contraindications • Patient should be stabilized and regulated before an anesthetic procedure • Preoperative, intraoperative, and postoperative fluid administration and glucocorticoids to avoid an Addisonian crisis
Hypothyroidism	• Respiratory difficulty • Delayed recovery	• Consider drugs that can be antagonized or are rapidly metabolized • Blood profile to monitor anemia
Gastrointestinal Gastric dilation/volvulus	• Cardiac arrhythmias • Septic shock	• Stabilize shock before anesthesia • Perioperative oxygen administration • Avoid the use of thiobarbiturates, halothane, nitrous oxide, and xylazine • Serum electrolytes before anesthesia • ECG to monitor for arrhythmias • IV fluid administration
Pancreatitis	• Hypotension	• Avoid the use of alpha-2 agonists and halothane • IV fluid and electrolyte administration • Complete blood panel to check for underlying diseases or conditions
Obesity	• Drug overdose • Respiratory difficulty • Hypoxemia • Hypoventilation • Airway obstruction	• Dose drugs on lean weight to prevent overdosing • Preoperative oxygen administration • Drugs that distribute to the body fat will have longer recovery times (halothane) • Complete blood panel to check for underlying diseases or conditions • IPPV • Maintain endotracheal tube as long as possible
Geriatric • A patient who has reached 75% of its expected life span	• Decreased organ function • Hypotension	• Decrease drug dose by 30%–50% • Allow longer time for response to drugs • Avoid xylazine and acepromazine • Blood profile • IV catheter • Maintenance fluids • Heat support

Table 2-27 Special Cases (Continued)

Condition	Potential Complications	Anesthetic Alterations	Special Surgical Care
Hepatic disease • portal–caval shunt, dehydrated, thin, icteric, and anemic	• Delayed recovery • Further hepatic disease • Hypothermia • Hypoglycemia • Pulmonary edema • Seizures • Hypotension	• Induction with isoflurane • Avoid preanesthetics • Avoid use of ketamine, tiletamine, or methohexital because of their seizure-inducing activity	• Complete preoperative blood panel, including coagulation panel • Heat support • Serial glucose values • Blood pressure measurement
Neonatal • A patient under 3 months of age	• Inadequate organ function • Hypothermia	• Decrease drug dose by 30%–50% • Allowing longer time for response to drugs	• Heat support
Renal disease	• Delayed recovery • Further renal disease • Hypotension • Renal hypoperfusion	• Reduce dosages of injectable agents (acepromazine, xylazine, diazepam, opioid agents, ketamine, and barbiturates) • Azotemic animals have increased CNS drug sensitivity • Acidotic animals have increased sensitivity to highly protein-bound anesthetics	• Complete blood panel and urinalysis preoperatively • Rehydration and IV diuresis before anesthesia • Avoid preoperative fasting • Blood pressure measurement • Red blood cell transfusion if PCV is <18% in cats and <20% in dogs • Proper positioning and padding is needed to avoid pressure necrosis • Careful positioning is needed in animals with urethral obstruction to avoid rupture • ECG on hyperkalemic animals (i.e., Acute renal failure)
Respiratory disease • pleural effusion, diaphragmatic hernia, pneumothorax, pulmonary contusions, pneumonia, tracheal collapse, and pulmonary edema	• Tachypnea, dyspnea, and/or apnea • Hypoxemia	• Avoid nitrous oxide • Preoperative and postoperative oxygen administration • Mild preanesthetic may be needed to reduce stress (acepromazine and butorphanol) • Rapid induction with an injectable anesthetic to obtain control of the airway	• Thorough physical and thoracic examination • Thoracic radiographs • Thoracocentesis (if necessary) • ECG • Arterial blood gases • Baseline complete blood count (CBC), serum electrolytes, and chemistry panel • Maintain endotracheal intubation as long as possible into the recovery period

Chapter 2 / Anesthesia

Condition	Signs	Management
Sighthounds • Greyhound, Saluki, Afghan Hound, Whippet, and Russian Wolfhound	• Death	• DO NOT use tranquilizers and barbiturates (i..e, thiopental); use agents such as diazepam and ketamine, methohexital, propofol, and inhalation agents • Heat support
Trauma • hit by car, head trauma, thoracic and abdominal trauma, thermal/burn trauma	• Respiratory difficulty • Cardiac dysrhythmias • Shock • Internal injuries • Tachycardia • Seizures (i.e., head trauma)	• Postpone any anesthesia for a few days if possible • Reduce drug doses • Avoid seizurogenic medications • Radiographs of affected area • Electrocardiogram • Oxygen therapy • IV fluid administration • Urinary catheter placement • Monitor body temperature
Urinary Obstruction	• Cardiac failure • Bradycardia • Cardiac dysrhythmias • Hyperkalemia	• Reduced dosages of ketamine-diazepam or isoflurane • IV fluid administration • Blood profile

VENTILATION

One of the key elements to successful anesthesia is providing adequate ventilation to the patient. Improper maintenance of ventilation may lead to hypoxia and then brain damage or even death. Even though respiration can be seen by the rising and falling of the chest, this does not always ensure adequate movement of air. Assisted ventilation or controlled ventilation can give peace of mind that the patient is receiving proper oxygen levels throughout its body.

Table 2-28 Ventilation—General Information

Uses	• Animals with compromised respiration (i.e., obese or debilitated animals) • Thoracic surgery (i.e., diaphragmatic hernia or pneumothorax) • Head, chest, or nerve trauma • Prolonged anesthetic procedures, >90 minutes • Drug overdose
Normal and Ventilator Values	
Tidal volume	• The amount of gas exchanged in one respiratory cycle • 5 mL/lb in awake animals • 7 mL/lb when ventilator in use
Inflation of the lungs	• 15–20 cm H_2O in awake animals and when ventilator in use • 20–30 cm H_2O when ventilator in use during thoracic surgery
Spontaneous ventilatory cycle	• 1 second in awake animals • <1.5 seconds when ventilator in use
Ventilator controls	
Volume preset	• Delivers a preset volume of gas • Delivers a constant volume despite changes in the lungs during anesthesia • Caution of developing high airway pressures • Caution of small leaks that cannot be compensated for; they will compromise the patient's tidal volume • Volume is variable and depends on the following: lung compliance, airway resistance, pressure within the thorax, and the number of functioning alveoli
Pressure preset	• Delivers a gas at a preset volume during the inspiratory phase • Does not allow a buildup of high pressure and compensates for leaks in the system • Pressure may need to be increased to compensate for volume variability
Time cycled	• Delivers gas at a preset frequency or respiratory rate, Inspiratory:Expiratory ratio (I:E), or inspiratory flow rate
Associated risks	• Decreased blood pressure and cardiac output • Hypoventilation or hyperventilation • Impaired sympathetic nervous system activity • Excessive ventilation rate; respiratory alkalosis • In-circle vaporizers can cause excessive amounts of vaporized anesthetics • Source of contamination to the breathing system • Improper setup of equipment or equipment malfunction

Skill Box 2-4 / Intermittent Positive-Pressure Ventilation (IPPV)

- Should be done every 5 minutes during an anesthetic procedure to provide adequate ventilation of the lungs
- Technique: close pop-off valve and gently squeeze the reservoir bag for ~1 second to a pressure reading of 20 cm H_2O, release bag and open pop-off valve

Table 2-29 Ventilation Administration

Types	Definition	Initiating Method	Frequency	Ending Method	Uses	Associated Risks
Manual Assist	• Animal's breathing is assisted by compressions of the reservoir bag.	• Intermittent Positive-Pressure Ventilation (IPPV) • The pop-off valve is closed and pressure is applied to the reservoir bag to a manometer reading of 20 cm H_2O to inflate the lungs and then released for exhalation • Vaporizer setting in an in-circle, nonprecision vaporizer should be turned to zero before an IPPV	• Every 5 minutes	• Normal procedure of discontinuing inhalant anesthetics	• Any healthy, anesthetized animal	• Overinflation of the lungs causing alveoli rupture • Constant pressure causing increased intrathoracic pressure (i.e., failure to reopen pop-off valve) • Decreased blood pressure and cardiac output because of maintenance of positive pressure, not allowing sufficient negative pressure to assist with blood flow • Impaired sympathetic nervous system activity • Hypoventilation and hyperventilation

Manual Controlled	• Animal's breathing is controlled by the anesthetist making compressions on the reservoir bag.	• 5–8 times per minute	• Reduce vaporizer setting initially and begin bagging (as described above) at a rate of 12–16 breaths/min. If the chest cavity is open, the manometer reading should be increased to 20–30 cm H_2O. Spontaneous breathing should cease after 3–5 minutes; if it does not, a neuromuscular agent may need to be used. Once control of respiration has been established, a rate of 8–12 breaths/min should be maintained. Inspiratory time should be 1–1.5 seconds with an expiratory time of twice as long. The pop-off valve should be closed during compressions, but should be opened every 2–3 breaths to allow escape of back pressure.	• Discontinue the use of the inhalant anesthetic and nitrous oxide while continuing to ventilate with O_2. If a neuromuscular agent was used, it should be reversed if possible. The rate of respiration should be gradually decreased to 5 breaths/min while the animal is observed for spontaneous breathing. Spontaneous breathing may take several minutes to resume, especially in older or debilitated animals or those undergoing a long anesthetic procedure. Once spontaneous respiration is seen, the amount of pressure placed on the reservoir bag can be reduced. Bagging can be stopped altogether when the rate and tidal volume are back to normal.	• Animals with compromised respiration (i.e., obese or debilitated animals) • Overinflation of the lungs, causing alveoli rupture • Constant pressure, causing increased intrathoracic pressure • Decreased blood pressure and cardiac output caused by maintenance of positive pressure, not allowing sufficient negative pressure to assist with blood flow • Impaired sympathetic nervous system activity • Hypoventilation and hyperventilation

Table 2-29 Ventilation Administration (Continued)

Types	Definition	Initiating Method	Frequency	Ending Method	Uses	Associated Risks
Mechanical Controlled	• The anesthetist sets the ventilator to control the rate and volume of the animal's respiratory cycle.	• There are many types of ventilators used in veterinary medicine each with varying complexity of controls. • Gases may be delivered by a pressure cycle, volume cycle, or time cycle. • Refer to the manufacturer's guidelines for instructions • Ventilation should be maintained at 8–12 breaths/min with inspiratory time of 1–2 seconds and expiratory time twice as long. • Oxygen rate should be 7–9 mL/lb	• 5–8 times per minute	• Discontinue the use of the inhalant anesthetic and nitrous oxide while continuing to ventilate with O_2. If a neuromuscular agent was used, it should be reversed if possible. The rate of respiration should be gradually decreased to 5 breaths/min while the animal is observed for spontaneous breathing. Spontaneous breathing may take several minutes to resume, especially in older or debilitated animals or those undergoing a long anesthetic procedure. Once spontaneous respiration is seen, the anesthetist should switch to manual-controlled ventilation. The rate can continue to be reduced to 1–4 breaths/min. Bagging can be stopped altogether when the rate and tidal volume are back to normal.	• Animals with compromised respiration; i.e. obese or debilitated animals • Thoracic surgery (i.e. diaphragmatic hernia or pneumothorax) • Head trauma • Animals with prolonged anesthetic procedures	• Improper setup of ventilator • Malfunction of equipment • Overinflation of the lungs causing alveoli rupture • Constant pressure causing increased intrathoracic pressure • Decreased blood pressure and cardiac output due to positive pressure that is maintained not allowing sufficient negative pressure to assist with blood flow • Impaired sympathetic nervous system activity • Hypoventilation and hyperventilation • Source of contamination to the breathing system
Assist/ Controlled	• The anesthetist sets a minimal respiratory rate which the animal may override by initiating spontaneous respiratory efforts at a faster rate.					

Skill Box 2-5 / Anesthetic Breathing Systems

Rebreathing—Circle System

- Patient rebreathes its own exhaled gases minus the carbon dioxide and with the addition of fresh oxygen and anesthetic gases

Types	Indications for use	Oxygen Flow Rates	General Information
Total Rebreathing/ CLOSED •Pop-off valve is completely closed	• Patients >15 lbs • Patients must have lungs strong enough to push gases through the machine	• 2-3mL/lb/min	• Do not use nitrous oxide • Relatively low gas rates can be used • Ventilation is readily observed and controlled by the rebreathing bag • Minimal heat loss and airway drying • Increased resistance to gas flow
Partial Rebreathing/ Semi-closed • Pop-off valve is partially open	• Patients >15 lbs	• 3(BW(kg) × 10) = ? mL/min • 5-20mL/lb/min	• Much higher gas rates need to be used • Ventilation can be observed by the rebreathing bag

Nonrebreathing System

- Patient receives fresh oxygen and anesthetic gases with each breath

Types	Indications for use	Oxygen Flow Rates	General Information
Open • Pop-off valve is completely open	• Any size patients, typically those <15 lbs • Minimal resistance to breathing	• 3(breaths/ min × 10) = ? mL/min • 0.5–4 L/min	• Much higher gas rates needed to eliminate exhaled gases • Minimal or no rebreathing of expired gases by patient • Resistance to gas flow is minimal

Rebreathing bag size

<15 lb = 1-liter bag

>15 lb and <40 lb = 2-liter bag

>40 lb and <120 lb = 3-liter bag

>120 lb and <300 lb = 5-liter bag

Compressed gas cylinders

Green tank = Oxygen

Blue tank = Nitrous oxide

Chapter 3

Basic Care

PHYSICAL EXAMINATIONS

A well-done physical examination gives the clinician invaluable information in the assessment of an animal's health. Technicians can assist the veterinarian by understanding the pertinence of each part of the examination and by being able to conduct an examination in an orderly, precise, and timely fashion. Physical examinations are conducted before immunizing, before an anesthetic procedure, and in conjunction with any visit to the veterinarian for a specific problem. The following charts will cover methods and specific areas of the physical examination in both pediatric and adult patients.

Table 3-1   Methods of Examination

Method	Definition	Technique
Visual	Using your eyes to check over an area	No explanation needed
Palpation	Using your hands to feel the contour of an area Tissue descriptions: • Doughy: soft tissue that can be impressed with fingertips • Firm: normal organ • Hard: bones • Fluctuant: soft, elastic, and undulates under pressure	Gentleness when palpating an animal is essential, because internal structures can be damaged if handled roughly.
	Abdominal palpation	*Gently* using 1 or 2 hands (for cats and small dogs, use 1 hand; for large dogs, use 2 hands), begin at the spine and move ventrally, allowing the abdominal viscera to slip through the fingers. Repeat throughout the abdomen. *Cranial abdomen* will allow palpation of the liver, spleen, and the small intestines. *Mid-abdomen* will allow palpation of the small intestines, kidneys, and spleen. *Caudal* abdomen will allow palpation of the colon, uterus, bladder, prostate, and small intestine.
Auscultation	Using a stethoscope to listen to the sounds produced by the functioning of various body organs	A stethoscope is placed so that it is flat against the area of interest on the animal's body.
	Cardiac auscultation	A stethoscope is placed against the thorax, and the number of heartbeats heard per minute are counted (one method is to use a 15-second count and multiply by 4). There are specific locations listed in Table 3-2 to hear specific valves of the heart.
	Respiratory auscultation	A stethoscope is placed flat against the sinuses, trachea, and thorax to hear the movement of air through the respiratory system. Various audible sounds may be heard in these areas and are detailed with each area of the body in Table 3-2.
	Abdominal auscultation	A stethoscope is placed flat against the abdomen to listen for normal gurgling sounds in the large intestines (borborygmus).
Percussion	Soft striking of the thorax	While listening with a stethoscope or your ear, thump the thorax gently.

When examining the oral cavity of an animal, handle the muzzle with care. Tongue depressors can assist in opening the mouth of an uncooperative animal.

Constant, gentle pressure will encourage relaxation of the abdominal musculature so that an organ may be palpated.

Table 3-2 Preliminary Examination

Method	Definition	Technique
Recent history	To ascertain the current issue for which the owner is bringing the animal to the clinic.	Current appetite, water intake, urination and defecation behavior, recent temperament, and current medications are noted. Recent activities to which the animal may have been exposed or a change in the home environment are also noted.
Past History	To note previous medical conditions that may exacerbate the current complaint.	Age, breed, sex, immunization dates as well as current medical therapies are noted.
Vital Signs	To note current physiologic status of the patient. Includes:	
Weight		Recorded in kilograms or pounds. Note whether animal is over or under typical weight guidelines for that breed (see Table 3-11, Body Conditioning Score); note the quantity and type of diet.
Temperature		Taken in the ear (ear thermometer) or rectally Normal temperatures: • Puppies/kittens: 100.5°–102.5° • Adult dogs/cats: 100.5°–102.5° Evaluated at the femoral artery in cats and dogs.
Pulse		• Count the number of beats you feel for 15 seconds and multiply by 4. Note pulse quality and strength. Evaluate for irregularities in rhythm as well as irregularities when compared with the auscultated heartbeat. Verify that the pulse is the same on both sides. Chart a pulse deficit if the pulse rate is less than the heart rate.
Heart rate		Auscultated: counting the number of beats of the heart you hear for 15 seconds and multiply by 4. Specific locations to hear specific valves: • Left 2nd–4th intercostal space above the sternal border = pulmonic valve • Left 3rd–5th intercostal space at mid thorax = aortic valve • Left 4th–6th intercostal space just above the sternal border = mitral valve • Right 3rd–5th intercostal space at mid thorax = tricuspid valve
Respiration		Evaluate: • Rate—auscultate and count number of breaths per minute • Depth—visual: watching the degree of chest movement • Character—abnormal lung sounds: "rales" (coarse to fine crackles), "rhonchi" (musical sounds—low or high pitched), or "wheezes" • Any difficulty with inspiration and/or expiration
General appearance	Visual assessment of the animal's overall health.	Condition of animal's coat, skin, and temperament is noted.

Table 3-3 General Physical Examination

Area	Specific Region	Method of Examination	Normal	Check For	Questions to Owner
Head and Neck	Head—general	Visual	Symmetrical	• Symmetry, alopecia, tumors or swellings, rashes, head tilt, and uniformed muscle mass on skull	• Head tilt or shaking? • History of seizures?
	Eyes Lids Eyeball Conjunctiva Sclera Pupil Cornea Lens	Visual and ophthalmic examination	Bright, clear, uniform, and responsive	• Cysts, conformity, lash growth, 3rd eyelid position and size, symmetry, ocular discharge, nystagmus, positioning within orbit: protruding vs. sunken, color, vascularity, uniformity of pupils, scars, ulcerations, pigmentation, and opacities	• Blinking or squinting? • Rubbing or pawing? • Discharge?
	Muzzle	Visual	Symmetrical	• Symmetry, inflammation, swelling, abscessed teeth and pain on opening mouth	• Rubbing or pawing?
	Nares	Visual	Symmetrical	• Symmetry, movement on inspiration—(should move laterally) and discharge	• Sneezing or heavy breathing? • Discharge?
	Oral cavity Lips Mucous membranes Teeth Hard and soft palate Tongue & Pharynx Tonsils	Visual	Symmetrical, pink and slightly moist	• Halitosis, inflammation, tumors or papillomas, anatomic defects, excessive salivation, crusting, pigment changes, color and capillary refill time, tacky, periodontal status, ulcerations, and foreign bodies	• Excessive salivation or dripping water after drinking? • Inappetance or difficulty eating?
	Ears	Visual and otoscopic examination		• Debris, exudate, odor, inflammation, response to sound, and sensitivity to canal massage or palpation	• Shaking head or scratching ears?
	Lymph nodes: Anterior cervical and submandibular	Palpation	Firm and freely movable	• Symmetry and size	

Table 3-3 General Physical Examination (Continued)

Area	Specific Region	Method of Examination	Normal	Check For	Questions to Owner
Head and Neck	Salivary glands: Mandibular and parotid	Palpation		• Symmetry and size (do not confuse with submandibular nodes)	
	Throat Trachea Larynx and thyroid Thoracic inlet	Palpation and auscultation	No coughing on palpation	• Coughing or sounds during examination, deviation or displacement, tumors, swelling, stridor, or jugular pulse waves	• Gagging, retching, difficulty swallowing? • If a cough is noticed, does the cough occur throughout the day? • Travel or exposure to other dogs?
Trunk and limbs	Trunk—general	Visual and palpation	• Visible sheen and completeness of coat	• Body form and weight, symmetry, tumors, alopecia, inflammation, ectoparasites or their residues, crusts, scales, pustules, and hydration status	• Scratching? • Changes in diet? • Did pruritus precede or coincide with lesions?
	Lymph nodes: Prescapular, axillary, and popliteal	Palpation		• Size and consistency	
	Limbs Muscle and bone Joints Paws	Visual and palpation		• Symmetry, inflammation, tenderness, tumors, range of motion, gait, atrophy, flexion and extension, interdigital, nails/nail bed, and knuckling	• Limping and/or favoring limb(s)? • Licking paws?
Thoracic cavity	Lungs	Auscultation and percussion	• Vesicular and bronchial (soft, rustling sounds) • On percussion, the lungs should sound clear and resonant	• Rate, depth and pattern of breathing (rales or rhonchi) and lung sounds (absence of lung sounds may indicate pleural effusion, and dull sound may indicate fluid filled or solid lungs)	• Fainting? • If cough is present, does it change throughout the day or worsen with exertion? • Recent travel?

Category	Structure	Method	Findings		Questions
Thoracic cavity	Heart	Auscultation	A short time gap should exist between these two sounds: S1 = loud, long, low-pitch (closure of atrioventricular valves) S2 = closure of semilunar valves	Dysrhythmias, murmurs, verify femoral and metatarsal pulses coincide with the heart rate (i.e., no pulse deficits)	• Any fainting, collapsing, or exercise intolerance? • Panting?
Abdomen	Kidneys	Palpation		Size, shape, and contours of surface	• Excessive drinking of water or urinating?
	Liver	Palpation with patient in lateral recumbency	Edges are normally sharp and well defined (nonpalpable in most pets)	Extension beyond costal arch is not normal	
	Urinary bladder	Palpation		Size, tone, and turgidity	• Frequency and amount of urine? • Foul odor, color change or blood? • Straining?
	Small intestines	Palpation		Tumors, foreign bodies, and pain on palpation	
	Mammary glands	Visual and palpation		Tumors, cysts, inflammation, temperature, and discharge	• If intact female, when last whelping occurred? • When was ovariohysterectomy performed?
Perineal	Perineal—general	Visual		Tumors, fistulas, exudate, and hernias	
	Vulva	Visual	Lochia	Size, inflammation, and discharge from or between perivulvar folds	• Last heat cycle or whelping?
	Penis	Visual and palpation	Preputial discharge	Tumors, inflammation, and discharge	• Normal urination? • Blood or urine color change?
	Scrotum	Visual and palpation		Descended testicles, swelling, and symmetry	

Table 3-4   Pediatric Physical Examination

This chart is designed to show the specific areas to note on puppies and kittens. A full examination should be conducted following Table 3-3, General Physical Examination.

Area	Specific Region	Method of Examination	Age Range	Puppy Normal	Kitten Normal	Check for
General Appearance	Temperament	Visual	Birth to 6 weeks	• First 2–3 weeks should consist of eating and sleeping • Nursing should be vigorous and active with a good "suckle reflex" • Active playtime with mother and littermates from 3 weeks on	• First 2–3 weeks should consist of eating and sleeping • Nursing should be vigorous and active with a good "suckle reflex" • Active playtime with mother and littermates from 3 weeks on	• Constant crying, extreme inactivity, and/or failure to gain weight can be signs of inadequate milk consumption • Separation from mother and littermates before 6 weeks of age can lead to numerous behavioral problems later in life
	Body Weight	Accurate scale, preferably a gram scale	Birth to 4 weeks	• Toy: 100–400 g • Medium: 200–300 g • Large: 400–500 g • Giant: >700 g • Birth weight should double in 10–12 days	• 100 g • Birth weight should double in 14 days	• Failure to gain weight is often the first sign of illness • Body weight should be checked initially, 12 hours after birth, and daily for 2 weeks; then checked weekly
			5 weeks to 6 months	• Should gain 1–2 g/day/lb of adult body weight	• Should gain 10–15 g/day on average (some days more, some less)	
	Skin	Visual Flea comb	Birth to 6 months	• Shiny hair coat • Complete hair coat		• State of hydration • Completeness of hair cover • Condition of foot pads • Wounds • Bacterial infections, external parasites, or dermatophytosis

General Appearance				
Temperature	• Rectal thermometer	Birth to 1 week	• 96°–97° F • Cannot regulate own body temperature for first 3 weeks • Newborn puppies and kittens should never be left unattended or warmed on electric heating pads, because their neuromuscular reflexes are not present until 7 days of age	• Cannot regulate own body temperature for first week	• Hypothermia or hyperthermia • Burns • Are owners using supplemental heat in any way (e.g., 75–100-watt bulb near crate/box)?
		2–4 weeks	• 100° F		
Head					
Eyes	• Penlight and handheld lens	Birth to 6 months	• Eyes open around 12–14 days • Iris is blue gray • Changes to adult color at approximately 4–6 weeks of age • Adult vision at 5–10 weeks of age • Pupillary light responses may not be evident until 21 days of age • Strabismus or deviation of eyeballs		• Discharge • Squinting or holding eye(s) closed • Rubbing or pawing at eye(s)
Ears	• Visual • Otoscope with infant-size cone	Birth to 6 months	• Complete hearing at 4–6 weeks of age • External ear canals open between 6 and 14 days and are completely open by 17 days • Canals may be full of desquamative cells and some oil droplets		• Size and position • Exudate and odor for possible bacterial or yeast infection or mites

Table 3-4 Pediatric Physical Examination (Continued)

This chart is designed to show the specific areas to note on puppies and kittens. A full examination should be conducted following Table 3-3, General Physical Examination.

Area	Specific Region	Method of Examination	Age Range	Puppy Normal	Kitten Normal	Check for
Head	Mouth	• Penlight • Tongue depressor or cotton swab	Birth to 3 months	• Sucking reflex is present at birth and disappears at 3 weeks of age • Deciduous tooth eruption		• Hairlip • Cleft palate • Sucking reflex • Occlusion or malfunction of jaw bones (malocclusion)
				• Incisors 2–4 weeks • Canines 3–5 weeks • Premolars 4–12 weeks	• Incisors 2–4 weeks • Canines 3–4 weeks • Premolars 3–8 weeks	
			4–6 months	• Permanent tooth eruption • Incisors 3–5 months • Canines 4–7 months • Premolars 4–6 months • Molars 4–7 months	• Incisors 3–5 months • Canines 4–7 months • Premolars 4–6 months • Molars 4–5 months	
	Nose	• Visual	Birth to 6 months	• Normal adult appearance		• Obstruction, stenosis, discharge, or abnormal shape • Swelling
	Skull	• Visual	Birth to 4 weeks	• Normal adult appearance		• Open fontanelle (soft spot on the forehead)
Thorax	General Appearance	• Visual	Birth to 6 months	• Symmetrical chest wall		• Wounds and rib fractures • Congenital sternal or spinal abnormalities

Region	System	Technique	Age	Normal findings	Abnormal findings
Thorax	Heart	• Visual • Stethoscope with 2 cm bell and 3 cm diaphragm	Birth to 4 weeks	• Heart rate = 220 beats/min • Normal heart rhythm is a sinus rhythm	• Heart rate and pattern • Murmurs (should be noted and DVM consulted, as some can be normal/physiologic)
			5 weeks to 6 months	• Heart rate: Dog: 70–180 beats/min Cat: 110–200 beats/min	
	Lungs	Same as Heart	Birth to 4 weeks	• Respiratory rate = 15–35 breaths/min	• Breathing rate and pattern • Asymmetrical or absent lung sounds
			5 weeks to 6 months	• Respiratory rate: Dog: 10–30 breaths/min Cat: 25–40 breaths/min	
Abdomen	General Appearance	• Visual	Birth to 4 weeks	• Umbilical cord falls off in 2–3 days	• Umbilical hernia • Umbilical inflammation or infection/ulceration
	Internal Organs	• Palpation	Birth to 6 months	• Kidneys are palpable in some dogs • Normal spleen sometimes palpable in an older puppy if foreleg is extended, allowing organs to fall caudally • Liver margins should not extend past the ribs • Stomach will feel like a large fluid-filled sac if full • Intestines are soft and freely movable without pain and may be fluid or gas filled. Thickened/"ropy" feel may indicate endoparasitism • Urinary bladder should have resistance to urine outflow • Intussusception—a sausage-like mass and very painful • Kidneys are palpable • Spleen only palpable if enlarged	• Enlarged or abnormally small organs • Pain on palpation • Masses

Table 3-4 Pediatric Physical Examination (Continued)

This chart is designed to show the specific areas to note on puppies and kittens. A full examination should be conducted following Table 3-3, General Physical Examination.

Area	Specific Region	Method of Examination	Age Range	Puppy Normal	Kitten Normal	Check for
Limbs	Forelimbs Hindlimbs	• Visual • Palpation	Birth to 6 months	• Normal adult appearance (breed-influenced)		• Deformities or absence of bones • Wounds, bruises, or swelling • Deformities or increased or decreased range of motion in joints
Perineum Genitals	Genitalia	• Visual • Palpation	Birth to 6 months	• Normal adult appearance • Descended testicles by 4–6 weeks of age (can take up to 16 weeks before declared cryptorchid)		• Cryptorchidism • Vaginitis • Congenital abnormalities
	Anus	• Visual • Palpation	Birth to 6 months	• Normal adult appearance		• Rectal prolapse • Inflammation or irritation
	Elimination for motherless neonates	• Rubbing	Birth to 3–4 weeks	• After each feeding, a cotton ball should be moistened with warm water and gently stroked over the genitals to stimulate urination and defection • A finger also can be gently rubbed in a circular pattern on the neonate's stomach		• Constipation

Table 3-5   Geriatric Physical Examination

This chart is designed to show the specific areas to note on geriatric animals. A full examination should be conducted, following Table 3-3, General Physical Examination. However, geriatric animals go through additional changes as a result of the natural aging process. Many of these changes cannot be visualized on a physical examination, but they may be inferred through the general examination and from discussion with the owner. These symptoms may contribute to or initiate more serious medical conditions, thereby making their determination valuable to the clinician.

Area	Specific Region	Effects	Associated with
General Appearance	Skin	• Decreased elastin and collagen • Decreased blood flow to skin • Thinning of skin and coat	• Ineffective barrier to pathogens • May require more maintenance by owner
	Toenails	• Increased length because of decreased activity • More fragile, crumble when trimmed	• Difficulty walking • Wounds in foot pads
	Musculature	• Decreased strength • Decreased tone	• Muscle atrophy and coordination
Head	Eyes	• Vision loss • Decreased pupillary light response • Change in lens opacity • Optic lens hardening	• Atrophy of the iris and ciliary muscles • Nuclear sclerosis
	Ears	• Hearing loss	• Loss of cochlear hair cells
	Nose	• Decreased sense of smell	• Decreased function of olfactory nerve endings
	Neck	• Thyroid nodules	• Hyperthyroidism (cats) • Tumor
Internal Organs	Brain	• Amyloid deposition	• Cognitive dysfunction disorder • Decreased glucose tolerance
		• Memory loss • Personality changes	• Cognitive dysfunction disorder

Table 3-5 Geriatric Physical Examination (Continued)

This chart is designed to show the specific areas to note on geriatric animals. A full examination should be conducted, following Table 3-3, General Physical Examination. However, geriatric animals go through additional changes as a result of the natural aging process. Many of these changes cannot be visualized on a physical examination, but they may be inferred through the general examination and from discussion with the owner. These symptoms may contribute to or initiate more serious medical conditions, thereby making their determination valuable to the clinician.

Area	Specific Region	Effects	Associated with
Internal organs	Lungs	• Loss of lung elasticity • Decreased tidal volume • Decreased expiratory reserve • Diminished cough reflex • Increased density on lung radiographs	• Rarely a cause of concern
	Heart	• Increased sternal contact • Tortuous, redundant aorta (cats) • Radiographic changes	• Rarely a cause of concern
	Kidney	• Decreased size • Decreased glomerular filtration rate • Decreased renal blood flow • Decreased ability to handle potassium • Increased mineralization of renal pelvis	• Kidney disease • PU/PD • No concern known
	Liver	• Decreased protein synthesis • Decreased metabolic function	• Liver disease
Limbs	Joints/cartilage	• Decreased production of chondroitin sulfate, keratin sulfate, and hyaluronic acid • Decreased proteoglycan content	• Degenerative joint disease
Genitals	Urethral sphincter	• Decreased tone	• Primary urethral sphincter incontinence
Neurological	Immune system	• Decreased function	• Chronic disease • Increased susceptibility to infections
	Blood	• Decreased ability to respond to needed red blood cell (RBC) increase • Hypertension	• Anemia • Renal or endocrine disease

IMMUNIZATIONS

Young animals receive a small amount of natural immunity from their mother's milk, exchanged in the form of colostrum, during the first few days of nursing. However, this temporary maternal protection wanes by 6–9 weeks. To continue and enhance this protection, vaccinations are available to protect the animal from contracting various highly contagious diseases. These diseases and their corresponding vaccinations are charted on the following pages.

Vaccines in general are meant for healthy animals, need to be stored in the refrigerator, and need to be shaken well before dispensing. A few guidelines to follow when vaccinating an animal are:

- *An animal should receive a complete physical examination and health evaluation by a veterinarian before any vaccination.*

- *Do not vaccinate pregnant animals with a modified live vaccine.*

- *Animals with a fever or in debilitated health should not be vaccinated until healthy.*

Because each animal and its environment is unique, vaccine recommendations will vary accordingly at the discretion of the veterinarian and in accordance with state laws.

> **Pinching the injection site before administration of the vaccine desensitizes the area. Changing to a 25-gauge needle also provides a less painful injection, because the new needle is not dull and is smaller.**

Table 3-6 Canine Disease

Disease	Corona virus	Distemper	Hepatitis	Infectious Tracheobronchitis
DEFINITION	Contagious viral disease affecting the gastrointestinal (GI) system, resulting in sporadic outbreaks of vomiting and diarrhea. Diarrhea is caused by virus invading the enterocytes of the villous tips.	An acute to subacute febrile and often fatal, highly contagious viral disease with respiratory, GI, and central nervous system (CNS) manifestations.	Viral disease caused by adenovirus type 1. Affects the liver, eyes, and endothelium.	Contagious respiratory disease often caused by the bacteria *Bordetella bronchiseptica*. It also can be caused by the viruses parainfluenza and adenovirus 1 and 2.
CLINICAL SIGNS	• Most infected dogs are asymptomatic • Anorexia, depression, vomiting and dehydration • Diarrhea; yellow-green to orange and malodorous • Mild respiratory effects • Puppies will exhibit more signs than adult dogs.	• Malaise, conjunctivitis, rhinitis, nasal discharge followed by pneumonia, vomiting, diarrhea, and fever • CNS signs: seizures, circling, pacing, ataxia, paresis, and myoclonus • Dental enamel hypoplasia, hyperkeratosis of foot pads, and abdominal pustules	• Fever, vomiting, diarrhea, depression, lethargy, pale mucous membranes, abdominal pain, hemorrhagic diathesis, tonsillitis–pharyngitis • CNS signs: disorientation, stupor, coma, and seizures • Hypoglycemia, hepatic encephalopathy, or nonsuppurative encephalitis • Corneal edema or anterior uveitis (i.e., "blue eye")	• Mild form = repetitive dry-sounding hacking cough (referred to as "seal-like") often followed by gagging and mild serous naso-ocular discharge • Severe form = productive cough, anorexia, fever, depression, naso-ocular discharge
GENERAL	• History • Clinical signs	• History • Clinical signs	• Clinical signs	• Cough easily elicited on palpation of trachea
CBC	• Normal	• Lymphopenia and leukopenia • Thrombocytopenia in early disease	• Neutropenia, lymphopenia, and thrombocytopenia	• Mild leukopenia • Neutrophilic leukocytosis with a left shift
BIOCHEMISTRY	• Normal	• Normal	• ↑ Alanine aminotransferase (ALT) and aspartate aminotransferase (AST) • ↓ Glucose	• N/A
URINALYSIS	• Normal	• Normal	• N/A	• N/A

DIAGNOSTICS

		Column 1	Column 2	Column 3	Column 4
DIAGNOSTICS	**RADIOLOGY**	• N/A	• Thoracic: interstitial or alveolar pneumonia	• Abdominal: hepatomegaly	• Thoracic: Mild form—N/A Severe form—interstitial density and alveolar pattern
	MISCELLANEOUS	• Electron microscope • Fluorescent antibody tests	• Fluorescent antibody test; detection of virus in intact cells (e.g., conjunctival scrapings)	• Bile acids: mild to moderately high • Coagulation tests: prolonged prothrombin time (PT), activated partial thromboplastin time (APTT), and hypofibrinogenemia • Abdominal ultrasound: hepatomegaly and abdominal effusion	• Airway cytology • Cultures of nasal swabs, transtracheal or bronchial washings for Bordetella and mycoplasma
TREATMENT	**GENERAL**	• Symptomatic • Supportive • Fluid therapy	• Supportive • Fluid therapy	• Symptomatic • Supportive • Fluid therapy with +/- potassium and dextrose supplementation	• Supportive
	MEDICATION	• Immodium	• Antibiotics • B vitamin supplementation	• Antibiotics for secondary pneumonia or pyelonephritis	• Antibiotics: chloramphenicol, tetracyclines, and gentamycin • Bronchodilators • Antitussives
	PATIENT CARE	• Typically none	• Humidification of airways • Clean discharge from eyes and nose • Nutritional support • Adequate fluid intake or therapy • Isolation to avoid infecting other patients	• Frequent feedings to avoid hypoglycemia • Restricted activity/cage rest	• Encourage outpatient care for uncomplicated disease • Airway humidification • Strict confinement • Nutritional support

Table 3-6 Canine Disease (Continued)

Disease	Corona virus	Distemper	Hepatitis	Infectious Tracheobronchitis
PATIENT CARE	• Typically none	• Monitor dehydration and electrolytes • Recheck thoracic radiographs if persistent cough	• Monitor blood chemistries • Monitor dehydration, acid–base balances, body weight, physical assessment, and electrolytes	• Adequate fluid intake • Airway humidification • Strict rest for 14–21 days
PREVENTION/ AVOIDANCE	• Vaccinate	• Vaccinate • Avoid infected dogs or wildlife	• Vaccinate	• Vaccinate • Prevent fomite spread • Isolate infected animals
COMPLICATIONS	• Persistent diarrhea for 10–12 days • Dehydration and electrolyte imbalances	• Occurrence of CNS signs may appear for up to 2–3 months after clinical signs • Seizures or CNS signs	• Hepatic failure or chronic active hepatitis • Acute renal failure • Disseminated intravascular coagulation (DIC) • Glaucoma	• N/A
PROGNOSIS	• Complete recovery expected	• Ranges from subacute to mortality • Mortality rate of 50%	• Guarded to good • Some with a complete recovery	• Complete recovery expected unless severe disease develops
NOTES	• Optional part of vaccine series • Consider vaccinating high-risk dogs: field trial dogs and kenneled dogs • Transmitted by fecal–oral route	• Unvaccinated puppies 6–12 weeks of age are most at risk • Transmitted through all body secretions and excretions and airborne • Easily destroyed by heat and most disinfectants; survives no more than a few days outside the host • Recovered dogs are not carriers	• Transmitted through oronasal exposure and shed in all secretions during acute infection • Shed for 6–9 months after recovery • Highly resistant to inactivation and disinfection, thus enabling spread by fomites and ectoparasites	• Highly contagious via aerosol spread and fomites • Disinfect with bleach, Nolvasan, or Roccal

FOLLOW-UP

Disease	Leptospirosis ZOONOTIC	Lyme Disease ZOONOTIC	Parvovirus	Rabies ZOONOTIC
DEFINITION	Acute and chronic bacterial disease affecting lungs, kidneys, and liver.	A multiorgan disease caused by the spirochete *Borrelia burgdorferi*.	Highly contagious disease causing severe enteritis and affecting the lymphatic system. Typically affects puppies between weaning and 6 months of age.	A virus that can infect almost all warm-blooded animals and is considered not treatable. It infects the nervous system, causing death of paralysis
CLINICAL SIGNS	• Fever, anorexia, conjunctivitis, dehydration, vomiting, myalgia, reluctance to move, or depression • Tachypnea, rapid irregular pulse, and poor capillary perfusion • Acute renal or hepatic failure • DIC: petechia, melena, and epistaxis	• Polyarthritis • Anorexia, lethargy, fever, and lymphadenopathy	• Anorexia, fever, depression, vomiting, and extreme dehydration • Diarrhea: profuse, liquid, hemorrhagic, and distinct metallic odor	• Three phases: *Prodromal phase (2–3 days)*—fever, slow corneal and palpebral reflexes, subtle behavior changes; *Furious phase (2–4 days)*—irritability, restlessness, barking, ataxia, seizures; *Paralytic phase (2–4 days)*—paralysis, depression, coma, and death of respiratory paralysis

DIAGNOSTICS

	Leptospirosis ZOONOTIC	Lyme Disease ZOONOTIC	Parvovirus	Rabies ZOONOTIC
GENERAL	• Clinical signs	• Joint palpation; lameness, swelling, and pain	• History • Clinical signs	• History • Clinical signs
Complete Blood Count (CBC)	• Leukopenia, Thrombocytopenia • Neutrophilia with left shift	• N/A	• Severe leukopenia and lymphopenia • Packed cell volume (PCV) is variable	• N/A
BIOCHEMISTRY	• ↑ Blood urea nitrogen (BUN), creatinine, AST, ALT, alkaline phosphatase (ALP), and bilirubin • Electrolyte imbalances; ↓ chloride, sodium, and potassium, ↑ phosphorus	• N/A	• ↑ Bilirubin, ALT, and AST • Electrolyte imbalances; ↓ potassium	• N/A
URINALYSIS	• Proteinuria, pyuria, bilirubinuria, isosthenuria	• N/A	• N/A	• N/A

Table 3-6 Canine Disease (Continued)

	Disease	Leptospirosis ZOONOTIC	Lyme Disease ZOONOTIC	Parvovirus	Rabies ZOONOTIC
DIAGNOSTICS	**RADIOLOGY**	• N/A	• Joints; ± effusion	• Abdominal; gas and fluid distention in gastrointestinal tract (GIT) • Often causing a misdiagnosis of GI obstruction	• N/A
	MISCELLANEOUS	• Microscopic agglutination test; + after 1 week, peaking at 3–4 weeks, fourfold rise in titer • Combined IgM–IgG enzyme-linked immunosorbent assay (ELISA) titers; IgM is + in first week and persists to 2 weeks; IgG + 2–3 weeks after infection and persists for months	• Immunofluorescent assay (IFA) tests and ELISA; 1:152 and up = highly positive • Synovial fluid analysis; suppurative and ± borrelia organisms within white blood cells (WBC)	• ELISA assay	• Cerebrospinal fluid (CSF); minimal ↑ protein and leukocytes • Postmortem virus isolation; fresh brain tissue
TREATMENT	**GENERAL**	• Supportive • Fluid therapy	• Supportive	• Symptomatic • Supportive • Fluid therapy; aggressive	• Supportive
	MEDICATION	• Antibiotic; penicillin for leptospiremia	• Antibiotics; tetracycline, ampicillin, doxycycline, and cephalexin • Aspirin or other nonsteroidal anti-inflammatory drugs (NSAIDs), or glucocorticoids for pain relief	• Antibiotics; ampicillin and gentamicin • Antiemetics; metoclopramide or H$_2$ blocker	• None
	PATIENT CARE	• Restrict activity/ cage rest • Nutritional support	• Encourage outpatient care	• Nothing by mouth for 24 hours after vomiting and severe diarrhea	• Strictly inpatient/quarantine • Runs and cages should be locked

FOLLOW-UP

PATIENT CARE	• Monitor blood chemistries and urinalysis	• Restricted activity	• Dogs should remain isolated for 1 week after complete recovery	• None
PREVENTION/ AVOIDANCE	• Vaccinate in highly infected areas	• Limit access to tick-infested areas • Use tick repellants/insecticides • Periodically check dogs for ticks	• Vaccinate out to 16–18 weeks • Isolate puppies as much as possible until vaccine series has been completed	• Vaccinate • Strict quarantine for those suspected of having rabies • Euthanize all animals known to have rabies
COMPLICATIONS	• DIC • Permanent renal and hepatic dysfunction	• CNS disorders • Fatal renal failure • Heart block (rare)	• Septicemia • Secondary bacterial pneumonia • Intussusception	• N/A
PROGNOSIS	• Most infections are subclinical, those that are acutely severe have a guarded prognosis	• Recovery expected, but possible recurrence within weeks to months	• Survival of 3–4 days is usually followed by rapid recovery • Immunity by natural infection is lifelong if the dog survives	• Almost 100% fatal
NOTES	• Spread in the urine of recovered animals for months to years after infection • Transmitted by food, water, bedding, soil, vegetation, or fomites • Disinfect with povidine–iodine	• Transmitted most commonly by the deer tick, *Ixodes dammini*, through a tick bite • Infected animals pose little risk to humans; they are more of a risk in passing ticks to humans	• Transmitted by the feco-oral route • Stable in the environment for months to years • Rottweilers, Doberman Pinschers, Pit Bull Terriers, and Labrador Retrievers seem to be at higher risk • Disinfect with 1:32 dilution of bleach and water or Parvocide®	• Transmitted in the saliva • Inactivated by disinfectants • Head should be chilled on wet ice (do not freeze) and sent to a lab for analysis

Table 3-7 Typical Canine Immunization Protocol

Vaccine	Age Given*/Frequency	Injection Site**	Vaccination Prevents	Your Clinic's Protocol
DHPP	• 6–9 weeks; then two more boosters 3–4 weeks apart • Puppies are given three shots in first 4 months and then boostered annually.	Subcutaneously	Canine distemper (D) Canine hepatitis (H) Canine parainfluenza (P) Canine parvovirus (P)	
Leptospirosis	1 year (because of high incidence of allergic reactions)/annually at DVM's discretion	Subcutaneously	Canine leptospirosis (L)	
Corona	1 year/annually at DVM's discretion	Subcutaneously	Canine corona virus (C)	
Bordetella	3–12 weeks/annually (can be given every 6 months)	Intranasally	Infectious tracheobronchitis	
Rabies	12–16 weeks/varies with state requirements: 1–3 years	Typically subcutaneously between shoulder blades, but other SC sites are acceptable	Rabies virus	
Lyme	2 vaccinations given 3 weeks apart/ annually in states with a high risk		Canine borreliosis	

*Injection site, age of administration, and booster protocol may vary depending on the manufacturer of the vaccination. Recommendations by the individual manufacturer should be followed. The frequency may vary depending on the state's requirements and the doctor's protocol.
**Possible reactions range from sensitivity at the injection site, a small bump or knot at the injection site, slight fever, hives, and lethargy to anaphylactic shock (vomiting, salivation, dyspnea, and incoordination).

Table 3-8 Feline Diseases

Disease	Calicivirus	Feline infectious peritonitis (FIP, feline corona virus)	Feline panleukopenia virus (FVP, feline parvovirus)
DEFINITION	One of the major causes of feline upper respiratory disease. An acute, highly contagious viral disease causing oral ulceration, pneumonia, and occasionally arthritis.	A systemic viral disease with high mortality. Two different forms: wet or effusive form or the dry or noneffusive, granulomatous form.	An acute, systemic, and enteric viral disease. It has a sudden onset, is highly contagious, and has a high mortality rate.
CLINICAL SIGNS	• Anorexia, depression, and fever • Mild sneezing, nasal discharge, and ulcerated tip of nose • Mild conjunctivitis • Oral ulcers and gingivitis • Dyspnea from pneumonia • Limping syndrome, enteritis, and interdigital paw ulcers • Possible arthralgia	• Fever, depression, inactivity, vomiting, diarrhea, pallor, poor condition, weight loss, and icterus • Abdominal or pleural effusion (wet form) • Dyspnea and exercise intolerance (dry form) • Ocular changes; iritis, chorioretinitis, irregular pupils and anterior uveitis • Neurologic changes: ataxia, seizures, behavioral changes, paresis, and urinary incontinence	• Anorexia, depression, fever, persistent vomiting, diarrhea, progressive dehydration • Rough and dull hair coat • Hypothermia (later) • Abdominal pain: crouching position and head between front paws
GENERAL	• History • Clinical Signs	• Clinical signs after other conditions have been ruled out	• History • Clinical signs
CBC	• Normal	• Leukopenia (early in disease) • Leukocytosis with neutrophilia and lymphopenia (late in disease) • Nonregenerative anemia	• Leukopenia
BIOCHEMISTRY	• Normal	• ↑ Bilirubin, ALP, ALT, globulins, and bile acids • ↑ BUN and creatinine	• ↑ Bilirubin and other liver enzymes • ↑ BUN and creatinine • Electrolyte imbalances
URINALYSIS	• Normal	• ↑ Bilirubin and protein	• N/A

DIAGNOSTICS

Table 3-8 Feline Diseases (Continued)

	Disease	Calicivirus	Feline infectious peritonitis (FIP, feline corona virus)	Feline panleukopenia virus (FVP, feline parvovirus)
DIAGNOSTICS	RADIOLOGY	• Thoracic: generalized ↑ density of the lungs	• Abdominal; effusion, organomegaly, lymphadenopathy, and ileocolic mass • Thoracic; effusion	• N/A
	MISCELLANEOUS	• Virus isolation; cell cultures of swabs from oropharynx, lung tissue, nasal cavity, conjunctiva, feces, and blood	• Abdominocentesis or thoracocentesis; straw-colored fluid, viscous, clots, fibrinous, and ↑ protein • Histopathologic examination; biopsy is the only definitive method for FIP diagnosis	• Virus isolation; feces • CITE test for canine parvovirus; detects FPV antigen in the acute stage
TREATMENT	GENERAL	• Self-limiting in 5–7 days • Supportive	• Therapeutic paracentesis • Fluid therapy	• Supportive • Fluid therapy
	MEDICATION	• Antibiotics; amoxicillin • Antibiotic (ophthalmic) • Pain medication	• Corticosteroids; prednisone • Immunosuppressive drugs; cyclophosphamide • Immunomodulatory drugs; interferon	• Antibiotics • Antiemetics; metoclopramide
	PATIENT CARE	• Oxygen supplementation if complicated pneumonia • Nutritional support	• Nutritional support	• Nothing by mouth until vomiting and diarrhea subside • Heat support if hypothermic
FOLLOW-UP	PATIENT CARE	• Keep eyes and nose clear of discharge • Support nutrition and fluid intake • Airway humidification • Provide soft foods if oral ulcers • Irrigate oral lesions with 0.2% chlorhexidine solution	• Confine to prevent exposure to other cats	• Heat support • Nutritional support once eating
	PREVENTION/AVOIDANCE	• Vaccinate • Prevent contact with FCV-infected cats	• Prevent contact with FIP-positive cats • Intranasal vaccine—very low efficacy • Routine disinfection • Control and prevent feline leukemia virus (FelV) infection	• Vaccinate • Prevent contact with infected cats

FOLLOW-UP (continued)

COMPLICATIONS	• Interstitial pneumonia • Secondary bacterial infections	• GI obstruction • Neurologic disease • Pleural effusion	• Hypothermia and shock • DIC • Mycotic infection • Jaundice
PROGNOSIS	• Excellent unless pneumonia develops • Recovered cats may shed the virus in their saliva for long periods	• Almost 100% mortality • Length of disease is a few days to months	• 50%–90% mortality in young kittens • Cats surviving 5 days typically have a rapid recovery
NOTES	• Transmission is through direct contact and fomites • Very resistant virus; disinfect with 1:32 dilution of bleach water • Cats that recover may remain subclinical carriers for months to years • Cats should be tested for FIV or FeLV to rule out underlying immunodeficiency syndromes • Occurs with FVR in most cases	• Transmitted through oral and respiratory secretions, feces, urine, and fomites • Survives in the environment for several weeks • Readily inactivated by commonly used disinfectants	• Transmitted through all body secretions for up to 6 weeks • Disinfect with 1:32 dilution of bleach water • Survives for up to 1 year in the environment • In utero transmission from infected queen leads to cerebellar hypoplasia in kittens

Disease	Feline Leukemia Virus (FELV)	Viral Rhinotracheitis (FVR, Feline Herpesvirus)	Bordetella Bronchiseptica
DEFINITION	A retrovirus causing immunodeficiency and neoplastic disease	One of the major causes of feline upper respiratory disease. A highly contagious viral disease causing rhinitis, conjunctivitis, and ulcerative keratitis	Bacteria causing a contagious respiratory disease Mortality : Kittens < 6 weeks—almost 100% Kittens > 6 weeks—around 50%
CLINICAL SIGNS	• Lymphadenomegaly • Rhinitis, conjunctivitis, and keratitis • Persistent diarrhea • Fever, wasting, skin infections • Gingivitis, stomatitis and periodontitis	• Anorexia, fever, and depression • Rhinitis, sneezing, nasocular discharge, hypersalivation, loss of voice, and cough (rare) • Ulcerative keratitis or herpetic ulcers, excessive lacrimation, conjunctivitis, and photophobia	• Asymptomatic • Cough (from a "hacking" type progressing to a "whooping" type cough) • Possible vomiting • Fever, lethargy • Ocular discharge • Mandibular lymphadenopathy

Table 3-8 Feline Disease (Continued)

	Disease	Feline Leukemia Virus (FELV)	Viral Rhinotracheitis (FVR, Feline Herpesvirus)	Bordetella Bronchiseptica
DIAGNOSTICS	GENERAL	• History • Clinical signs	• Clinical signs	• Clinical signs
	CBC	• Nonregenerative anemia • Lymphopenia and neutropenia • Thrombocytopenia and immune-mediated hemolytic anemia	• Transient leukopenia followed by leukocytosis	• Neutrophilic leukocytosis w/left shift
	BIOCHEMISTRY	• Will often show abnormalities depending the system affected	• Normal	• Normal
	URINALYSIS	• Will often show abnormalities, depending the system affected	• Normal	• Normal
	RADIOLOGY	• N/A	• Skull; chronic disease shows changes in the nasal cavities and frontal sinuses	• Thoracic: diffuse or mixed interstitial lung pattern
	MISCELLANEOUS	• ELISA test for virus antigen detection • Bone marrow aspirate or biopsy • IFA test	• Virus isolation; cell cultures of swabs from the pharynx, nasal epithelium or conjunctiva	• Tracheal wash w/ culture and sensitivity
TREATMENT	GENERAL	• Symptomatic	• Supportive • Fluid therapy	• Supportive • Fluid therapy w/ complicated disease
	MEDICATION	• Antibiotics; especially with *Haemobartonella* infection • Immunomodulatory drugs; interferon	• Antibiotics; amoxicillin and enrofloxacin • Antibiotics (ophthalmic) • Antiviral eye medications; Vira-A • Immunomodulatory drugs; interferon	• Antibiotics: Clavamox, Baytril, Tetracycline, Antirobe; 14–21 days
	PATIENT CARE	• Blood transfusions; many may be necessary. Using blood from FeLV-vaccinated cats may reduce the level of FeLV antigenemia in some cats	• Nutritional support • Keep eyes and nose clear of discharge • Support nutrition and fluid intake • Airway humidification • ↑ Environmental temperature; herpesvirus is temperature sensitive	• Rest

FOLLOW-UP

PATIENT CARE	• Symptomatic	• Confine indoors to decrease environmentally induced stress • Symptomatic
PREVENTION/ AVOIDANCE	• Vaccinate outdoor cats and those living with an FeLV-positive cat • Quarantine and test all new cats to the household or local environment • Prevent contact with FeLV positive cats	• Vaccinate • Prevent contact with FHV-infected cats • Canine vaccinations have been used in catteries; researchers have been looking into a feline-specific vaccine.
COMPLICATIONS	• Lymphoma • Fibrosarcoma • Glomerulonephritis • Toxoplasmosis • Haemobartonellosis	• Chronic rhinosinusitis • Persistent nasal discharge • Herpetic ulcerative keratitis • Permanent closure of nasolacrimal duct • Pneumonia—death
PROGNOSIS	• >50% of cats die from related diseases in 2–3 years	• Good; 7–10 days • Uncomplicated: 10–14 days • Complicated: 2–6 weeks
NOTES	• All FeLV-positive cats MUST remain indoors to prevent further spreading of the disease • Test each cat before first vaccine or if there has been a long period without vaccines • More false-positive cats when using whole blood on the ELISA test • Do not use modified live vaccines • Transmission is through cat-to-cat bites, grooming, and shared dishes and litter boxes	• Transmission is through direct contact and fomites • Very resistant virus; disinfect with 1:32 dilution of bleach water • Readily inactivated by commonly used disinfectants • Cats should be tested for FIV and FeLV to rule out underlying immunodeficiency syndromes • Bacteria shed for at least 19 weeks

Table 3-9   Typical Feline Immunization Protocol

Vaccine	Age Given*/Frequency	Injection Site**	Vaccination Prevents	Your Clinic's Protocol
FVRCP	7–12 weeks; booster 3–4 weeks later (at least 1 booster after 12 weeks old)/ booster 1 year later; then good for 1–3 years, depending on manufacturer or clinic.	Typically subcutaneously on right lower shoulder or intranasal, depending on manufacturer.	Feline viral rhinotracheitis (FVR) Feline calicivirus (C) Feline panleukopenia (P)	
FELV	FELV test should be performed before vaccinating. 9–12 weeks; booster 3–4 weeks later Annually	Left hind lower thigh area (having a designated site is important in monitoring development of sarcomas).	Feline leukemia (FELV)	
RABIES	12–16 weeks/Varies with state requirements: 1– 3 years	Right hind lower thigh area	Rabies virus (RV)	
FIP	16 weeks; then 3–4 weeks later/Annually	Intranasally	Feline infectious peritonitis (FIP)	

*Injection site, age of administration, and booster protocol may vary depending on the manufacturer of the vaccination. Recommendations by the individual manufacturer should be followed. The frequency may vary depending on the state's requirements and the doctor's protocol. Each animal should be assessed for potential risk/exposure before vaccination.
**Possible reactions range from sensitivity at the injection site, a small bump or knot at the injection site, slight fever, hives, lethargy to anaphylactic shock (vomiting, salivation, dyspnea & incoordination) and injection site sarcomas. Any bump found at the injection site should be checked by a doctor.

GENERAL NUTRITION

Proper nutrition is as important as physical examinations, vaccinations, and dental care in maintaining a healthy pet. Unfortunately, not much time is usually given to the subject during client education. Obesity still remains the biggest nutritional challenge; it is estimated that 40% of dogs and 30% of cats in the United States are obese. Understanding how to feed a pet according to its life stage, how to determine the current condition as well as how this changes with disease, and how to get a pet back to its ideal condition are the keys to proper clinical nutrition.

Table 3-10   General Life Stage Feeding Guidelines

Each stage of an animal's life presents changes in nutritional needs. The overall goal of nutrition is to obtain an optimum body conditioning score. (See Table 3-11)

	Diet	Frequency/Amount	Avoid	Obesity	Thin
Puppy	• Begin introducing puppy growth food at 3 weeks of age • Weaning at 6–8 weeks of age	• Free choice for kittens and small breed puppies • Time-limited 3–4 meals daily for large breed puppies	• Adult foods • Poor-quality, unbalanced, commercial food • Homemade diets of single-food items • Indiscriminate mixtures of single-food items • Supplements that may cause dietary imbalances • Overfeeding and extra vitamins during rapid growth phase	• Large breed—developmental orthopedic disease	• Small breed—hypoglycemia
Adult	• High-quality adult food • Homemade diets made from approved published recipes	• 2–3 meals daily • See Box 3-1 on calculating the appropriate amount of food	• Poor-quality, unbalanced, commercial food • Homemade diets of single food items • Indiscriminate mixtures of single food items • Supplements that may cause dietary imbalances	• Diabetes • Osteoarthritis • Skin problems • Surgical risk	• Hypoglycemia • Hypothermia • Muscle disorders

Table 3-10   General Life Stage Feeding Guidelines (Continued)

Each stage of an animal's life presents changes in nutritional needs. The overall goal of nutrition is to obtain an optimum body conditioning score. (See Table 3-11)

	Diet	Frequency/Amount	Avoid	Obesity	Thin
Pregnancy	• Diet should gradually be changed during the last 3 weeks to a puppy growth diet to provide additional nutrients	• During the first 6 weeks, the feeding schedule should not change, and the dam should maintain her normal weight • During the last 3 weeks, the dam's weight should increase by 25%	• Carbohydrate-free meat-type diets should be avoided during gestation and whelping to prevent hypoglycemia and decreased survival at birth	• Dystocia	• Trouble conceiving
Lactation	• High-quality puppy growth food • Homemade diets made from approved published recipes	• Free-choice • Nutrients increase approximately 3×	• Low-calorie diets (e.g., weight-reducing diets)		• Insufficient amount of milk supply
Geriatric	• High-quality adult food • Homemade diets made from approved published recipes • Supplement with Vitamin E may be warranted • Increase protein	• 2–3 meals daily • See Box 3-1 on calculating the appropriate amount of food • Many recommend reducing the caloric intake by 20% to avoid obesity	• Placing the bowl in hard-to-reach places (e.g., arthritic cat having to jump onto a table to eat)	• Diabetes • Osteoarthritis • Skin problems • Surgical risk	• Hypoglycemia • Hypothermia • Muscle disorders

Dams must supply all nutrients needed to litter whose weight will double in 10 days

Table 3-11   Body Conditioning Score

The Body Conditioning Score standardizes the interpretation of the overall physical appearance of the animal. It should be a basic part of every examination and should be noted in the record for future comparison.

Canine	Body Conditioning Score	Feline
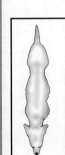	**1- Very Thin** *Ribs: Easily visible and felt with no cover* *Waist: Severe waist* *Tail Base: Lumbar vertebrae and pelvic bones are raised with no fat between the skin and bone* *Side View: Severe abdominal tuck* *Overhead View: Accentuated hourglass shape*	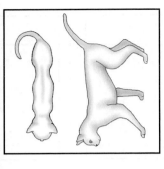
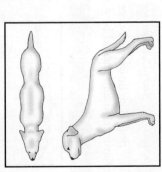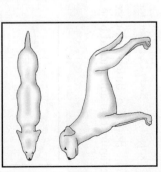	**2- Underweight** *Ribs: Easily felt with minimal fat cover* *Waist: Easily noted* *Tail Base: Bones are raised with minimal fat between the skin and bone* *Side View: Prominent abdominal tuck* *Overhead View: Marked hourglass shape*	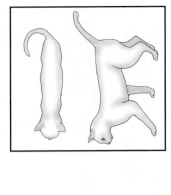

Table 3-11 Body Conditioning Score (Continued)

The Body Conditioning Score standardizes the interpretation of the overall physical appearance of the animal. It should be a basic part of every examination and should be noted in the record for future comparison.

Canine	Body Conditioning Score	Feline
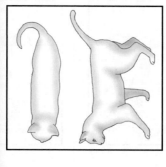	**3- Ideal** *Ribs: Easily felt with slight fat cover* *Waist: Observed behind ribs* *Tail Base: Smooth contour but bones can be felt under a thin layer of fat* *Side View: Abdominal tuck* *Overhead View: Well proportioned waist*	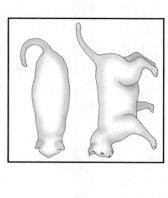
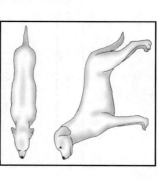	**4- Overweight** *Ribs: Difficult to feel with moderate fat cover* *Waist: Poorly discernible* *Tail Base: Some thickening but bones can be felt under a moderate layer of fat* *Side View: No abdominal tuck* *Overhead View: Back is slightly broadened*	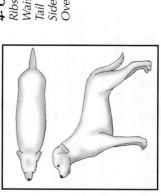

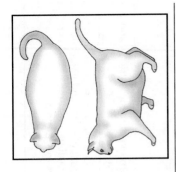

5- Obese
Ribs: Difficult to feel under thick fat cover
Waist: Absent
Tail Base: Thickened and difficult to feel bones beneath prominent layer of fat
Side View: Fat hangs from the abdomen
Overhead View: Markedly broadened and prominent paralumbar fat deposits

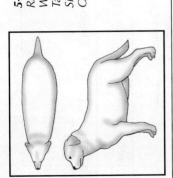

Table 3-12 Diseases And Their Nutritional Requirements

Disease	Objective	Dietary Considerations	Comments
Cardiology *Heart Failure*	• Control sodium retention • Maintain optimum body weight	• ↓ Sodium, chloride, protein, and phosphorus, ↓ Magnesium (cats) • ↑ B-complex vitamins, Taurine (cats)	• Softened water contains a significant amount of sodium
Dermatology *Food Allergy*	• Avoid offending food item	• No gluten (wheat, barley, rye, buckwheat, and oats) • No previously introduced protein source; substitute with rabbit, venison, or tofu • No previously introduced carbohydrate source; substitute with rice or potato • ↓ Additives (azo-dyes, non-azo dyes, antioxidants, BHA, and sodium nitrate) • Hydrolyzed ingredients to reduce molecular weights (e.g., hypoallergenic diets)	• Feed exclusively for 6 weeks • Canned food contains the least amount of additives
Endocrinology *Diabetes mellitus*	• Correct obesity • Minimize postprandial fluctuations in blood glucose • Consistent feeding times and caloric intake	• ↑ Fiber and high-complex carbohydrates (>40%) • ↓ Fat • Supplement with additives that aid in glycemic control (chromium and acarbose)	• Avoid semi-moist foods • Weigh animal frequently • Feed small frequent meals
Hyperthyroidism	• Correct cachexia	• Highly digestible diet with high bioavailability of protein	• Poor absorption of many nutrients and ↑ metabolism
Pancreatitis	• ↓ Pancreatic secretions	• Initially ↓ protein and fat, gradually add in carbohydrates (boiled rice, pasta, potatoes), and then add in a protein source (cottage cheese or lean meat) • ↑ Digestibility	• NPO for 3–5 days, then begin with small amount of water and gradually move to small frequent meals of ↑ carbohydrates to ↑ protein

Condition	Objectives	Nutritional Factors	Comments
Pancreatic exocrine insufficiency (EPI)	• Correct malnutrition • Reduce requirements for digestive enzymes	• Supplement with pancreatic enzymes • ↓ Caloric density • ↓ Fiber and fat • +/- Supplement of medium-chain triglycerides • +/- Supplement with tocopherol, cobalamine, and fat-soluble vitamins	• Avoid high-fiber diets • Supplementation with tocopherol, cobalamine, and fat-soluble vitamins is best done parenterally, initially
Gastroenterology *Constipation*	• Normalize GI motility • ↑ Hydration • ↑ Bulk	• ↑ Laxatives and fiber (canned pumpkin, coarse bran, or psyllium) • ↑ Water intake • ↓ Ingestion of constipating materials (bones, hair, cat litter, or cloth)	• ↑ Exercise and prevent obesity • Maintain a clean litter box to encourage frequent defecation • Check anus/rectum for causes for poor defecation habits
Diarrhea	• Normalize GI motility • ↑ Hydration • ↑ Bulk • Provide GI rest • ↑ Caloric intake due to catabolism	Dogs: • ↓ Fat, lactose, and additives • Highly digestible diet, 80% carbohydrates Cats: • ↑ Protein • ↓ Carbohydrate	• No food for 24–48 hours (fast) • No restriction on water, if no vomiting • Gradually reintroduce normal diet after diarrhea is resolved (2–3 normal stools in a row) • Small, frequent meals to prevent gluttony
Flatulence	• ↓ Intestinal gas production • ↓ Aerophagia • ↓ Bacterial fermentation of nutrients	• ↓ Soy, whole wheat products, fiber, and fat • Avoid all milk products • Highly digestible diet	• Small, frequent meals • Discourage gluttony; provide a noncompetitive environment • ↓ Stress • ↑ Exercise
Hepatic lipidosis	• Correct anorexia • ↑ Caloric intake/density	• ↑ Protein and carbohydrates • ↓ Fat • +/- Supplement with thiamine, taurine, arginine, L-carnitine, and a multi-	• Recovery is directly related to early diagnosis and treatment via enteral tube feeding

Table 3-12   Diseases And Their Nutritional Requirements (Continued)

Disease	Objective	Dietary Considerations	Comments
Liver Disease	• Maintain body weight • Promote hepatic regeneration • ↑ Caloric intake/density	• Initial ↓ protein, then gradual ↑ protein • +/- Supplemental vitamins K1, E, A, B, C, and D • Control sodium intake • ↑ Levels of aromatic amino acids and methionine • ↓ Levels of branched-chain amino acids, copper, and arginine • Easily digested carbohydrates (rice, pasta, and potato) • Highly digestible ingredients	• Small meals • Slowly increase amount over a few days
Vomiting	• Correct hydration • Provide GI rest • ↓ Gastric secretions	• Highly digestible, bland diet of single carbohydrates and protein sources (low-fat cottage cheese, boiled chicken or hamburger, rice, pasta, or potato) • ↓ Fat	• No food for 24 hours, then small amounts fed frequently (every 2–4 hours) • Small amount of water or ice
Hematology/ Immunology *Anemia*	• Support RBC production	• ↑ Iron, cobalt, copper, B-complex vitamins, and protein	• Iron deficiency is usually due to excessive loss (e.g., hemorrhage, GI ulcers, and ectoparasitism) versus inadequate intake
Musculoskeletal *Bone loss and fracture repair*	• Correct deficiency of energy and protein	• ↑ Protein and energy	
Debilitation	• Replete tissue, plasma, and nutrients	• Extremely digestible diet • ↑ Protein, fat, B-complex vitamins, Vitamin E, n_3 fatty acids, branch-chain amino acids, zinc, potassium, Glutamine/glutamate, and arginine • ↓ Carbohydrates	• Assist with feeding if needed

Condition	Goals	Key Nutritional Factors	Comments
Obesity	↓ Body weight; Control caloric intake; Maintain omega 3 and 6 fatty acids in proper ratio to maintain skin and coat conditioning	↓ Caloric density (fat); ↑ Bulk to control hunger (fiber); Supplement arginine to aid in muscle strength and tone while losing weight	Prevention is easier than treatment of obesity
Oncology	Prevent cancer cachexia; ↑ Nutrient intake	Highly digestible and palatable diet; ↓ Simple carbohydrates; +/- Supplement with arginine, cysteine, and glutamine, and vitamin E; ↑ Omega-3 fatty acids, fat, and fiber	Nutritional intervention must begin early in disease to prevent cachexia; Many vitamins and minerals may be added; further research should be done
Renal/Urology *Kidney Disease*	↓ Amount of nitrogenous waste; Delay progression of renal failure; Prevent malnutrition; Nitrogen trap—excess nitrogenous waste into colon via feces	↓ Protein, phosphorus, and sodium; ↑ Potassium, non-protein calories, and B-complex vitamins; Supplement n-3 Fatty acids	Do not ↓ protein until moderate to severe renal failure; Protein recommendations: Dogs: 2.0–2.2 g/kg/day Cats: 3.3–3.5 g/kg/day; Restrict sodium gradually over 2–4 weeks
Urolithiasis-Canine *Struvite*	Maintain acidic urine (pH of 6.2–6.4); Resolve underlying infection	↓ Protein, calcium, phosphorus, and magnesium; ↑ Sodium to increase water intake to produce dilute urine	Dissolution on average takes 36 days
Ammonium urate	Maintain alkaline urine (pH of 7.0–7.5); Dissolution and prevention of uroliths; ↑ Water consumption to ↓ urine concentration	↓ Purine, protein, sodium, and phosphorus; +/- Supplement with sodium bicarbonate; +/- Supplement with allopurinol if diet ineffective alone	Meat-based diets tend to have increased purine; vegetable-based diets may be more suitable

Table 3-12   Diseases And Their Nutritional Requirements (Continued)

Disease	Objective	Dietary Considerations	Comments
Calcium oxalate *Cystine*	• Maintain alkaline urine (pH of 7.1–7.7) • ↑ Water consumption • Bind calcium in urine to prevent crystal precipitate	• ↓ Potassium • ↓ Sodium, protein, and phosphorus	• Medical dissolution is not possible for Calcium oxalate stones, once formed
Urolithiasis-Feline			
Struvite	• Maintain acidic urine (pH of <6.4) • Dissolution and prevention of uroliths	• Highly digestible diet • ↑↓ Potassium, taurine • Supplement with urine acidifier	• Average dissolution is 35 days after negative radiographs
Calcium oxalate	• Maintain alkaline urine (pH of 6.6–6.8) • Dissolution and prevention of uroliths	• ↓ Protein, sodium, calcium, and oxalic acid • Discontinue supplementation with vitamin C or urine acidifier • +/- Supplementation of vitamin B_6	• Medical dissolution is not possible for calcium oxalate stones, once formed

Skill Box 3-1 / Daily Caloric Requirement Worksheet for a Healthy Animal

Many factors affect the energy requirements of animals. Understanding these factors may prevent an animal from becoming obese. Daily caloric requirements are altered by the physiologic state (e.g., adult maintenance, pregnancy, lactation, and growth), activity level, temperament, environmental temperature, and the diet's digestibility.

Step 1: Calculate Daily Caloric Requirement
  –as provided by the National Research Council for maintenance of an adult animal

  Dog: (Body weight kg)$^{0.75}$ $\times$132 = _____ Kcal/day

(This has been shown to be 5%–6% higher than what is actually needed to maintain optimum weight. Adjust Kcal based on visual and manual examination of animal.)

  Cat: 70–80 Kcal $\times$_____kg = _____ Kcal/day

  Pregnancy:
      Weeks 1–4 = (Body weight kg)$^{0.75}$ $\times$132 = _____ Kcal/day
      Week 5 = Maintenance $\times$1.1
      Weeks 6–9 = Maintenance $\times$1.2
  Lactation:
      Week 1 = Maintenance $\times$1.5
      Week 2 = Maintenance $\times$2
      Weeks 3–5 = Maintenance $\times$3
  Growth:
      Weaning to 50% of adult body weight =
          (Body weight kg)$^{0.75}$ $\times$264 = _____ Kcal/day
      51% of adult body weight to adult body weight =
          (Body weight kg)$^{0.75}$ $\times$198 = _____ Kcal/day

(These calculations do not take into consideration the type of breed and their differences in growth requirements. Adjust Kcal based on visual and manual examination of animal.)

  Step 2: Calculate Volume of Food Required
      _____ Kcal/day / _____ Kcal/cup of food = _____ cup(s) of food/day
  Step 3: Calculate Amount of Each Feeding
      _____ cup(s) of food/day / 2–3 feedings per day = _____ cup(s) of food/feeding

Table 3-13 Pediatric Feeding Guidelines

Age	General Nutritional Facts	Diet	Weaning	Methods
Birth to Weaning	• Body fat stores are only at 1%–2% at birth, presenting the risk of hypoglycemia, starvation, and hypothermia • Adequate glycogen reserves do not develop until after first few days of nursing • All neonates need to receive colostrum in the first 24 hours of life to ensure transfer of passive immunity • Hypothermia can lead to poor nursing • Energy requirement is 22–26 kcal/100 g	• Dam's milk • Commercial formulations • Temporary canine diet of 1 qt whole cow's milk, four egg yolks, and 1 tbsp corn oil • Temporary feline diet of 3 oz condensed milk, 3 oz water, 4 oz plain yogurt (not low fat), and 3 large or 4 small egg yolks • Neonates should receive 13 mL/100 g/day of replacement diet for the first week, 17 mL/100 g/day the second week, 20 mL/100 g/day the third week, and 22 mL/100 g/day the fourth week	• Food introduction begins at 3–4 weeks • Mix growth food with warm water to moisten or make into a slurry • Neonates should be encouraged to eat by placing their feet in the food, smearing food on their lips, or introducing food into their mouth • Weaning (complete weaning should not start before 6 weeks of age and close human contact has occurred) 1. The dam/queen should be separated from the neonates the day before weaning. The neonates should be fed, and food should be withheld from the dam/queen. Water not removed 2. The neonates should be reunited with the dam/queen overnight and be allowed to nurse to drain the mammary glands. Food only should be withheld from both the dam/queen and the neonates overnight. 3. The neonates are removed from the dam/queen the next morning and weaned.	• Nursing • Orogastric tube (refer to Chapter 8: Table 8-11) • Bottle feeding 1. Hold the neonate in a small towel or washcloth with its back placed in the palm of your hand and your fingers placed under its forelimbs 2. Hold the bottle with the nipple pointing downward at an angle that restricts air from getting into the nipple 3. Squeeze a drop of milk on the nipple and then introduce the nipple into the side of the mouth roughly behind where the canine teeth would be 4. Do not squeeze the bottle while in the neonate's mouth to avoid laryngotracheal aspiration
Weaning to 6 months	• Supplementation with table scraps, meats, or other items may lead to a finicky eater, nutritional deficiencies, or excesses • Puppies should be fed time-limited meals 3 times daily • Kittens should be fed free-choice, or at least 3 times daily	• High-quality puppy/kitten growth food	• Does not apply	• Eating on their own

Chapter

4

Dentistry

ANATOMY

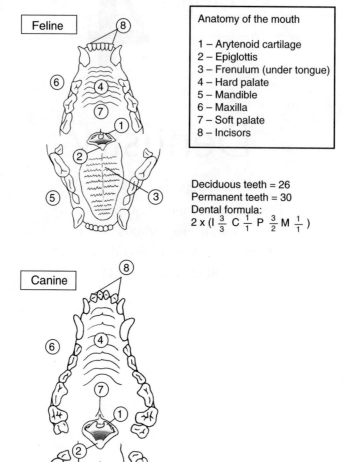

Feline

Canine

Anatomy of the mouth

1 – Arytenoid cartilage
2 – Epiglottis
3 – Frenulum (under tongue)
4 – Hard palate
5 – Mandible
6 – Maxilla
7 – Soft palate
8 – Incisors

Deciduous teeth = 26
Permanent teeth = 30
Dental formula:
$2 \times (I\ \frac{3}{3}\ C\ \frac{1}{1}\ P\ \frac{3}{2}\ M\ \frac{1}{1})$

Deciduous teeth = 28
Permanent teeth = 42
Dental formula:
$2 \times (I\ \frac{3}{3}\ C\ \frac{1}{1}\ P\ \frac{4}{4}\ M\ \frac{2}{3})$

Fig. 4-1 Dentition: Feline and canine.

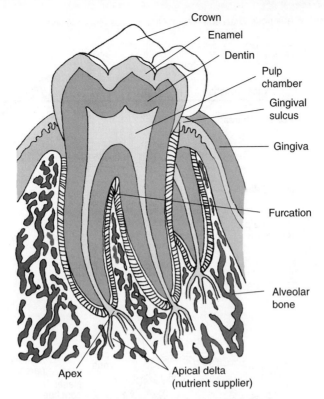

Fig. 4-2 Cross section of a triple-rooted tooth.

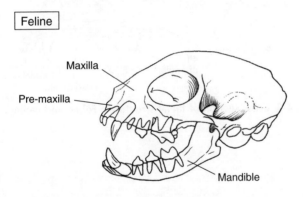

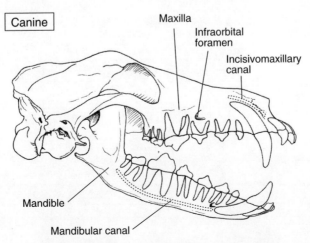

Fig. 4-3 Skeletal structure: Feline and canine.

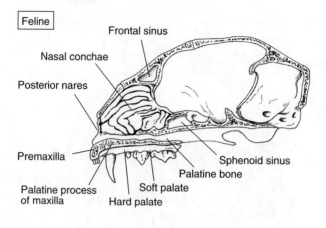

Feline

Frontal sinus

Nasal conchae

Posterior nares

Premaxilla

Sphenoid sinus
Palatine bone

Palatine process
of maxilla

Soft palate
Hard palate

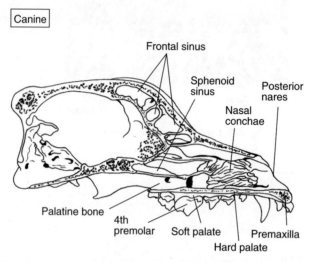

Canine

Frontal sinus

Sphenoid
sinus

Posterior
nares

Nasal
conchae

Palatine bone

4th
premolar   Soft palate

Premaxilla

Hard palate

Fig. 4-3 Cross section of facial structures: Feline and canine.

DENTAL INSTRUMENTS/ EQUIPMENT

Table 4-1   Hand-Held Instruments

Instrument	Usage
Curette scalers	Used beneath the gingiva to remove calculus and to root plane
Dental claw	Used to remove large amount of calculus supragingivally
Dental elevators	Used to displace the tooth from its support structures
Dental extraction forceps	Used to remove tooth from jaw and to clean heavy calculus off teeth
Dental hoe	Used to remove large amounts of calculus supragingivally
Explorer	Used to examine the tooth's surface subgingivally and check tooth mobility
Periodontal probe	Used to measure the depth of the gingival sulcus in millimeters
Periosteal elevators	Used to reflect and retract mucoperiosteum
Scaler	Used on the exposed tooth to remove calculus above the gingiva {NOT USED SUBGINGIVALLY}

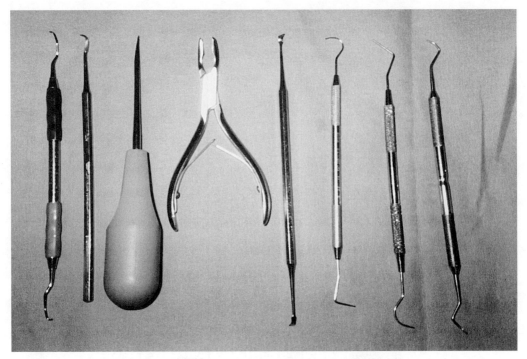

Fig. 4-4 Hand-held non-mechanical dental instruments.

Table 4-2 Maintenance of Hand-Held Instruments

Hand-held instruments need to be sharpened on a regular basis with a stone and oilstone oil.

Sharpening Stones	Type/lubricant required	Usage
India	Fine/medium— oil lubricant	To sharpen extremely dull instruments
Arkansas	Fine—oil lubricant	To finish sharpening after a medium coarse stone was used
Ceramic	Fine/medium—water lubricant or dry	Same as other two, but uses water as its lubricant
Conical	A round Arkansas stone—oil lubricant	To sharpen curved instruments; can shorten the life of an instrument because it damages the face of the instrument.

Skill Box 4-1 / Sharpening Technique

Flat Stone

1. Place small amount of oil onto the stone and wipe to cover the stone face.
2. Hold stone between thumb and index finger slightly off perpendicular to the floor.
3. Place instrument to be sharpened on the oiled stone with the tip facing the operator and the face of the instrument parallel to the ground.
4. Move the instrument up and down on the stone, ending with a down stroke.
5. Check for sharpness by visual inspection or by using a plexiglass rod. Dull edges look rounded and reflect light. Sharp edges gives off no light reflection.
6. Disinfect instrument after sharpening.

Conical Stone

1. Place instrument in hand with tip pointing outward, wrapped around the oiled conical stone.
2. As you rotate the stone, slide the stone toward the tip of the instrument.

Table 4-3 Mechanical Instruments

Decision on dental equipment should be a clinic-directed process, reviewing many of the types of equipment available, with assessment of who will be using it and what procedures will be performed. Manufacturer's care and maintenance instructions should be made a part of the clinic's routine.

Always use a light touch to avoid heat buildup on the tooth, and never remain on one tooth for more than 10–15 seconds.

Equipment	Description
Scalers: 1. Ultrasonic:	Converts energy to sound waves, which result in a mechanical vibration of the handpiece. When water passes over the tip, a scouring property known as cavitation is produced. Follow manufacturer's maintenance guidelines.
Magnetostrictive	Tip vibrates in an elliptical motion and has a working tip on all sides; uses metal stacks
Piezoelectric	Tip vibrates in a linear motion; only one side of the tip is used against the tooth; uses crystals in handpieces
2. Sonic	Converts air to mechanical vibration. Follow manufacturer's maintenance guidelines.
3. Rotary	Tartar and calculus removal. Caution must be used because these instruments can easily damage the enamel, dentin, and soft tissue. For this reason, they are not recommended
Polishers/Drilling Units	Two types are available, electric or air driven. Various heads are available. Follow manufacturer's maintenance guidelines.

DENTAL PROPHYLAXIS

Table 4-4 Dental Cleaning Process

Step	Method	Purpose/Notes
1. SETUP Technician: • Face shield or glasses, gloves, surgical mask, smock for dental use only, and surgical cap • Dental equipment/supplies • Adjustable stool Patient: • Appropriate measures to maintain patient's temperature • Appropriate monitoring equipment • IV catheter/fluids if necessary • Pre-planned pain management protocol by veterinarian • Anesthesia protocol to anesthetize patient • Appropriate-size mouth gag • Gauze sponges in back of throat to absorb excess water and debris • Head positioned downward to permit proper drainage	Not applicable.	• Proper setup reduces risk of cumulative trauma disorders (CTD) to technicians. CTDs include carpal tunnel syndrome and any trauma caused by repetitive motions. • Heating pad w/proper cover to decrease chance of burning, towels and warmed fluid bags • Doppler or other blood pressure device, pulse oximeter, electrocardiogram (ECG), and/or apnea monitor
2. ORAL EXAMINATION The technician should perform a thorough examination of the animal's mouth; charting any abnormal conditions. The veterinarian should be consulted on any abnormality noted.	**External examination:** • Check the symmetry of the animal's head and face. • Check for halitosis. • Note any nasal or ocular discharge or swelling. • Check occlusion. • Check lips, mouth, and tongue for any anomalies. **Internal examination:** Chart degree of plaque/calculus, missing teeth, and any abnormalities that can be visualized at this time.	• Be gentle with any manipulation of the tongue so as not to injure the nerve supply or muscle attachments. • Follow a routine to ensure that all teeth are checked, cleaned, and charted.

Table 4-4   Dental Cleaning Process (Continued)

Step	Method	Purpose/Notes
3. BRUSH TEETH	Brush with chlorhexidine toothpaste and irrigate with 0.1%–0.2% chlorhexidine solution.	To get rid of excess bacteria before cleaning
4. REMOVAL OF GROSS CALCULUS	Use forceps (calculus or extraction) to remove large accumulations of calculus. Using a modified pen grasp, place the scaler at a 45–90-degree angle on the tooth such that the tip conforms to the curve of the tooth, and the cutting edge of the scaler is beneath the calculus. Use a pull stroke away from the gumline. This stroke should use the shoulder muscles and not the wrist. This is to only be used supragingivally. Ultrasonic scalers can be used to complete the removal of any remaining calculus.	To decrease the overuse of the ultrasonic scaler
5. ULTRASONIC CLEANING	Using the same grasp as on a scaler, use light brush stroke touches on the tooth. Keep the tip moving to prevent overheating of the tooth and remain no longer than 10–15 seconds on any tooth. Use only on those teeth with plaque/calculus.	Cleaning teeth absent of any plaque/calculus is not recommended because of the damaging effects on the cementum.
6. SUBGINGIVAL CLEANING AND ROOT PLANING	Preliminary removal of subgingival calculus can be achieved with perio-shaped rotosonic, sonic, or subsonic scalers. Use hand curettes to complete the job. Use a 45–90-degree angle and a sharp, firm, pulling stroke. Check removal effectiveness with an explorer. Root plane, using a curette, on teeth with pocketing of 4–6 mm. 10–20 short overlapping strokes (horizontal, vertical, and oblique) will achieve a glassy smooth surface. This can be accomplished without surgery in some cases (pocketing of 4–5) and is noted as root plane closed (RPC); in other cases (pocketing of 5–6 mm), the root will need to be exposed by cutting a flap in the gingiva, which is considered surgery and noted as root plane open (RPO).	Used when pocket depths are: Dog: 3–5 mm Cat: 2–4 mm Cementum is beneficial to the reattachment process, and therefore care must be given not to be too aggressive in these techniques.
7. AIR DRY TEETH or USE A PLAQUE DISCLOSING SOLUTION	Direct a stream of compressed air to each tooth to inspect for remaining plaque.	To double check for plaque. Plaque will show up as white specks.

Step	Procedure	Notes
8. POLISH TEETH	Using plenty of medium to fine paste with a light touch (enough to make the cup flare) and a setting in accordance with the manufacturer guidelines, place the prophylaxis cup on the tooth at the gumline and move smoothly downward. Do not let the prophylaxis cup remain on the tooth longer than 5 seconds. If a coarse paste must be used, be sure to finish with a fine paste.	A smooth surface deters plaque accumulation. Polish ALL teeth.
9. IRRIGATION	Use 0.1%–0.2% chlorhexidine solution and flush each tooth.	15 cc chlorhexidine to 1 gallon of distilled water
10. TOOTH EVALUATION	Measure and chart the gingival sulcus for each tooth, tooth mobility, and general gingival health. Radiograph any suspect teeth for further evaluation by the veterinarian.	Refer to Table 4-5, Dental Health Charting Components, and Table 4-10, Techniques for Standard Dental Radiographic Procedures.
11. ADJUST PATIENT TO OTHER SIDE AND REPEAT STEPS 3–10.	Disconnect endotracheal tube. Turn patient over with legs facing down (do not flip patient over on its back), reconnect the endotracheal tube, and start the dental routine on this side.	
12. EXTRACTIONS	Check with your state's policy on technicians performing extractions. Proper training is extremely important.	Extractions are recommended to follow step #9 (irrigation), to ensure that the least amount of bacteria is present.
13. FLUORIDE TREATMENT	Apply 1.23% acidulated phosphate fluoride gel to dried teeth and let sit for 4 minutes. Depending on the manufacturer's guidelines, rinse or wipe thoroughly.	Decreases tooth sensitivity, decreases rate of plaque formation, and is believed to be beneficial on cervical line lesions in cats.
14. CLEAN UP ANIMAL AND CONTINUE WITH PROPER CLOSURE OF ANESTHETIC PROTOCOL	Inspect the animal's mouth for blood and debris or gauze, and remove if found. Dry off the animal's head with a towel or hairdryer.	Each clinic should set up and follow a cleaning routine for the dental area and equipment.
15. HOME CARE INSTRUCTIONS	Depending on what the dental prophylaxis revealed and the veterinarian's diagnosis, the owner should be appropriately advised of home care to include next recheck, daily brushing, and food recommendations.	

Table 4-5 Dental Health Charting Components

Below are some of the generally used charting symbols. Your clinic may have adapted its own. There are currently two numbering systems used when charting an animal's teeth, anatomic and triadan systems. Each clinic will decide which system best serves their dental services.

Area of Concern	Method	Charting Symbol	Description
PLAQUE/CALCULUS Plaque Index = PI	Visual examination	PI0	No plaque
		PI1	Thin film at gingival margin
		PI2	Moderate amount at gingival margin
		PI3	Heavy accumulation with overlapping into interdental space
Calculus Index = CI		CI1	Calculus covers $1/2$ of the crown
		CI2	Calculus covers $3/4$ of the crown
		CI3	Calculus covers all of the crown and is found subgingivally
GINGIVAL HEALTH/ PERIODONTAL DISEASE INDEX Gingival Index = GI	Visual examination and periodontal probe	GI0	Normal : Gum tissue is shrimp colored; sharp gingival margins
		GI1	Marginal gingivitis: Mild inflammation, slight color change, mild alteration of gingival surface, halitosis
		GI2/PDI1	Moderate gingivitis: Moderate inflammation, tissue is ruby red, plaque, bleeding
Periodontal Disease Index = PDI		GI3/PDI2	Severe gingivitis/early periodontitis: Severe inflammation, tissue has red and purple margins, pockets are forming, bleeding and ulceration; <25% alveolar loss
		PDI3	Moderate periodontitis: Severe inflammation and edema with deep pus-forming pockets, slight tooth mobility and early bone loss around alveolar socket; 25%–50% alveolar loss
		PDI4	Severe periodontitis: Tooth mobility and loss of teeth, pus, >50% bone loss, and presence of anaerobic gram-negative rods
GINGIVAL SULCUS POCKETING	Periodontal probe placed in gingival sulcus and walked around the tooth	P + the mm depth	1–4 is considered normal for dogs; 0.5–1 mm for cats; pocketing depths over these generally require more than a standard prophylaxis, and the veterinarian should be consulted.
GINGIVAL HYPERPLASIA	Periodontal probe	+ With the mm of tissue above the gingival line	

GINGIVAL RECESSION	Periodontal probe placed on the free gingival margin	Drawn line on tooth to reflect recession	If complete attachment is gone, note "AL" as complete attachment loss
LESIONS	Periodontal probe	Circled on the chart L1 L2 L3 L4 L5	Stage 1—enamel only affected; pits/fissures on occlusal surfaces Stage 2—enamel and dentin affected; PM & M proximal surface Stage 3—exposed pulp; I & C proximal surface included Stage 4—includes root fracture; I &C incisal surface included Stage 5—unstable tooth
TOOTH MOBILITY	Periodontal probe Radiograph	M1 M2 M3	Slight mobility Moderate mobility: 1 mm of movement Marked mobility: > 1mm of movement
FURCATION EXPOSURE	Visual examination Periodontal probe Radiograph	FE1 FE2 FE3	Minimal detection of an entrance Probe enters furcation, but does not extend through Probe passes through the furcation
MALPOSITIONED TEETH	Visual examination Radiograph	Curved arrow to signify how tooth is positioned	
MISSING TEETH	Visual examination	Circled on chart	Radiograph to see whether tooth exists
ODONTOCLASTIC RESORBTION LESIONS (Neck lesions or cervical line lesions)	Visual examination Periodontal probe Radiograph	ORL or CLE	Graded I–V: I = enamel only affected; edges can be felt with an explorer, but generally not seen II = enamel and dentin affected; lesion seen and felt III = pulp penetration IV =tooth unstable V = crown is gone, root(s) remaining
RETAINED ROOTS	Visual examination Periodontal probe Radiograph	Rtr	Tooth crown is missing, but roots are still present
ROOT PLANING		RPC RPO	Closed root planing Open root planing

Table 4-5 Dental Health Charting Components (Continued)

Below are some of the generally used charting symbols. Your clinic may have adapted its own. There are currently two numbering systems used when charting an animal's teeth, anatomic and triadan systems. Each clinic will decide which system best serves their dental services.

Area of Concern	Method	Charting Symbol	Description
SLAB FRACTURES/ FRACTURES	Visual examination	FxC FxO + "V" or "N"	Closed fracture; only through the enamel Open fracture; damage extends into the pulp cavity/canal; V = vital tooth (alive); pulp chamber bleeds If awake—animal flinches when tooth is touched; if anesthetized—the lower jaw will chatter NV = nonvital tooth (dead); dark pulp chamber
SUPERNUMERARY TEETH	Radiograph	Drawn tooth	Mark on chart where the extra teeth are located and radiograph to see whether any unerupted teeth are present
WORN TOOTH	Visual	W	Brown in the center with no access to the pulp cavity by an explorer
EXTRACTIONS		X XS XSS	Simple extraction (one root) Sectioned extraction (two or three roots) Surgical extraction (requires gingival retraction)

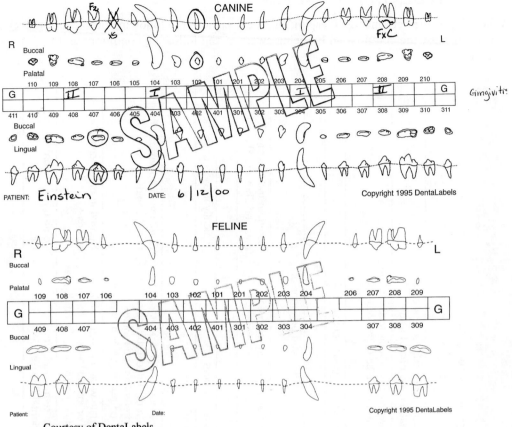

PATIENT: Einstein   DATE: 6|12|00   Copyright 1995 DentaLabels

Gingivitis

Copyright 1995 DentaLabels

Courtesy of DentaLabels

Address:
DentaLabels
19 Norwood Avenue
Kensington, CA 94707
510-524-6162 or 800-662-7920

Fig. 4-5 Sample of a patient's dental health chart.

This particular chart uses the triadan numbering system.

COMMON DENTAL DISORDERS

Although it is the veterinarian's responsibility to diagnose the following problems, the technician can assist the veterinarian by being aware of the following conditions and their presentation.

Table 4-6   Anatomic Disorders

Disorders	Description	Concern	Notes
Anterior crossbite	• Maxilla is shorter than mandible • Upper incisors are caudal to the lower	Inappropriate wear on teeth	
Base narrow lower canine teeth	Permanent canine teeth are lingually or mesially displaced	Soft or hard tissue damage and possibly formation of oronasal fistula	
Brachygnathism	• Maxilla is longer than mandible • Overshot jaw (parrot mouth)	Overcrowded mandibular teeth; resulting increased chance of periodontal disease	
Dental interlock	Abnormal eruption of deciduous teeth	Prevents forward growth of mandible	
Fusion	2 tooth buds grow together		
Gemination	1 root with 2 crowns	Plaque accumulation and periodontal disease	
Impacted upper canine teeth	Teeth are not able to erupt	Formation of inapparent oronasal fistula	Common in Miniature Poodles and Shetland Sheepdogs
Level bite	End-to-end bite of the incisors		
Oligodontia	Less teeth than considered normal	Cosmetic/show dogs	Typically incisors or premolars
Polydontia (supernumerary)	More teeth than considered normal	Periodontal disease	
Posterior crossbite	Mandible is wider than maxilla at the premolars	• Heavy amounts of calculus can develop on the buccal surface of the lower premolars and molars • Increased home care is a necessity	Common in boxers and long nosed breeds
Prognathism	• Mandible is longer than maxilla • Undershot jaw • Associated with anterior crossbite	Inappropriate wear on teeth and overcrowded or rotated teeth, resulting in increased chance of periodontal disease	Normal in brachycephalic breeds
Retained deciduous	Permanent teeth erupt lingually to deciduous (except upper canines)	• Can cause malocclusion • Periodontal disease	Common in toy breeds and cats
Wry mouth	One quadrant develops unevenly from other quadrants		

Table 4-7   Pathologic Disorders

Disorders	Description	Concern/Notes
Caries	Rare, but can occur. Odontoclastic resorption lesions are often mistaken as caries	Upper 1st and 2nd molars and lower 1st molar are most commonly affected
Contact ulcers	Ulcer caused by continual contact of mucosa and teeth	Requires consistent home care
Enamel hypoplasia	Sections of enamel are reduced or missing, typically caused by the animal having had distemper, high fevers, nutritional deficiency, or heavy parasitism as a puppy	Client education is needed, typically including a brushing and stannous fluoride routine
Eosinophilic ulcers	"Rodent ulcer" is a slowly growing cancer that destroys soft tissues and bones on the lips of cats. Round, well-defined, reddish brown lesions. Occasionally found on tongue and hard palate	Usually benign
Fractures	Typically involves the canines, upper 4th premolars, and incisors, but can occur with any tooth	Chronic exposure to infection Infraorbital swelling
Gingival hyperplasia	Thickening of gingiva caused by chronic inflammation; overgrowth of gingival tissue	
Inapparent oronasal fistula	Abscess of maxillary canine tooth Clinical signs: nasal discharge with possible presence of swelling over the root. A periodontal probe will extend from the palatal aspect of the maxillary canine to the nasal cavity	Infection
Nasopharyngeal polyps	Polyp attached to a long, thin stalk found in cats	Can cause respiratory distress or interfere with swallowing
Odontoclastic resorption lesions (ORL)	Decay of enamel at the neck of the tooth. Also known as EORs (external odontoclastic resorption), cervical line lesions, or neck lesions (CLE).	Painful to animal. Radiographs should be taken before restoration. Typically graded I–V.
Periodontal disease	Caused by a lack of daily dental care, which results in excess bacteria in the mouth and causes plaque accumulation, which results in calculus formation.	
Stomatitis foreign body, chemical-caused, thermal-caused, or immune-related	An inflammation of the soft tissue of the oral cavity	Infection

Table 4-7 Pathologic Disorders (Contiued)

Disorders	Description	Concern/Notes
Tetracycline staining	Stains on teeth of young dogs caused by administration of tetracycline to a pregnant dog or young pups	Cosmetic only
Tumors: benign Epulides:	Tumor that involves the periodontal ligament and can be bone invasive Fibromatous: generally smooth, pink, and originating from gingival sulcus. Rarely displaces teeth Ossifying: gingiva covers new bone growth Acanthomatous: large and invasive	Biopsy
Tumors: malignant melanoma	Slow-spreading, bone-invasive tumor; metastasizes quickly	Most common malignant tumor in dogs. Rare in cats
Squamous cell carcinoma	Slow-spreading, bone-invasive tumor. Typically red, irregularly surfaced, friable, and very vascular.	2nd most common malignant tumor in dogs. Common in cats
Malignant fibrosarcoma		3rd most common malignant tumor in dogs. Rare in cats, but if it does occur it is usually located under the tongue

RADIOLOGY

Radiology is an analysis tool used by the veterinarian in the evaluation of the health of an animal's mouth. Radiographs assist in the evaluation of complete removal of all root remnants after extraction, identification of unerupted/impacted teeth, the status of periodontal disease, or the progress of a therapeutic program. Radiographs also assist in the diagnosis of fistulas, cysts, tumors, and neoplasms.

Equipment

Clinics should invest in a dental X-ray machine if they plan to provide thorough dental diagnostic services and therapy to their clients. The clinic's medical X-ray machine can be used, but the radiograph will not be as diagnostic, and its use is usually more time consuming. Other accessories useful in the taking of dental radiographs are foam wedges, sandbags, syringe cases (1-cc and 3-cc protective syringe cases cut to various lengths = radiolucent mouth gags), and appropriate safety apparel. Each clinic should assess their particular needs and research the variety of equipment available.

Table 4-8   Starting Ranges For Creation Of Technique Charts

Machine Type	Animal Size	kVp	MA	Focal Distance	Time
Dental X-ray	Small dogs and cats:	40–50 kVp	8–10 MAs	10–12-inch focal distance	$^1/_{10}$–$^2/_{10}$ seconds
	Medium dogs	50–65 kVp	10 MAs	10–12-inch focal distance	$^1/_{10}$–$^2/_{10}$ seconds
Veterinary X-ray		60–64 kVp	100 MAs	10–12 inch focal distance	$^1/_{15}$–$^1/_{20}$ seconds

Table 4-9 Film

Stippled side always faces the X-ray beam. Place the raised dot corner with the same orientation.

Type of File	Usage	Sizes
Periapical	Small dogs and cats	Sizes: 0 = $^7/_8 \times 1^3/_8$ in. for smallest dogs and cats 1 = $^{15}/_{16} \times 1^9/_{16}$ in. used when narrow film is needed 2 = $1^1/_4 \times 1^5/_8$ in. routine use
Occlusal	Medium and large dogs	4 = $2^1/_4 \times 3$ is used intraorally or extraorally to show location of cystic lesions, impacted teeth, salivary duct stones, and bone fractures

When developing film, follow manufacturer's guidelines. Fixer time is typically twice the developing time. The temperature of the room will affect the developing time. Agitation of chemicals is important to remove air bubbles from the liquids. Film should be left in final water rinse between 5 and 60 minutes.

Table 4-10 Techniques For Standard Dental Radiographic Procedures

Technique	Description	Usage
Parallel	Patient is placed in lateral recumbency, with affected arch closest to X-ray tube and film positioned parallel to the long axis of the tooth, but as close to the tooth as possible. The X-ray beam is positioned perpendicular (90-degree angle) to the film and the axis of the tooth.	• Evaluating mandibular premolars, molars, or nasal cavity • Positions at which the angle between the film and the long axis of structure is <15 degrees
Bisecting angle of maxillary teeth	Patient is placed in dorsal, sternal, or lateral recumbency. Film is placed intraorally. The beam is placed over the root of the tooth of interest AND perpendicular to an imaginary bisecting line between the plane of the tooth axis and the plane of the film. **A tongue depressor used as the bisecting angle will help with visualization of the bisecting angle technique.**	**Technique of choice,** because it minimizes distortion of the teeth. • Evaluating maxillary premolars and molars, and both maxillary/mandibular canines and incisors.

Table 4-11 Typical Radiographic Positions

View	Description of Positioning	Visualization Diagram	Radiograph
INCISORS AND CANINES: Rostral maxillary view	*Patient:* sternal recumbency *Film:* placed against the canine and premolar tips *Beam:* centered over midline of nose and perpendicular to bisecting line. On cats and small dogs, the beam will need to be centered more over the nose	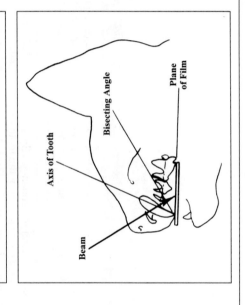	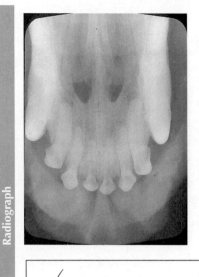

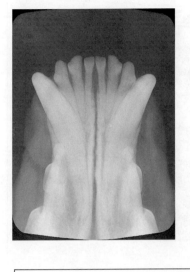

No radiograph

Beam

Axis of Tooth

Bisecting Angle

Plane
of Film

No diagram

Rostral mandibu-
lar view

Patient: dorsal recum-
bency with pad under maxilla
for support
Film: placed against the canine
and premolar tips of the maxilla
with part of the film extending
out of the mouth and the tongue
pushed toward the back of
mouth, off the film
Beam: directed rostro-caudally,
centered over the chin perpendicular to the bisecting line

Rostral oblique

Patient: dorsal recumbency
Film: resting on the maxilla
Beam: closer to ventral than rostral with bisecting technique,
but move approximately 30 degrees from midline to the side of
the canine

Table 4-11 Typical Radiographic Positions (Continued)

View	Description of Positioning	Visualization Diagram	Radiograph
PREMOLARS AND MOLARS: Caudal mandibular view Dogs: 4th premolars and molars Cats: Mandibular premolars and molars	*Patient:* lateral recumbency *Film:* placed between tongue and jaw; parallel to the axis of the tooth roots *Beam:* as close as possible and perpendicular to the long axis of the tooth. The beam may need to be moved more ventrally, and a support may be needed to keep the film in place	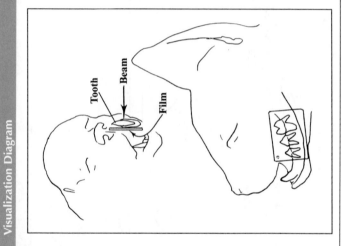	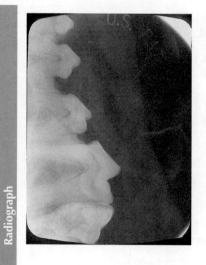

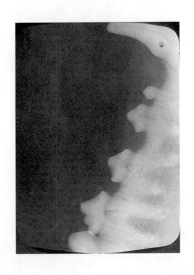

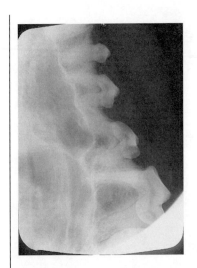

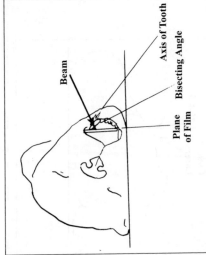

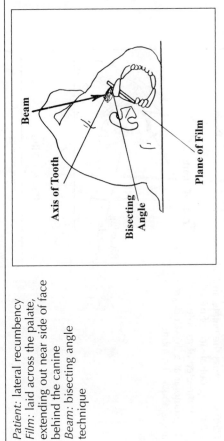

Rostral mandibular view
Dogs: premolars

Patient: lateral recumbency
Film: vertical to table in mouth, placed at the crown of near lower canine and base of opposite lower canine.
Beam: centered over premolars and bisecting lower canine

Rostral maxillary view
Dog: premolars and canines

Patient: lateral recumbency
Film: laid across the palate, extending out near side of face behind the canine
Beam: bisecting angle technique

Table 4-11 Typical Radiographic Positions (Continued)

View	Description of Positioning	Visualization Diagram	Radiograph
Caudal maxillary view Dog – 4th premolar, molars	*Patient:* lateral recumbency *Film:* laid across the palate and extending out of side of mouth *Beam:* directed at middle of 4th premolar at a 30–45-degree angle above the tooth	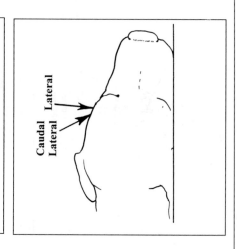	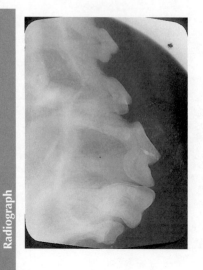

Maxillary view
Cat: premolars
and molars

Patient: lateral or sternal recumbency with mouth propped open
Film: vertically in mouth, resting on the far side lingual teeth; parallel to tooth roots
Beam: modified parallel technique, directed at the base of root in question

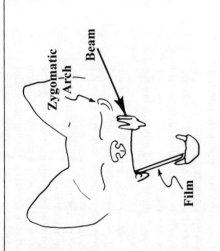

No radiograph

EXTRACTIONS

Depending on the laws governing technicians in your state, extractions may only be performed by a veterinarian. Table 4-12 indicates the instruments typically used and the general procedure so that the technician will be better able to assist the veterinarian. If technicians in your state are allowed to perform these procedures, proper training in this area is critical. General extraction complications include fractured socket or jaw, fractured or broken root tips, hemorrhage, endocarditis, secondary infection, oronasal fistula, soft tissue trauma, alveolitis, and gingival laceration.

Table 4-12 General Extraction Procedures

Extraction	Instruments	General Procedures	Cautions
SIMPLE: involves elevation of the tooth Dog and cats: incisors, upper 2nd premolar, upper molars, Possibly canines	Dental elevators Surgical blade (#15) with scalpel handle Extraction forceps Periosteal elevators Needle holder Thumb forceps Scissors: periodontal and suture Absorbable suture (3–0 or 4–0) Curettes Excavators Gauze sponges Senn retractor Surgical towels Disinfectant solution Synthetic packing material : {Consil™, Collaplug™}	1. Sever gingival attachment sharply with a no. 15 blade angled at a 45-degree angle to the long axis of the tooth. 2. Elevate gingiva from tooth, then insert the elevator between the tooth and the alveolar crest/bone to begin loosening the periodontal ligament fibers. Elevator is placed tight to the tooth neck, pointing to the tip of the root and rotated around the tooth. Use short rotating movements to sever periodontal ligament fibers and advance apically. 3. Use twisting motions to add leverage; applied carefully and held for several seconds. 4. Using the extraction forceps, grasp the tooth gently but firmly close to the gumline and twist. If no movement is noted, use the elevators again. Once the tooth is extracted, check for any retained roots. 5. Clean alveoli of necrotic or infected debris with bone curette. 6. Assess for sharpness, and, if it exists, smooth the excess alveolar crest with the dental drill. 7. X-ray if any retained root tips are suspected. 8. A root tip pick, small elevator, or surgical retrieval techniques may be required to extract a broken root. 9. Lavage extraction site. 10. The pocket can be filled with a synthetic material. 11. Compress extraction area with gauze. 12. Suture if necessary—absorbable (chronic gut) with tapered or cutting needle depending on gingival tissue consistency.	*Elevation:* Gingival damage and bone damage. Root breakage caused by improper use or force (especially on deciduous or feline teeth). *Suturing:* Extra trauma may be caused by suturing small extraction sites; may not be the ideal approach on every extraction

SECTIONED: target tooth is cut between the roots to the surface of the bone.	Same as the simple PLUS: Dental drill with tapered fissure type cutting burs or general purpose pear-shaped burs Root tip picks Bone implant material	1. Incise gingival attachment 2. Radiograph teeth to be extracted 3. Elevate gingiva with a periosteal elevator 4. Section tooth with drill 5. Elevate between crown sections, one root at a time 6. Follow simple extraction steps 2–13.	Do not use adjacent teeth for leverage. Avoid getting air from drill into the bone; it can cause an air embolus in the animal's system.
SURGICAL: cutting to the bone to extract roots The upper 4th premolar, canines, and a dog's upper 1st and 2nd premolar must be given special consideration and extracted appropriately.	Same as Sectioned	1. Radiograph the tooth/teeth 2. Incise gingival attachment 3. Creation of a buccal mucoperiosteal flap 4. Elevation of the flap if necessary 5. Reduction of the alveolar crest with cutting bur 6. Follow Sectioned extractions steps 4–13.	Done when there is no access to the root, a danger to the adjacent structures exists, tooth root fragility exists, or ankylosis of the bone to the root is present.

Post Extraction Care: Pain management and antibiotic requirements must be addressed and prescribed by the veterinarian. The client is typically asked to rinse the site daily and have the surgical sites rechecked after a 2-week period.

Chapter 5

Emergency Care

Emergencies typically happen at the most inconvenient times. A well-stocked clinic and a staff trained in handling emergencies will make your team more efficient and each emergency therefore less stressful. Each member of the clinic should have a specific job during emergencies. Understanding the basics of what constitutes an emergency as well as being able to perform stabilizing and monitoring techniques is essential to assisting the veterinarian. This chapter covers the basic supplies, support, and monitoring techniques necessary to handle an emergency. It also gives a very general coverage of emergencies by body system.

All diagnoses and treatment prescriptions can be done only by the veterinarian. These tables are to assist the technician in monitoring the patient. The technician then will be able to alert the veterinarian of abnormalities and to carry out the doctor's treatment therapy where applicable. Please note that this chapter is not meant to be "all inclusive," and we would urge each clinic to have a thorough emergency resource library in the clinic.

EMERGENCY SUPPLIES

Having the following supplies and equipment ready will assist the veterinarian and staff in handling most emergencies. Each clinic will have preferences regarding supplies and should set up an emergency cart/area to suit their needs. The drugs that are listed are examples of what may be needed and are not meant to be inclusive.

Table 5-1   Emergency Supplies

Equipment	General Supplies	Cardiac Drugs
AMBU bag	Aspirator bulbs or 60-mL syringes	*Antidysrhythmics:* Diltiazem, dexamethasone sodium phosphate, esmolol, lignocaine, procainamide, propranolol, verapamil
Blood gas analysis	Bandage materials	*Diuretics:* Furosemide
Crash cart	Colon tubes	*Inotropes:* Digoxin, dobutamine, dopamine, isoprenaline, isoproterenol
Defibrillator	Endotracheal tubes	*Vasodilators:* Acepromazine, hydralazine, nitroglycerin ointment, nitroglycerin patch, captopril, diltiazem, sodium nitroprusside, amlodipine besylate, enalapril
Doppler	Enema can with tubing	*Sedatives:* Morphine, butorphanol, buprenorphine
Electrocardiogram (ECG)	IV catheters	
Heat source	IV fluids (crystalloids, colloids, blood, plasma, etc.)	
Nebulizer	Oxygen	
Oxygen cage	Stomach tubes	
Pulse oximeter	Thoracocentesis pack	
Rapid infusor	Venostomy set	
Respirator		

Table 5-1   Emergency Supplies

	Other: Aspirin (antithrombotic therapy) Atropine (sinus bradycardia) Calcium chloride (ventricular asystole) Calcium gluconate (hyperkalemia therapy) Dextrose (hyperkalemia therapy and hypoglycemia therapy) Epinephrine (ventricular asystole and hypoglycemia therapy) Glycopyrrolate Heparin (antithrombotic therapy) Insulin (hyperkalemia therapy) Lidocaine Potassium chloride (chemical defibrillator) Sodium bicarbonate (hyperkalemia therapy)
Respiratory Drugs	*Antitussive:* Butorphanol tartrate, hydrocodone bitartrate, codeine, dextromethorphan, Temaril-P *Bronchodilators:* Cholinergic blockers, antihistamines, beta-2-adrenergic agonists (e.g., epinephrine, isoproterenol, albuterol), Methylxanthines (e.g., aminophylline) *Stimulants:* Doxapram hydrochloride, naloxone, yohimbine
Gastrointestinal Drugs	*Antidiarrheals:* Narcotic analgesics *Antiemetics:* Chlorpromazine, prochlorperazine, anticholinergics, metoclopramide *Antiulcer:* H$_2$ receptor antagonists (e.g., cimetidine, ranitidine), antacids (e.g., magnesium hydroxide), gastromucosal protectants (e.g., sucralfate) *Emetics:* Apomorphine, xylazine, ipecac syrup *Protectants/Adsorbents:* Bismuth subsalicylate, kaolin/pectin, activated charcoal
Neurologic Drugs	*Antiseizuring:* Diazepam, barbiturates, potassium bromide *Muscle Relaxant:* Methocarbamol
Ophthalmic Drugs	*Reduces Intraocular Pressure (IOP):* Carbonic anhydrase inhibitors, timolol maleate, mannitol, glycerol *Topical Anesthetics:* Proparacaine hydrochloride, tetracaine *Stains:* Fluorescein strips
Renal/Urinary Drugs	*ACE inhibitors:* Captopril, enalapril *Antidiuretics:* Vasopressin *Calcium channel blockers:* Diltiazem, verapamil *Diuretics:* Furosemide, mannitol 20%, glucose *Urinary Alkalizers:* Potassium citrate, sodium bicarbonate (oral) *Vasodilators:* Hydralazine, dopamine, dobutamine
Reproductive Drugs	*Oxytocin*

Toxicologic Drugs

Adsorbent: Activated charcoal
Antidotes: Acetylcysteine (against acetaminophen)
  Dimercaprol (against arsenical compounds)
  Ethanol (against ethylene glycol)
  Fomepizole/Antizol-Vet (against ethylene glycol—dogs only)
  Penicillamine (against copper-associated hepatopathy and long-term lead poisoning)
  Pralidoxime (against organophosphates)
Antihistamine: Diphenhydramine
Anti-ulcer: Misoprostol—Famotidine/sucralfate/ranitidine
Bronchodilator: Aminophylline
Calcium Supplement: Calcium gluconate
Diuretic: Mannitol
Emetic: Apomorphine, hydrogen peroxide, syrup of ipecac, xylazine
GI Protectant: Oral kaolin, sucralfate
Hemostatic Agent: Vitamin K_1
Inotropic Agent: Epinephrine
Laxative: Enemas, milk of magnesia
Muscle Relaxant: Methocarbamol

Solutions/Other

Dextrose
Hetastarch
LRS
Normosol-R
Oxyglobin
Saline
Whole blood

MONITORING/NURSING EQUIPMENT

Any person involved in supportive care of patients must know their equipment (usage and maintenance). Operator's manuals should be kept either near or on the equipment or in one central binder, where they can be easily referenced.

Table 5-2 Monitoring/Nursing Equipment

Equipment	Technique/Types of Machine	Notes
Capnography	Dependent on the specific machine	• High respiration rates and panting can result in false readings
Blood pressure	Peripheral pulse palpation	• Evaluate both sides for symmetry • Auscultate heart and palpate pulse together for comparison. Identify any pulse deficits
	Oscillometry	• Operator errors are frequent • Cuff size is important (should be 20% wider than the limb diameter) • Cuff placement should be at same level as the heart • Common sites are: dorsal metatarsal, dorsal metacarpal, or ventral tail
	Doppler	• Shave area of sensor placement • Operator errors are frequent • Cuff size is important: 2.5-cm premature infant cuff for cats and small dogs 4.0-cm neonatal cuff for medium to large dogs
	Aneroid manometer with intra-arterial cannula	• Flush cannula frequently with heparinized saline to prevent thrombus formation

Pulse oximeter	Dependent on the specific machine	• Normal >95% • Best on pink/moist mucosal tissue
ECG	Dependent on the specific machine	

Blood gas analyzer	See Box 5-1	• Body temperature and hematocrit are essential
		• Assesses need for intermittent positive-pressure ventilation (IPPV)/ oxygen therapy:
		  (PaO_2 < 50 mm Hg; normal = 90–100 mm Hg)
		  ($PaCO_2$ >50 mm Hg; Normal = 35–45 mm Hg)

Humidifier	Water reservoir through which gas is bubbled	
	Heated water vapor supplier	
	Heat and moisture exchanger (HME)	• Use with caution in small dogs and cats
	Nebulizer	• Watch for overhydration or airway flooding • Use sterile water in the nebulizer

TELEPHONE ASSESSMENT AND EMERGENCY TRANSPORTATION RECOMMENDATIONS

When a client calls with an emergency situation, asking very specific questions and advising the owner on how to move the animal are very important. It is also good to have the client place a plastic tarp or heavy blanket/towel in their car for protection from the animal's bodily fluids.

Table 5-3   Telephone Assessment And Emergency Transportation Recommendations

Pre-Clinic Questions to Client	Transportation Recommendations
Nature of injury	Dependent on injury; see below
Breathing difficulty/heart rate	Minimize stress
MM (mucous membrane) color	None
Consciousness of animal	If conscious, muzzle before moving unless there is a respiratory problem; minimize stress; use a carrier
Bleeding	Wrap bleeding area in towel or blanket and apply direct pressure
Wounds	Apply muzzle before moving; wrap in towel or blanket
Ambulation	Nonwalking: Place animal on board or heavy cardboard before moving. Be extremely careful in the movement, because it could exacerbate any existing condition.
Fractures	Apply muzzle; wrap fractured area with a roll of newspaper or tie limb to board or cardboard
Vomiting/diarrhea	Transport on towel/blanket/carrier
Urination difficulty	Transport on towel/blanket/carrier
Abdominal distention	If nonambulatory, have the owner place animal on board before moving; Do NOT put pressure on the abdomen
Coughing	Transport on towel/blanket/carrier
Expected arrival time	Drive safely

Skill Box 5-1 / Emergency First Step/CPR

These steps should be assigned to various team members so that the animal is examined and critical issues can be resolved quickly.

A	**A**lert the emergency team of upcoming arrival of patient **A**ssess the patient **A**irway accessibility/functionality must be assessed
B	**B**reathing must be stabilized (tracheal intubation → resuscitation bag) If the animal is not breathing, give 2 breaths, go to step C, and continue breathing at a rate of 6–20 breaths/min. • Using an anesthesia machine: 6–20 breaths/min and a flow rate of 100% oxygen at 150 mL/kg/min • Manometer pressure: Canine pressure ≤20 cm H_2O Feline pressure ≤15 cm H_2O
C	**C**irculatory function must be stabilized (Chest compressions/hemostasis/ECG) • Check for femoral or carotid artery pulse repeatedly throughout this process • If *no pulse* and animal is *<7 kg,* lay animal in lateral position and start compressions with thumb over the 4th and 5th intercostals • If *no pulse* and animal is *>7 kg,* keep animal supported in dorsal position and start compressions with the palm of the hand over the distal $\frac{1}{3}$ portion of the rib cage and the second hand over the first • *One person:* **15 compressions then 2 ventilations** at a rate of 60 (large animal) to 120 (small animal) compressions/min • *Two people: 1 compression, 1 ventilation* at a rate of 60–120 compressions/min. • *Three people:* **1 compression, 1 ventilation, 1 abdominal compression** between chest compressions
D	**D**rugs to assist in the patient's stabilization (fluids, IV catheter)
E	**E**valuation of the patient with a thorough examination

TRIAGE

Triage is the assessment of the five major organ systems to ascertain the level of priority for treatment. Immediate steps are taken as each problem is identified. The systems in Table 5-4 are listed from left to right in order of priority.

Table 5-4 Triage

Respiratory	Cardiovascular	Neurologic	Abdominal/Renal	Musculoskeletal
1. Initial Assessment				
Viable airway	Hemorrhage	Mentation	Distention	Fractures
Respiratory distress	MM	Ambulation	Micturition ability	Bruising
Respiration rate and type	CRT	Seizuring	Urine production (color, character, and amount)	Wounds
Physical stance	Pulse rate and type	Pain response	Palpation of bladder	Burns
Paradoxical respiration	Temperature	Pupillary response/position		
Auscultation of both sides of the body		Motor reflexes		
		Head posture		
		Ear examination—exudate and tympanic membrane		
2. Stabilization of Life-Threatening Conditions				
During the survey examination, the animal is treated for any life-threatening conditions as they are diagnosed.				
3. Full Physical Examination with Comprehensive Diagnosis and Therapeutic Plan by Veterinarian				
Once the animal is stable, a thorough examination is conducted by the veterinarian, and a comprehensive diagnosis and therapeutic plan are established.				

MONITORING

Table 5-5 lists the various attributes that can be used to monitor a patient. The attributes are designated by each system that may be in a state of emergency. For example, glucose monitoring would be of value for an animal in an endocrine or renal emergency but does not provide diagnostic information in a respiratory emergency.

Table 5-5 Monitoring: Physical, Clinical, and Electronic Attributes

MONITORING: Attribute	Respiratory	Cardiovascular	Endocrine	Gastrointestinal	Nervous	Renal	Reproductive	Toxic Substance
PHYSICAL ATTRIBUTES								
Respiratory Rate	X	X	X	X	X	X	X	X
Respiratory Effort	X	X	X	X	X	X	X	X
MM	X	X	X	X	X	X	X	X
CRT	X	X	X	X	X	X	X	X
Heart Rate	X	X	X	X	X	X	X	X
Pulse	X	X	X	X	X	X	X	X
Rectal Temperature	X	X	X	X	X	X	X	X
Ambulation					X			X
Nystagmus					X			X
General Behavior	X	X		X	X	X	X	X
Pupillary Reflexes and Size					X			X
Vomitus	X			X		X		X
Diarrhea				X				X
Abdominal Pain				X		X		X
Defecation				X				X
Urination/Micturition		X	X	X		X	X	X
CLINICAL ATTRIBUTES								
PACKED CELL VOLUME (PCV)	X	X				X		
TOTAL PROTEIN (TP)		X				X		
GLUCOSE			X			X		
BUN/ CREAT.		X				X		
SERUM SODIUM CONCENTRATION		X				X		
ELECTROLYTE ANALYSIS	X	X	X	X	X	X	X	X
BLOOD GAS ANALYSIS	X							
URINALYSIS						X		X
BLOOD SMEAR							X	X
ACTIVATED CLOTTING TIME	X						X	X
ELECTRONIC ATTRIBUTE								
CENTRAL VENOUS PRESSURE (CVP)		X					X	X
ELECTROCARDIOGRAPHY (ECG)	X	X	X	X			X	X
BLOOD PRESSURE (BP)		X				X		
PULSE OXIMETRY	X	X						
END TIDAL CAPNOGRAPHY	X							
CARDIAC OUTPUT		X						
OXYGEN DELIVERY AND CONSUMPTION	X	X						

SHOCK

Table 5-6   Shock

Type	Cardiogenic	Hypovolemic	Septic/Neurologic
CAUSES	Dilated cardiomyopathy, hypertrophic cardiomyopathy, cardiac tamponade, acute heart failure, congestive heart failure (CHF) (decompensated)	Hemorrhage, severe epistaxis, fluid loss caused by burn injury, severe vomiting or diarrhea, Addisonian crisis	GI compromise/rupture, urinary tract infection (UTI), septic peritonitis, pneumonia, bacterial endocarditis, bite wounds, myelosuppression

CLINICAL SIGNS

Type	Cardiogenic	Hypovolemic	Septic/Neurologic
BEHAVIORAL	• Mental dullness • Cough	• Extreme weakness	• Mental depression • Dyspnea • Extreme weakness Decompensatory stage: • Cool extremities
PHYSIOLOGIC	• Pale MM; cyanotic color • Prolonged CRT • Weak femoral pulses; pulse deficits • Tachycardia w/weak pulses (cardiac tamponade) • Possible arrhythmias • Cool extremities/hypothermia • Variable HR and RR • Harsh lung sounds/crackles • Hepatomegaly (cardiac tamponade) • Jugular distention (cardiac tamponade) • Muscle weakness/collapse • Dyspnea/tachypnea	Compensatory stage: • Tachycardia • Possible high arterial blood pressure • Bounding pulses • Pale or hyperemic MM • Rapid CRT • Tachypnea • Cool extremities Decompensatory stage: • Tachycardia or bradycardia • Poor peripheral pulses • Pale MM and prolonged CRT • Hypothermia • Oliguria	Compensatory stage: • Tachycardia • Possible high arterial blood pressure • Bounding pulses • Hyperemic MM • Rapid CRT • Tachypnea • Pyrexia Decompensatory stage: • Tachycardia or bradycardia • Poor peripheral pulses • Pale MM and prolonged CRT • Petechiation (skin, gums, sclera) • Peripheral edema • Tachypnea • GI bleeding (hematemesis, hematochezia)

DIAGNOSIS

Type	Cardiogenic	Hypovolemic	Septic/Neurologic
GENERAL	• Blood pressure • ECG	• Blood pressure • ECG	• Blood pressure • ECG
CBC	X*	X	X
BIOCHEMISTRY	X	X	X

		Column 1	Column 2	Column 3
DIAGNOSIS	URINALYSIS	X	X	X
	RADIOLOGY	When stable	When stable	When stable
	MISCELLANEOUS	• Blood gas analysis • Pulse oximetry	• Blood gas analysis • Activated coagulation time (ACT)/coagulation panel • Endoscopy/ultrasonagraphy • Central venous pressure (CVP)	• Blood gas analysis • ACT/Coagulation panel • Endoscopy/ultrasonagraphy • CVP
TREATMENT	GENERAL	• Oxygen supplementation • IV catheter • Fluid support	• Oxygen supplementation • IV catheter(s)	• Oxygen supplementation
	MEDICATION	Varies on presenting/diagnostic symptoms: • Positive inotropes • Calcium channel blockers • Beta-blockers • Diuretic therapy • Vasodilator therapy	Varies on presenting/diagnostic symptoms: • Fluid therapy/colloid therapy/blood • Positive inotropes • Steroid therapy (short-acting)	Varies on presenting/diagnostic symptoms: • Fluid therapy • Positive inotropes • Antibiotics • Sodium bicarbonate • Steroid therapy
	PROCEDURES	Varies on presenting/diagnostic symptoms: • Pericardiocentesis (cardiac tamponade) • Echocardiography	Varies on symptoms: • Blood plasma transfusions • Control source of hemorrhage • Chest/abdominal tap • Bandaging wound	Varies on symptoms: • Surgery • Blood plasma transfusions • Clean wounds • Abdominocentesis, arthrocentesis
	PATIENT CARE	*Monitor:* *Respiratory:* Respiratory rate (RR), lung sounds *Cardiovascular:* Blood pressure (BP), heart rate (HR), MM, CRT, body temperature, CVP, ECG *Central nervous system (CNS):* General behavior *Musculoskeletal:* Muscle strength *Urinary:* Urine production	*Monitor:* *Respiratory:* RR, lung sounds *Cardiovascular:* BP, HR, MM, CRT, body temperature, CVP, ECG, packed cell volume (PCV), TP *CNS:* General behavior *Musculoskeletal:* Muscle strength *Urinary:* Urine production, blood urea nitrogen (BUN), and creatinine	*Monitor:* *Respiratory:* RR, lung sounds *Cardiovascular:* BP, HR, MM, CRT, body temperature, CVP, ECG, PCV, TP, blood chemistries *CNS:* General behavior *Musculoskeletal:* Muscle strength *Urinary:* Urine production, BUN, and creatinine

*An "X" reflects that this testing would be done.

CARDIAC EMERGENCIES

Table 5-7 Cardiac Emergencies

CLINICAL SIGNS	DEFINITION	An incident that results in a decrease in the heart's capability to maintain an adequate blood flow to meet the body's oxygen requirements
	CAUSES	Cardiogenic shock: Acute congestive heart failure, cardiac tamponade; hypovolemic, septic, neurologic, or anaphylactic shock; dysrhythmias, canine cardiomyopathy
	BEHAVIORAL	May include: weakness/collapse, cold extremities, dyspnea with or without the cough or muffled sounds, head extended, possible bubbles out of the mouth/nose (often bloody), lethargy, exercise intolerance, open-mouth breathing, abdominal respiration, resistance to restraint/movement, jugular distention, depression, anxiety, acute blindness, sudden lameness or paralyzed limbs, pallor
	PHYSIOLOGIC	May include: Pale mucous membranes, slow CRT, cyanosis, dysrhythmias, dilated pupils, tachycardia with weak pulses, bounding pulse, abdominal swelling, harsh lung sounds, decreased blood pressure, dehydration, decreased urine output, pulmonary edema, hepatomegaly, ascites, blood loss
DIAGNOSIS	GENERAL	Thorough physical examination with minimum additional stress
	COMPLETE BLOOD COUNT (CBC)	X
	BIOCHEMISTRY	X; possible thyroid panel
	URINALYSIS	X
	RADIOLOGY	Thoracic radiographs ONLY when patient is stable – DV view
	MISCELLANEOUS	ECG; CVP; arterial blood gases (ABG); blood culture (endocarditis)
TREATMENT	GENERAL	• MINIMUM STRESS AND HANDLING • Heat supplementation • Support patient in sternal position
	MEDICATION	Varies, depending on condition: • Oxygen therapy • Fluid therapy (cautious) • Vasolidators • Positive inotropes • Diuretic therapy • Mild tranquilization (opioids)

PROCEDURES

Vary, depending on condition:
- Bilateral thoracocentesis with ECG monitoring
- Monitor ABG and CVP

PATIENT CARE

Monitor:
Respiratory: RR
Cardiovascular: HR, pulse, blood pressure, MM, body temperature
Metabolic: Electrolytes
Renal: Renal status, hydration, body weight
Normal pulse rate: Dogs: 70– 160 beats/min (toys → 180; puppies → 220)
                             Cats: 110–220 beats/min

Blood pressure:
1. Systolic pressure: Period of most pressure (the contraction) in the heart; this is when vascular sounds can be heard
2. Diastolic pressure: Period of least pressure (the resting phase) in the heart; this is when the vascular sounds change in character or intensity
3. Pulse pressure: The difference between the systolic and the diastolic
   Normal blood pressure:* (rates are dependent on method used to obtain measurement; 3–5 measurements should be taken)

	Dogs	Cats
Systolic	= >180 mm Hg	Systolic: >170–180 mm Hg
Diastolic	= >100 mm Hg	Diastolic: >120 mm Hg

TREATMENT

*Tilley, Larry P., and Smith, Francis, W.K., The 5-Minute Veterinary Consult, Canine and Feline, 2nd Edition. Philadelphia: Lippincott Williams & Wilkins, 2000

Skill Box 5-2 / Blood Gas Analysis

Setup	Prepackaged kit or Heparinized syringe Rubber cork to seal off needle after the blood draw Prepare the artery/vein to be used (femoral artery, dorsal metatarsal, brachial, aural, or lingual) Arterial catheter if continuous monitoring is necessary
Technique	1. With an assistant maintaining adequate restraint (arterial blood draws may be more painful to the patient than venipuncture), palpate the artery (veins can be used if the clinician only needs acid–base information. Oxygenation information can be obtained only with an arterial blood sample.) Prepare the area. 2. Hold finger on palpated artery. 3. Insert the needle of your heparinized syringe at a 45–90-degree angle into the artery, aiming needle toward your finger 4. Once blood flashes in the hub, draw your sample of 1 mL (1 mL will avoid heparin dilution of sample) 5. Tap out any air bubbles and immediately seal the needle with a cork or rubber stopper (air bubbles will affect your results) 6. The assistant should apply pressure to the artery for up to 3–5 minutes to prevent formation of a hematoma. A bandage also may be needed.
Handling	Follow manufacturer's directions regarding setup of the sample. If the sample cannot be read in 10 minutes, place it in an ice bath.

*Analysis***				
Oxygenation	(PO_2 a):	Normal:	Dog: 85–95 mm Hg	Cat: N/A
	(PO_2 v):		Dog: 40–57 mm Hg	Cat: 35–40 mm Hg
Ventilation	(PCO_2 a):		Dog: 29–36 mm Hg	Cat: N/A
	(PCO_2 v)		Dog: 35–46 mm Hg	Cat: 29–45 mm Hg
Blood pH	(pH a):		Dog: 7.38–7.45	Cat: N/A
	(pH v):		Dog: 7.31–7.50	Cat: 7.24 –7.40
Bicarbonate	• (HCO_3^- a):		Dog: 17–25 mEq/L	Cat: N/A
	• (HCO_3^- v):		Dog: 25–35 mEq/L	Cat: 24–34 mEq/L
Base excess			Dog: >−4 and < 4	Cat: >−4 and <4

** I-STAT NORMALS, Heska (a = arterial; v = venous; • = calculated values) (Reproduced under permission of Heska Corporation, copyright 2001)

Table 5-8 Pleural Cavity Emergency Techniques/Skills

Technique	Setup	Positioning/Preparation	Comments
Needle Thoracocentesis	• 14–16-gauge IV cannula or 18–22-gauge needle or 19-gauge butterfly catheter • 20–60-mL sterile syringe • Extension tubing • 3-Way stopcock • ±Local anesthesia • ±Surgical blade • Sterile gloves • Oxygen	*Position:* Lateral or sternal recumbency *Preparation:* Intercostal spaces: 5th–8th if air filled; 7th–11th if fluid	• Save extracted fluid for analysis and total protein • Performed by a veterinarian
Chest Drain	• surgical blade • thoracostomy tube (trocar) –or– 12-20 Fr red rubber catheter • curved forceps (e.g., Carmalt) • syringe/chest drain valve • suture • blunt forceps • sterile dressing • sterile gloves • scissors • local anesthesia • oxygen • ± suction	*Position:* Lateral recumbency *Preparation:* Intercostal spaces 4 – 10th	• Save extracted fluid for analysis and total protein • Immediately occlude trocar catheter to prevent pneumothorax • Performed by a veterinarian
Pericardiocentesis	• 14–18-gauge 5 –15cm over or through the needle catheter • 30–60-mL syringe • 3-Way stopcock • Local anesthesia ± sedation • ECG monitor • Oxygen • Ultrasound	*Position:* Lateral right recumbency *Preparation:* One side of thorax; sternum to costochondral junction (3rd–7th intercostals)	• ECG monitoring is important with this procedure; should the catheter or needle touch the epicardium, ventricular premature complexes will be seen • Ultrasound-guided method is method of choice • Performed by a veterinarian

GASTROINTESTINAL EMERGENCIES

Table 5-9 Gastrointestinal Emergencies

DEFINITION		An incident that results in the injury or blockage of the gastrointestinal system at any point from the mouth to the rectum and the supportive organs
CAUSES		Foreign bodies/obstructions, gastric dilation—volvulus (GDV) (canines), acute intussusception, hemorrhagic gastroenteritis, acute pancreatitis, acute hepatic failure, bowel perforation, rectal prolapse, acute gastritis, poisons, colitis, constipation, parasitic infections
BEHAVIORAL		May include pawing at the mouth, drooling/hypersalivation, restlessness, abdominal distention/pain, nonproductive retching, vomiting, anxiety, painful or difficult defecation, diarrhea with/without blood; excessive water intake, lethargy
PHYSIOLOGIC		May include halitosis, cyanosis, weak or rapid pulse, reduced femoral pulses (bloat/GDV), decreased CRT, dehydration, fever
GENERAL		Thorough examination and clinical signs
CBC		X
BIOCHEMISTRY		X
URINALYSIS		X
RADIOLOGY		X; abdominal films ± contrast dyes
MISCELLANEOUS		Endoscopy; stomach tube; laparotomy; abdominocentesis; ultrasound; parvovirus test; fecal analysis; feline leukemia virus (FeLV)/FIV test; bile acids test

CLINICAL SIGNS

DIAGNOSIS

GENERAL

Intravenous catheterization

MEDICATION

Varies according to presenting/diagnostic symptoms:
- Sedation/pain therapy
- Gastric protectants
- Antidiarrheal
- Antacids
- Fluid therapy
- Antiemetics
- Antibiotics
- Plasma therapy

PROCEDURES

Varies according to presenting/diagnostic symptoms:
- Surgery

PATIENT CARE

- Monitor:
  Respiratory: RR, respiratory effort
  Cardiovascular: HR, pulse, CRT, MM
  Metabolic: Serum electrolytes, white blood cells (WBC), amylase/lipase
  Renal: Hydration, urine output, bodily excretions
- NPO for several hours to gradual introduction of bland or regular food depending on emergency

TREATMENT

Table 5-10   Gastrointestinal Emergency Techniques/Skills

Technique	Setup	Positioning/Preparation	Comments
Stomach tube (nasogastric or gastric)	• Local anesthetic • Lubricant • Nasogastric or gastric tube • Tape • Suture • Elizabethan collar • Mouth speculum/roll of tape (gastric only) • Sterile saline	*Position:* Sternal *Preparation:* none	• Mark proper placement on the tube before insertion (from nose to 8th–9th rib) • Verify placement of a *nasogastric tube* by flushing tube with sterile saline (1 mL). If animal coughs, replace tube. • Verify placement of *gastric tube* by palpating the neck • Flush tube with sterile saline after food or water is administered
Enema	• Glycerin type -OR- • Enema can; tubing; examination gloves	*Position:* Lateral or sternal *Preparation:* none	• Do not use phosphate enemas in cats or small dogs
Gastric lavage	• Endotracheal tube (if anesthesia is used) • 2 stomach tubes (1 large; 1 small) • Mouth speculum • Saline or water	*Position:* Lateral *Preparation:* none	• Measure stomach tube from nose to the 13th rib • Verify placement of stomach tube by blowing into the tube or administering a small amount of water • Warm lavage fluids to body temperature
Abdominocentesis	• 18–20-gauge needle • 3-Way stopcock • 60 mL syringe • IV extension set • Lavender & sterile red top tubes	*Position:* Lateral *Preparation:* Up to all four abdominal quadrants	• Performed by a veterinarian • Save sample for analysis
Peritoneal lavage	• 10–14-gauge over-the-needle catheter • Scalpel • Blade • Tape • Suture • 44 mL/lb warm normal saline	*Position:* Lateral *Preparation:* Wide area between bladder area and the umbilicus	• Performed by a veterinarian

METABOLIC EMERGENCIES

Table 5-11   Metabolic Emergencies

DEFINITION		An incident in which the balance of the animal's metabolic system is disrupted, placing the patient in a medical crisis
CAUSES		Diabetes mellitus, diabetic ketoacidosis, hypoglycemia, hypoadrenocorticism (Addison's), hyper- or hypocalcemia, hyper- or hyponatremia, hyper- or hypokalemia, metabolic acidosis, metabolic alkalosis, hypoproteinemia, thyrotoxicosis
CLINICAL SIGNS	**BEHAVIORAL**	May include hypersalivation, vomiting, polyuria/polydipsia, acetone breath, diarrhea, panting, ataxia, muscle tremors, restlessness, coma
	PHYSIOLOGIC	May include dehydration, hypotension, severe depression, epigastric pain, weight loss, blindness, hyperthermic or hypothermic
DIAGNOSIS	**GENERAL**	Thorough physical examination
	CBC	X
	BIOCHEMISTRY	X
	URINALYSIS	X
	RADIOLOGY	N/A
	MISCELLANEOUS	ECG
TREATMENT	**GENERAL**	Intravenous catheterization
	MEDICATION	Varies, depending on presenting/diagnostic symptoms: • Insulin therapy • Fluid therapy (± sodium bicarbonate, glucose, or electrolytes) • Diuretic therapy • Antiemetic
	PROCEDURES	Adrenocorticotropic hormone (ACTH) stimulation test (Addisonian crisis)
	PATIENT CARE	Monitor: Temperature, attitude *Respiratory:* RR *Cardiovascular:* Pulse *Metabolic:* Blood pH, electrolytes, blood glucose *Renal:* Urine output, urine pH, glucose and ketones (every hour with diabetic cases)

NEONATAL EMERGENCIES

Table 5-12   Neonatal Emergencies

	DEFINITION	Conditions that can endanger the lives of newborn kittens or puppies
CLINICAL SIGNS	CAUSES	Hypoxia, hypothermia, dysphagia
	BEHAVIORAL	Not breathing on their own
	PHYSIOLOGIC	Cyanotic MM
DIAGNOSIS	GENERAL	N/A
	CBC	N/A
	BIOCHEMISTRY	N/A
	URINALYSIS	N/A
	RADIOLOGY	N/A
	MISCELLANEOUS	N/A
TREATMENT	GENERAL	Oxygen supplementation
	MEDICATION	Doxapram hydrochloride
	PROCEDURES	Resuscitation (See Skill Box 5-3)
	PATIENT CARE	• Monitor body temperature (recommended room temperature, 25–30° C [77-86° F] for first few days; then 22° C [71.6° F] without draft) Keep animal warm; provide heat supplementation as needed. • Supplemental nutrition (orogastric intubation—soft polythene tube (2 mm) measured from the mouth to a level with the 9th rib; syringe feeders (2 mL) for 2–5 days, eye droppers, sucking devices, or stomach tube; feed every 2–4 hours for first 5 days; formula warmed to body temperature (39° C [102.2° F]). Wipe perineal area with warm moist towel. Refer to Table 3-13 for feeding guidelines.

Skill Box 5 -3 / Neonatal Resuscitation

1. Clear fluid from nostrils/oropharynx with syringe bulb, plastic pipette, or cotton swabs.
2. Supporting the head and neck, swing the neonate slowly downwards in a large arc. Make sure neonate is well supported to avoid whiplash or concussive injury.
3. Dry neonate vigorously/gentle compression of chest/rubbing thorax
4. Place 1–2 drops doxopram hydrochloride sublingually to establish respiratory effort.
5. Holding the neonate with its head elevated above its heart and its neck extended, use acupuncture to stimulate respiration. Place a 25-gauge needle into the midline just below the nose (philtrum) at acupuncture point governing vessel (GV) 26. Penetrate the skin and subcutaneous tissue from 2–4 mm. Rotate the needle up and down at this point to stimulate the site.
6. Artificial respiration: 20-gauge catheter to endotrachea or blow gently into the nose and mouth (Normal =15–40 breaths/min)
7. Warm water bath

NEUROLOGIC EMERGENCIES

Table 5-13 Neurologic Emergencies

CLINICAL SIGNS	
DEFINITION	An incident in which the capabilities of the brain, spinal cord, or other neural elements are debilitated
CAUSES	Head injuries, spinal cord injuries, comas, seizures, vestibular syndrome, cancer/tumors, toxins, bacterial infections, parasitic infestations, and metabolic imbalances
BEHAVIORAL	May include seizures, loss of motor ability to various limbs, loss of balance/coordination, head tilting, nystagmus, depression, disorientation, blindness, hyperventilation, circling, vomiting, mastication, salivation
PHYSIOLOGIC	May include Cheyne-Stokes respiration, Schiff-Sherrington's posture, decreased facial sensation, pain on palpation, hyperthermia, anorexia, anisocoria **Abnormal Neurologic Postures:** ***Schiff-Scherrington:*** Extensor rigidity in both forelimbs; hindlimbs are flaccid or paralyzed with possible loss of superficial and pedal reflex (severed spinal injury between T2 and L4 or dislocation of vertebra) ***Decerebellate rigidity:*** Extensor rigidity in forelimbs; hindlimbs are flexed (trauma to cerebellum) ***Decerebrate rigidity:*** Extensor rigidity in fore and hind limbs (severe trauma to the brain stem)
DIAGNOSIS	
GENERAL CBC	Thorough physical examination; neurologic examination X
BIOCHEMISTRY	X
URINALYSIS	X
RADIOLOGY	X
MISCELLANEOUS	• Arterial blood gases; ear smear; otoscopic examination of tympanum

GENERAL
- HANDLE WITH EXTREME CARE and provide a quiet, dimly lit area
- Oxygen supplementation
- Intravenous catheterization
- Cold water baths or cool enemas (if hyperthemic)
- Keep body elevated at 30–45-degree angle (if head injury)

MEDICATION
Varies, depending on presenting/diagnostic symptoms:
- Fluid therapy: Hypertonic saline or hetastarch
- Anticonvulsant therapy (diazepam, phenobarbital)
- Antibiotic therapy
- Diuretic therapy (Lasix, mannitol)
- Steroid therapy (rapid-acting type—e.g., Solu-Medrol, dexamethasone SP)
- Minimal sedation (except in status epilepticus, which may require pentobarbital anesthesia)

PROCEDURES
Myelography, spinal tap

PATIENT CARE
Monitor:
Respiratory: RR, effort and pattern
Cardiovascular: Body temperature, pulse, auscultate rate and pattern
Metabolic: Blood glucose level (maintain between 100 and 200 mg/dL)
Neurologic:
- State of consciousness: Alert, depressed, confused, delirious, coma
- Pupils: Response, size
- Voluntary motor activity versus reflexive
- Loss of motor coordination and head tilting
- Sense of deep pain reflex of limbs and tail

TREATMENT

Table 5-14   Neurologic Emergency Techniques/Skills

Technique	Setup	Positioning/Preparation	Comments
CSF collection	• General anesthesia • 20–22-gauge spinal needle • 6-mL sterile syringe • Sterile sponges • Sterile test tubes (lavender and sterile red top) • Spinal fluid manometer and 3-way stopcock (optional)	*Position:* Lateral/sternal with head @ 90 degree flexion *Preparation:* Sterile preparation of the extraction site (typically the dorsal base of the skull) with nose parallel to table top	Performed by a veterinarian

OPHTHALMIC EMERGENCIES

Table 5-15 Ophthalmic Emergencies		
DEFINITION	An incident in which the vision of the animal is in danger of loss	
CAUSES	Corneal laceration/abrasion/perforation/ulcers, hyphema, foreign bodies, lens luxation, glaucoma, proptosed globe, uveitis, descemetocele, orbital cellulitis, chemical burns, bite wounds/scratches	
CLINICAL SIGNS **BEHAVIORAL**	May include pain, squinting, pawing or rubbing the eye, fear of light, running into objects	
PHYSIOLOGIC	May include ocular discharge, dilated pupil, negative menace response, absent papillary light reflex, corneal edema, blepharospasm, aqueous flare, increased or decreased intraocular pressure, prolapsed nictitans, miotic pupil, lacrimation, loss of visual acuity	
DIAGNOSIS **GENERAL**	Ophthalmic examination; Shiotz tonometer (normal = 15–25 mm Hg); Tonopen; Schirmer Tear Test; Fluorescein	
CBC	N/A	
BIOCHEMISTRY	N/A	
URINALYSIS	N/A	
RADIOLOGY	N/A	
MISCELLANEOUS	N/A	
TREATMENT **GENERAL**	Referral to ophthalmologist	
MEDICATION	Varies, depending on presenting/diagnostic symptoms: • Antiglaucoma therapy (e.g., timolol maleate, daranide) • Diuretic therapy (e.g., mannitol) • Miotic therapy—papillary constriction (e.g., piloccarpine) • Mydriatic therapy—papillary dilation (e.g., epinephrine, atropine) • Topical anesthetics • Topical antibiotics • Steroids	
PROCEDURES	Varies, depending on presenting/diagnostic symptoms: • Cold/warm compresses • Proptosed: Cover with saline gauze; anesthesia and reinsertion ASAP • Surgery	
PATIENT CARE	Elizabethan collar	

Table 5-16 Ophthalmic Emergency Techniques/Skills

Technique	Setup	Positioning/Preparation	Comments
Schirmer Tear Test: Test I: basal and reflex tear production Test II: assesses basal tear production only	Schirmer Tear Test Strips Ophthalmic anesthetic for Test II only	*Position:* Sternal *Preparation:* None	Evaluate strip after 60 seconds of being in the patient's eye. Normals: Dog: 19.8 ±5.3 mm/min Cat: 16.9 ±5.7 mm/min
Intraocular pressure measurement	Schiotz tonometer/Tonopen Ophthalmic anesthetic	*Position:* Sternal; hold head back *Preparation:* ophthalmic anesthetic	Typically performed by a veterinarian
	Applanation tonometer	*Position:* Sternal; hold head back *Preparation:* ophthalmic anesthetic	Typically performed by a veterinarian

RENAL/URINARY EMERGENCIES

Table 5-17 Renal/Urinary Emergencies

CLINICAL SIGNS	**DEFINITION**	An incident that results in the debilitation of the capabilities of the urinary system
	CAUSES	Azotemia, obstructions, feline lower urinary tract disease, bladder ruptures/ureter or urethra, abdominal trauma, acute renal failure, uroliths, pyelonephritis, severe cystitis, bacterial infection, toxins
	BEHAVIORAL	May include dysuria, lethargy, vomiting, decreased appetite, crying, painful abdominal palpation
	PHYSIOLOGIC	May include distended bladder, dehydration, anorexia, hematuria, anuria, polyuria/polydipsia, halitosis
DIAGNOSIS	**GENERAL**	Clinical signs and physical examination
	CBC	X
	BIOCHEMISTRY	X, (BUN, creatinine, potassium, protein, TCO_2)
	URINALYSIS	X
	RADIOLOGY	X
	MISCELLANEOUS	Ultrasonography, blood pressure, central venous pressure (CVP)

Table 5-17   Renal/Urinary Emergencies (Continued)

TREATMENT	**GENERAL**	Varies, depending on presenting/diagnostic symptoms: • Intravenous catheter • Urethral catheterization • Hydropropulsion (retrograde, normograde) • Cystocentesis
	MEDICATION	Varies, depending on presenting/diagnostic symptoms: • Fluid therapy • Diuresis therapy • Antibiotic therapy
	PROCEDURES	Varies, depending on presenting/diagnostic symptoms: • Possible surgery (e.g., urethrotomy/ostomy, exploratory laparotomy)
	PATIENT CARE	• Elizabethan collar • Possible diet change • Monitor: *Renal:* Urine production (every 2–4 hours), pH, and specific gravity • Bladder size • Hydration status and body weight • BUN, creatinine, phosphorus *Metabolic:* Serum electrolytes, PCV, TP • Urethral catheter should be removed between 24 and 48 hours

Table 5-18	Genitourinary Emergency Techniques/Skills		
Technique	Setup	Positioning/Preparation	Comments

Urethral catheterization	• *Female:* Vaginal speculum
	• *Both sexes:* Sterile gloves; urinary catheter; tape; suture; Elizabethan collar
		Position: Female—Lateral or dorsal
		           Male—Lateral or standing
		Preparation: Female—Vaginal area
		           Male—Prepuce area
			Refer to Chapter 7, Laboratory, for step-by-step instructions

Cystocentesis	• 21–23-gauge 1–2-inch needle; 5–10-mL syringe	Position: Dorsal or lateral Preparation: Varies with clinic	Enter patient's skin at a 45-degree angle caudally with a slight negative pressure on the syringe (Refer to Skill Box 7-18)
Urohydropropulsion	• Flexible catheters; 60-mL syringe; sterile saline	Position: Lateral Preparation: Clean appropriate areas	Performed by a veterinarian

REPRODUCTIVE/GENITAL EMERGENCIES

Table 5-19 Reproductive/Genital Emergencies

CLINICAL SIGNS	**DEFINITION**	An incident in which the genital organs are damaged or a pregnancy/delivery has become difficult or life threatening
	CAUSES	Male: Acute scrotal dermatitis, scrotal neoplasia, testicular torsion, infectious orchitis, acute prostatitis, laceration of the penis, fractures of the os penis, paraphimosis Female: Dystocia, pyometra, eclampsia, uterine prolapse/torsion/rupture, acute metritis, vaginal prolapse/neoplasia, septic mastitis
	BEHAVIORAL	May include: Male: Licking genital area, pain, vomiting, walking difficulties, depression, difficulty urinating/defecating Female: Restlessness, panting, salivation, unproductive labor/delivery, licking genital area, pain, vomiting, walking difficulties, depression
	PHYSIOLOGIC	May include: Male: Unilateral swelling of testicles, extended penis, abdominal pain, inappetence Female: Fever, anorexia, foul-smelling or purulent vulvar discharge, hot/swollen/painful mammary glands, muscle weakness, continuous contractions without production of a neonate within 20 minutes, time delay between pups/kittens > 4–5 hours
DIAGNOSIS	**GENERAL**	Thorough physical examination
	CBC	X
	BIOCHEMISTRY	X
	URINALYSIS	X
	RADIOLOGY	X
	MISCELLANEOUS	Ultrasonography (torsion, pyometra), vaginal smears

TREATMENT

GENERAL
Varies, depending on presenting/diagnostic symptoms:
- Intravenous catheter
- Elizabethan collar if animal is inflicting trauma to the affected area
- Hot/cold compresses, depending on problem
- Keep animal quiet if problem is dystocia

MEDICATION
Varies, depending on presenting/diagnostic symptoms:
- Antibiotic therapy
- Fluid therapy
- Calcium therapy
- Oxytocin

PROCEDURES
Varies, depending on presenting/diagnostic symptoms:
- Surgery (e.g., ovariohysterectomy, cesarean, prostatic abscess)

PATIENT CARE
- Monitor: General temperament, temperature
- *Renal:* Urine output

RESPIRATORY EMERGENCIES

Table 5-20 Respiratory Emergencies

DEFINITION	An incident that compromises the animal's breathing ability
CAUSES	Trauma, disease, smoke inhalation, collapsing trachea, laryngeal paralysis, foreign bodies, soft tissue swellings, feline asthma, brachycephalic occlusive syndrome, lung parenchymal issues, lung contusions, pulmonary edema, pneumothorax, pleural effusion, diaphragmatic rupture, cancer, aspiration pneumonia
BEHAVIORAL (CLINICAL SIGNS)	May include open mouth breathing, neck extended, abduction of elbows, head straightened, a preference to stand or lie in sternal recumbency, lips drawn back, cough

PHYSIOLOGIC (CLINICAL SIGNS)	• Increased respiration rate and effort
	• Irregular patterns:
	  • **Kussmaul:** Very deep sighing/gasping movements typically secondary to metabolic or diabetic acidosis and renal disease
	  • **Cheyne-Stokes:** Periods of apnea followed by increasing depth and frequency of respirations, then decreasing depth and frequency; associated with disorders affecting the respiratory center or control
	  • **Biot's:** Faster, deeper breaths than normal with abrupt pauses between the cycles
	  • **Diaphragmatic:** The diaphragm assumes all control for ventilatory movement; associated with lower cervical damage or CNS respiratory centers
	• MM color: pale or cherry red mucous membranes
	  • Pale = Anemia or peripheral vasoconstriction
	  • Cherry red = Toxins; cyanide or carbon monoxide
	  • Chocolate = Toxins; paracetamol; acetaminophen
	  • Cyanosis = Severe hypoxemia/airway obstruction
	• delayed CRT (CRT > 3)

GENERAL (DIAGNOSIS)	Thorough examination and clinical signs
CBC (DIAGNOSIS)	X
BIOCHEMISTRY (DIAGNOSIS)	X
URINALYSIS (DIAGNOSIS)	X
RADIOLOGY (DIAGNOSIS)	Thoracic radiographs ONLY when patient is stable.
MISCELLANEOUS (DIAGNOSIS)	ABG; heartworm test; pH analysis; laryngeal/oropharyngeal examination

TREATMENT

GENERAL
- MINIMAL RESTRAINT, HANDLING, AND STRESS
- Oxygen supplementation
- Intravenous access

MEDICATION

Varies according to presenting/diagnostic symptoms:
- Fluid therapy
- Drug therapy (bronchodilators, corticosteroids)
- Diuretic therapy
- Antibiotic therapy

PROCEDURES

Varies according to presenting/diagnostic symptoms:
- Thoracocentesis
- Endoscopic assessment of area in question
- Lung wash/bronchioalveolar wash/lavage with sodium chloride
- Nasal catheter
- Transtracheal oxygen catheter
- Tracheostomy
- Transtracheal aspirate
- Surgery to remove obstruction/correct rupture
- Artificial respiration/ventilator therapy (anesthesia and endotracheal intubation—e.g., laryngeal paralysis)

PATIENT CARE
- Monitor:
  Respiratory: RR, respiratory effort, auscultate lungs
  Cardiovascular: MM, HR, Pulse, PO_2
- Nebulization (saline or water misted into a closed cage every 4–6 hours)
- Coupage (firm patting of the chest to stimulate coughing)
- If patient is not sternal, change positioning every 4 hours
- Watch for signs of vomiting or regurgitation

Table 5-21 Respiratory Emergency Techniques/Skills

Oxygen therapy's purpose is to increase hemoglobin saturation and to improve tissue oxygen tensions. Not creating more stress to the patient is of extreme importance, and continual assessment of patient's temperament is essential. The techniques are listed from no anesthetic used progressing to anesthetic procedures. These techniques can be performed by a technician unless specifically noted.

Technique	Setup	Positioning/Preparation	Comments

Mouth-to-nose	• Clean cloth	*Position:* Sternal	• Place clean cloth over the animal's nose and mouth. Inhale deeply and then exhale into the clothed nostrils of the animal.
			• Rates: 15–20 breaths/min large dogs
			   20 breaths/min medium dogs
			   30–40 breaths/min small dogs and cats

Flow by oxygen	• Oxygen access	*Position:* Sternal or lateral	• Flow rate: 5–6 L/min • Less stress; but also less % oxygen to patient than other methods
Mask	• Oxygen • Appropriately sized mask	*Position:* Sternal or lateral	• Flow rate: 5–6 L/min • May agitate animal • Be sure mask is not too tight
Incubator	• Oxygen • Humidifier	*Position:* Sternal	• Good for small animals
Oxygen cage		*Position:* Sternal	• Provides isolation • Difficult to monitor • Humidification, carbon dioxide and internal cage temperature must be monitored
Elizabethan collar w/plastic cling wrap	• Oxygen access and tubing • Humidifier • Elizabethan collar • Cling wrap • Adhesive tape	*Position:* Sternal	• Flow rate: 50–200 mL/min/kg • Vent hole in cling wrap is needed to prevent condensation

Procedure	Equipment/Supplies	Position/Preparation	Notes
Nasal catheter	• Local anesthetic (tetracaine) • Oxygen and extension tubing • 3–8 nasal tube or • 8–12-Fr urinary catheter with extra holes placed in the tube • Lubricant • Adhesive tape, suture, staples, or glue • Elizabethan collar	*Position:* Sternal	• Flow rate: 110–440 mL/min/lb • Oxygen must be humidified • Nasal oxygen prongs for humans also can be used • Not best method for brachycephalic dogs • Can be used in combination with the wrapped E-collar • See Skill Box 5-4 for step-by-step procedure
Endotracheal tube	• Oxygen access	*Position:* Sternal or lateral	• Must be comatose or anesthetized
Ambu bag	• Typically used with an endotracheal tube	*Position:* Lateral	• Transfer to oxygen delivery system as soon as possible; the Ambu bag only provides about 16% oxygen • Observe chest during inhalation/exhalation
Tracheostomy	• Oxygen • Scalpel • #10, #11 or #15 surgical blade • Thumb forceps • Hemostats • Suture • Fenestrated drape • Tracheostomy tubes • Sterile dressing (telfa pad) • Umbilical tape	*Position:* Lateral	• Performed by a veterinarian • Humidified flow rate: 22 mL/min/lb • Clean tube and wound every 2 hours with a saline flush and suction tube using sterile technique • Single lumen tubes should be replaced every 24 hours • Do not use soft fluffy dressing as it can be inhaled into the tube
Transtracheal catheter	• Oxygen • Red rubber catheter or nasal catheter • Sedation may be required	*Position:* Sternal	• Use humidified oxygen • Must pass the arytenoids and advance 2 inches into the trachea
Translaryngeal/transtracheal wash	• Oxygen • Warmed sterile saline • 12–18-gauge through the needle catheter • Local anesthesia or • General anesthesia with a sterile endotracheal tube • Culture medium, lavender and sterile red-top tubes	*Position:* Lateral *Preparation:* Ventral midline of neck	• Performed by a veterinarian • Take samples (culture medium, lavender and sterile red-topped tubes)

Skill Box 5-4 / Nasal Catheter Placement

Equipment: Topical Anesthesia (2% lidocaine for dogs; proparacaine HCl for cats)

Extension tubing

3–8-Fr soft rubber nasal catheter (8–12-Fr urinary catheter or red feeding tube with multiple holes would also work or human nasal oxygen prongs)

Lubricant

2–0 to 3–0 silk suture

Tape

Oxygen source with humidifier setup (an infusion bottle or a sterile bottle filled with sterile water or saline can be used)

Procedure:

1. Set up oxygen source.
2. Place animal in sternal position.
3. Elevate the animal's muzzle slightly and apply a few drops of anesthetic into the nare that will be used.
4. Pre-measure (between the medial canthus of the eye and the most rostral aspect of the nare), and mark the catheter.
5. Lubricate the end of the catheter.
6. Slowly insert the catheter to the marked line.
7. Bring the outside portion of the catheter up between the eyes and suture (with butterfly tape and suture) on the top of the head.
8. Place an Elizabethan collar on the animal.
9. Hook animal up to the humidified oxygen source. Flow rate: 110–165 mL/min/lb

TOXICOLOGIC EMERGENCIES

Table 5-22 Toxicologic Emergencies

DEFINITION	An incident in which ingestion of a toxin or exposure to a toxin has occurred	
CAUSES	Pesticides, insecticides, herbicides, rodenticides, household compounds/chemicals, household plants, bacterial/fungal toxins, medication overdoses	
CLINICAL SIGNS — **BEHAVIORAL**	May include progressive depression, vomiting, diarrhea, weakness, hyperexcitability, muscle tremors, seizures, hypersalivation, dyspnea, stupor, ataxia, anuria	
PHYSIOLOGIC	May include specific odor from mouth, edema of face, arrhythmias, abdominal pain, hyperthermia	
DIAGNOSIS — **GENERAL**	Thorough physical examination and history regarding plants/compounds in the animal's environment and recent activity.	
CBC	X; draw blood samples before administering drugs	
BIOCHEMISTRY	X; draw blood samples before administering drugs	
URINALYSIS	X	
RADIOLOGY	X	
MISCELLANEOUS	• Special blood tests: Ethylene glycol testing; coagulation screen • ECG	

Table 5-22   Toxicologic Emergencies (Coninued)

GENERAL	Varies, depending on	
	• Stabilize patient's vital signs (respiration, cardiovascular, CNS, body temperature)	
	• Intravenous catheter	
	• Dependent on toxin:	
	• Urinary catheter (aids in monitoring urine output)	
MEDICATION	Varies, depending on presenting/diagnostic symptoms:	
	• Antidote	
	• Emesis therapy	
	• Fluid therapy	
	• Gastrointestinal protectants (demulcent, adsorbents, cathartics, chelators)	
	• Antiemetic therapy	
PROCEDURES	Varies, depending on presenting/diagnostic symptoms:	
	• Gastric lavage	
	• Enemas	
	• Baths	
PATIENT CARE	Monitor:	
	Respiratory: RR, respiration effort	
	Cardiovascular: HR, pulse, body temperature, CVP (every 2 hours)	
	Neurologic: General behavior, attitude, tremors, seizures	
	Metabolic: Serum electrolytes (every 6 hours)	
	Renal: Urine output hourly, bodily excretions	

TREATMENT

Skill Box 5-5 / Enema Administration

I. Warm Water Method:

Equipment: Canister

Extension tubing with clamp

Red rubber catheter

Warm water with salt (1 Tbsp. salt/1 liter warm water)

Lubricant

Examination gloves

Gown

General anesthesia

Procedure: (This procedure can sometimes induce emesis. If using light anesthetic, keep the animal's head lowered and watch for any airway problems associated with vomiting. A general anesthetic with endotracheal intubation may provide a safer method.)

1. Set up the canister, extension tubing, and rubber catheter. Fill the canister with warm water. Suspend the canister high enough to permit gravity to initiate the flow of water and prime the tubing/catheter by allowing the water solution to run through the tubing to evacuate the air. Once the solution is flowing from the tubing, clamp off the tube.

2. Put on examination gloves. Place animal on a flat surface, preferably a wet bench.

3. Lubricate the end of the catheter.

4. Gently insert the catheter into the rectum of the animal.

5. Release the clamp and move the catheter into the animal with a forward/backward motion to lubricate.

6. Reset the clamp and extract the catheter out of the rectum. Wait for a backflush of water and feces. Manual/digital manipulation is often necessary to break up the pieces of feces and verify progress.

7. Repeat as necessary.

II. Glycerin Enema (two types: glycerin suppositories and liquid glycerin)

1. Place animal on a flat surface. Gently insert the tip of the enema into the animal's rectum. Dispense to appropriate amount as directed by the veterinarian.

2. Place the animal in a cage and supply frequent opportunities to defecate (litterbox or walks) and check every 10–20 minutes for excretion.

Skill Box 5-6 / Charcoal/Barium Administration

Equipment: Mouth speculum

Feeding tube (measure feeding tube from mouth to the 13th rib)

Charcoal or barium

60-mL catheter-tipped syringes

Gowns and several towels

Procedure:

1. Place animal on a flat surface. Have your syringes filled and ready to administer. With proper restraint, insert the mouth speculum.

2. Insert the feeding tube into the esophagus. Verify that you are not in the trachea. Verify placement of stomach tube by blowing into the tube or administering a small amount of water and monitoring for coughing.

3. Using the prepared syringes, place the specified amount of charcoal or barium into the feeding tube. Flush the tube with water to empty the feeding tube.

4. Remove the feeding tube, being sure to hold off the exposed end so as not to drip any remaining contents as you are exiting the animal and then the mouth speculum. Be alert for vomiting.

5. Place the animal back in its kennel or begin radiographic series.

TRAUMA EMERGENCIES

Table 5-23 Trauma Emergencies

	DEFINITION	An incident (environmentally caused or inflicted injury) that results in physiologic trauma to the animal
CLINICAL SIGNS	CAUSES	Hit by car, burns, electrocution, hypothermia, frostbite, heatstroke, fractures, animal attack, lacerations
	BEHAVIORAL	May include shock, pain, depression, seizures, panting, shivering, limping
	PHYSIOLOGIC	May include increased or decreased temperature, bradycardia or tachycardia, petechiae, hemoptysis, dyspnea, moist rales, localized burns, necrosis of lips/tongue, pulmonary edema, loss of consciousness, pneumothorax, hemorrhage, diaphragmatic hernia
DIAGNOSIS	GENERAL	Thorough physical examination
	CBC	X
	BIOCHEMISTRY	X
	URINALYSIS	X
	RADIOLOGY	X
	MISCELLANEOUS	ECG

Table 5-23 Trauma Emergencies (Continued)

TREATMENT	**GENERAL**	Varies, depending on presenting/diagnostic problems: • IV catheterization • Hypothermia: Wrap in warm blankets; incubator; on heating pad; warm compresses; immerse in warm water DO NOT RUB! • Hyperthermia: Cool baths, alcohol baths, enemas • Heatstroke victims: Lower temperature gradually and only to 103.5° F with cold towels draped around the patient; DO NOT IMMERSE IN COLD WATER. • Oxygen supplementation
	MEDICATION	Varies, depending on presenting/diagnostic problems: • Pain management • Fluid therapy (colloid therapy) • Antibiotic therapy • Blood transfusions
	PROCEDURES	Varies, depending on presenting/diagnostic problems: • Burns: If burn is < 2 hours old, apply cold compress for at least 30 minutes • Surgery • Abdominal tap/abdominal wrap • Fracture stabilization
	PATIENT CARE	Monitor: • Cardiovascular: shock, temperature • Neurologic: pain management Prevent further self-trauma

Chapter 6

General Medicine

The purpose of this chapter is to provide a general understanding about specific disease processes and how they affect the animal patient. The charts provide information that the veterinary technician can use to better care for the animal and to discuss with the owner the main causes, progression, and follow-up care needed by the patient. The charts are meant as a general overview with the common protocol for a condition, not as the sole diagnostic source. The diagnostic procedures, treatments, and medications will not apply to all animals. Each animal reacts and responds to a disease in their own individual way, giving varying degrees of blood values and varying responses to medications and treatments.

This chapter is well supported by the other charts found in this book. By referring to the nutrition charts, pharmacology chapter, laboratory chapter, etc., a thorough understanding of a disease and its progression can be gained.

Table 6-1 Cardiopulmonary

DISEASE	Asthma and Bronchitis (feline)	Brachycephalic Airway Syndrome	Bronchitis (canine)
DEFINITION	Asthma and bronchitis are secondary to inflammation and airway disorders causing bronchoconstrictive episodes. The distress is often seen on expiration or as coughing fits. The causes may be allergic, bacterial, infection, pulmonary parasites, heartworm disease, or inhaled irritants.	Brachycephalic breeds have a congenital condition of obstructive airways where the soft palate overlaps the tip of the epiglottis. Common contributing causes are stenotic nares and elongated soft palate; secondary everted laryngeal saccules are a sequela.	Bronchitis is usually a progressive condition leading to permanent damage. Less frequently it can be acute with reversible damage. The causes include viral, bacterial, mycoplasma, infection, pulmonary parasites, heartworm disease, allergic, inhaled irritants, or foreign bodies.
CLINICAL SIGNS	• Respiratory distress, coughing, dyspnea, wheezing, gagging, vomiting, and sneezing (variable)	• Stertor, stridor, coughing, change in voice, and gagging • ↓ exercise tolerance • Cyanosis and dyspnea • Enlarged tonsils	• Coughing, tachypnea, shortness of breath, gagging, and wheezing • Exercise intolerance • Cyanosis and syncope • Pulmonary crackles
GENERAL	• History • Clinical Signs	• History • Clinical signs • Airway examination	• History • Clinical signs • Airway examination
CBC	• Neutrophilia • Monocytosis and eosinophilia (variable)	• Normal	• Neutrophilia or monocytosis • Eosinophilia • ↑ PCV
BIOCHEMISTRY	• Normal	• Normal	• Normal
URINALYSIS	• Normal	• Normal	• N/A
RADIOLOGY	• Thoracic: pulmonary hyperinflation, aerophagia, flattened diaphragm, peribronchial or interstitial infiltration, atelectasis of middle lung or lung collapse, or pronounced bronchial pattern	• Thoracic: tracheal stenosis or aspiration pneumonia • Cervical/pharyngeal: thickened and lengthened soft palate and tracheal stenosis	• Normal in acute disease • Thoracic: ↑ cardiac size (variable), ↑ interstitial density, peribronchial infiltrates, lung lobe atelectatic, flattening diaphragm, dilated airways, hyperinflation, or bronchial pattern

DIAGNOSIS

		Condition 1	Condition 2	Condition 3
DIAGNOSIS	MISCELLANEOUS	• Fecal analysis: parasites (e.g., *Aelurostrongylus abstrusus*) • Heartworm serology: heartworm • Tracheal wash fluid analysis: eosinophils, activated macrophages, nongenerative neutrophils, bacteria and parasites • Electrocardiogram (ECG) to rule out heart disease • Bronchoscopy: tumors and airway pathology	• Tracheoscopy: location and severity of stenotic tracheal lesions and pharyngeal abnormalities	• Transtracheal/bronchial wash fluid analysis: bacteria, parasites, and fungi • Bronchoscopy: sputum sample, tumor, inflammation, foreign bodies, and parasites • Fecal analysis: parasites • Heartworm tests: microfilaria and adult antigen • ECG: sinus arrhythmia, peaked P waves, and a wandering atrial pacemaker
TREATMENT	GENERAL	• Symptomatic • Oxygen therapy	• Surgery: nasal wedge resection, laryngeal sacculectomy, or staphylectomy	• Supportive
	MEDICATION	• Antibiotics: chloramphenical, clavamox, trimethoprim-sulfa, tetracycline, or quinolones • Bronchodilators: aminophylline, theophylline or terbutaline • Corticosteroids: prednisolone	• No specific medications	• Antibiotics: clavamox, trimethoprim-sulfa, cephalothin, or quinolones • Antitussives: hydrocodone or butorphanol • Bronchodilators: aminophylline, theophylline, or terbutaline • Corticosteroids: prednisone • Corticosteroids (inhalers): fluticasone • Tranquilizers
FOLLOW-UP	PATIENT CARE	• Handle cats gently to avoid added stress	• Intensive monitoring postoperatively for signs of airway collapse (e.g., hypoxia)	• Airway humidification • Chest wall coupage
	PATIENT CARE	• Monitor clinical signs	• Monitor for several days postoperatively for signs of aspiration while eating • Do not encourage exercise and limit exercise in ↑ environmental temperatures	• Weight loss

Table 6-1 Cardiopulmonary (Continued)

FOLLOW-UP

DISEASE	Asthma and Bronchitis (feline)	Brachycephalic Airway Syndrome	Bronchitis (canine)
PREVENTION/ AVOIDANCE	• Early detection of recurrent infections • Eliminate any contributing environmental factors (e.g., cigarette smoke, dirty furnace filters, or certain cat litters)	• Maintain appropriate weight control • Selective breeding	• Maintain appropriate weight control • Use a harness instead of a collar • Eliminate any contributing environmental factors (e.g., cigarette smoke and dirty furnace filters) • Humidifier followed by light exercise to encourage expelling of sputum • Maintain oral health • Heartworm prevention
COMPLICATIONS	• Progression of disease • Bronchiectasis	• Death of hypoxia during or after an anesthetic procedure • Incisional hemorrhage leading to laryngeal occlusion	• Pneumonia • Bacterial infection • Bronchiectasis
PROGNOSIS	• Guarded • Excellent with determination of environmental allergen	• Fair • Guarded if severely affected	• Good • Poor with irreversible changes from chronic bronchitis
NOTES		• **Caution:** Endotracheal tubes should be left in place as long as possible after an anesthetic procedure to prevent tracheal occlusion	• **Caution:** Equipment used (e.g., nebulizer) needs to be thoroughly cleaned to prevent bacteria contamination

DISEASE	Cardiomyopathy, Dilated		Cardiomyopathy, Hypertrophic
	Canine	Feline (systolic dysfunction)	Feline (diastolic dysfunction)
DEFINITION	Dilated cardiomyopathy is a disease of the ventricular muscle. Advanced cases of disease show dilation of all chambers. Causes are typically idiopathic but have been linked in some cases to nutritional deficiencies, viral, protozoan, and immune-mediated mechanisms.	Dilated cardiomyopathy is a disease of the ventricular muscle. Advanced cases of disease show dilation of all chambers. It is most commonly caused by taurine deficiency and is typically reversible. It also can be idiopathic, often the end stage of another disease. This disease leads to congestive heart failure or low cardiac output.	Hypertrophic cardiomyopathy is a disease that occurs independently of other cardiac diseases. It is characterized by concentric hypertrophy of the ventricular free wall or intraventricular septum. This leads to decreased ventricular compliance and ventricular diastolic dysfunction.

CLINICAL SIGNS	• Weakness, lethargy, anorexia, weight loss, muscle wasting, exercise intolerance, syncope and collapse • Tachypnea, dyspnea, coughing, muffled lung sounds, wheezes, crackles, cyanosis, pulmonary edema and pleural effusion • Arrhythmia, pulse deficits, ↑ capillary refill time (CRT), murmur, gallop, or atrial fibrillation • Abdominal distension, hepatomegaly, and ascites	• Anorexia, weakness, inactivity, vomiting, depression, hypothermia, ↓ skin turgor, pallor, ↑ CRT, and pulse deficits • Murmur, soft heart sounds, ventricular gallop, summation gallop, or arrhythmia • Tachypnea, dyspnea, quiet lung sounds, crackles, pulmonary edema, pleural effusion, or labored breathing • Abnormalities of ocular fundus • Pain, posterior paresis, and constant crying	• Anorexia, depression, inactivity, reluctance to move, collapse, and possible sudden death • Tachypnea or dyspnea • Pain and constant crying • Atrial gallop rhythm, systolic murmur, sinus tachycardia, and muffled heart sounds • Weak femoral pulse, pelvic limb paralysis, cold limbs, and cyanotic pads and nailbeds
GENERAL	• History • Clinical signs • Cardiac auscultation • Pulmonary auscultation	• History • Clinical signs • Cardiac auscultation	• History • Clinical signs • Cardiac auscultation
CBC	• Normal	• Leukocytosis • Anemia • ↓ PCV: <18%	• Normal
BIOCHEMISTRY	• ↑ Blood urea nitrogen (BUN), creatinine, and alanine aminotransferase (ALT) • ↓ Sodium, chloride, potassium, protein, taurine, and l-carnitine	• ↑ creatine kinase (CK), aspartate transaminase (AST), ALT, BUN, creatinine, and glucose • ↓ Potassium	• ↑ CK, AST, ALT • Azotemia
URINALYSIS	• Normal	• Normal	• Normal
RADIOLOGY	• Thoracic: ↑ cardiac size, left atrial (LA) and left ventricle (LV) enlargement, pleural effusion, and pulmonary edema	• Thoracic: ↑ cardiac size, rounding of cardiac apex, engorged pulmonary veins, ascites, pleural effusion, or pulmonary edema	• Thoracic: ↑ cardiac size, valentine-shaped heart, elongated heart shadow, LA enlargement, pulmonary edema, and pulmonary vein dilation

DIAGNOSIS

Table 6-1 Cardiopulmonary (Continued)

DISEASE		Cardiomyopathy, Dilated		Cardiomyopathy, Hypertrophic
		Canine	Feline (systolic dysfunction)	Feline (diastolic dysfunction)
DIAGNOSIS	MISCELLANEOUS	• Echocardiogram: chamber enlargement, and speed of velocity and flow • ECG: atrial fibrillation, arrhythmias, low voltages (variable), ↑ QRS duration, tachycardia, ventricular premature contractions (VPCs) and LV enlargement	• Plasma taurine: <40 nmol/L • Echocardiogram: anatomic abnormalities, dilation of LA and LV, ↓ LV contractility, valvular regurgitation, low aortic outflow velocity, or LV muscle thinning • ECG: arrhythmias, ↑ amplitude and duration of P waves, left atrial or ventricular enlargement patterns or sinus bradycardia (variable) • Pleural effusion analysis: total protein (TP) <4.9g/dL and nucleated cell count <2,500/mL	• Echocardiogram: hypertrophy of the intraventricular septum, LV posterior wall, papillary muscles, left atrial enlargement, and hyperdynamic myocardium • ECG: sinus tachycardia, atrial premature contractions (APCs) and VPCs, ↑ P wave duration, ↓ R wave amplitudes, or ↑ QRS width • Blood pressure: ↓ pressure
TREATMENT	GENERAL	• Symptomatic	• Symptomatic • Fluid therapy • Oxygen therapy • Thoracocentesis	• Symptomatic • Fluid therapy • Oxygen therapy • Thoracocentesis
	MEDICATION	• Angiotensin-converting enzyme (ACE) inhibitors: enalapril • Antiarrythmias: lidocaine or procainamide • Bronchodilators: aminophylline • Ca channel blockers: diltiazem • Diuretic: furosemide • Positive inotropes: digoxin and dobutamine • Vasodilator: nitroglycerin ointment	• ACE inhibitor: enalapril • Arterial dilators: hydralazine • Aspirin • Bronchodilator: aminophylline • Diuretic: furosemide • Positive inotropes: digoxin and dobutamine • Sedation: acepromazine or milrinone • Vasodilator: nitroglycerin ointment	• β-blockers: propanolol or atenolol • ACE inhibitor: enalapril • Aspirin • Bronchodilator: aminophylline • Ca channel blocker: diltiazem • Diuretic: furosemide • Sedation: acepromazine • Vasodilator: nitroglycerin ointment • Warfarin
	PATIENT CARE	• Treated as outpatient	• Heat support • Low-stress environment • Taurine supplementation: 250 mg bid	• Heat support • Restricted activity

FOLLOW-UP

PATIENT CARE	• Monitor PE, radiographs, and ECG at regular intervals • Sodium-restricted diet • Taurine or L-carnitine supplementation	• Monitor taurine, electrolyte, and renal levels • Check thoracic radiographs after 1 week of initiating treatment • Repeat echocardiogram after 3–6 months of initiating treatment • Sodium-restricted diet	• Observe closely for return of clinical signs • Monitor blood values, depending on medical treatment chosen • Repeat echocardiogram after 4–6 months of initiating treatment • Sodium-restricted diet
PREVENTION/ AVOIDANCE	• N/A	• Feed a high-quality diet with adequate taurine supplementation	• Avoid stressful situations
COMPLICATIONS	• Sudden death • Hypothyroidism	• Hyperthyroidism • Thromboembolism	• Mitral valve regurgitation • Left heart failure • Cardiac arrhythmias • Disseminated intravascular coagulation (DIC) • Thromboembolism
PROGNOSIS	• Grave: 6–24 months after diagnosis	• Good with taurine supplementation after survival of first 2 weeks • Poor for idiopathic causes	• Fair to good with some forms if diagnosed and treated early • Poor with progressive heart failure
NOTES	• Great Danes, Irish Wolfhound, Saint Bernard, Doberman pinschers, Springer spaniel, and Cocker spaniel	• **Caution:** Aggressive fluid therapy must be monitored closely for overload and worsening disease • Pain and crying may indicate thromboembolism to posterior aortic branches • Burmese, Abyssinian, and Siamese	• **Caution:** Aggressive fluid therapy must be monitored closely for overload and worsening disease • Pain may indicate thromboembolism

Table 6-1 Cardiopulmonary (Continued)

	DISEASE	Cardiomyopathy, Restrictive (feline diastolic dysfunction)	Congenital Heart Disease	Endocardiosis (Chronic Valvular Heart Disease, Chronic Mitral Valve Insufficiency)
	DEFINITION	Restrictive cardiomyopathy is a group of myocardial diseases that result in impaired ventricular filling. This impairment is unknown but might be caused by delayed myocardial relaxation or endocardial fibrosis.	Congenital heart disease is the most common heart condition in animals < 1 year of age. It is malformation of the heart or great vessels. The following is a list of congenital heart defects: patent ductus arteriosus, pulmonic stenosis, subaortic stenosis, ventricular septal defect, atrial septal defect, mitral dyplasia, tricuspid dyplasia, and tetralogy of Fallot	Endocardiosis is the most common cardiovascular disease in dogs. It accounts for >75% of cases of congestive heart failure in dogs. The disease is an alteration in a structure of the mitral valve complex causing malfunction and progressive secondary cardiac changes, ultimately resulting in chronic heart failure.
	CLINICAL SIGNS	• Lethargy, anorexia, depression, hypothermia, and cachexia • Murmur, gallop, or arrhythmia • Tachypnea, dyspnea, panting, cyanosis, open mouth breathing, crackles, pulmonary edema, or pleural effusion • Ascites • Pain	• Exercise intolerance, fainting, collapse, weakness, and stunted growth • Respiratory distress, cyanosis, tachypnea, and anoxia • Murmurs • Abdominal swelling • Seizures	• Weight loss, cough, tiring, and syncope • Tachypnea, wheezing, congestion, crackles, chronic small airway disease, cyanosis, or pleural effusion • Tachycardia, systolic murmur, pulse deficits, arrhythmias, cardiac tamponade, or muffled heart sounds
DIAGNOSIS	**GENERAL**	• History • Clinical signs • Cardiac auscultation	• History • Clinical signs • Cardiac auscultation	• History • Clinical signs • Cardiac auscultation • Pulmonary auscultation
	CBC	• Normal	• ↑ PCV	• Normal
	BIOCHEMISTRY	• ↑ CK, AST, and ALT • Azotemia	• Normal	• ↑ BUN, creatinine, phosphorus, ALT, and AST
	URINALYSIS	• Normal	• N/A	• Normal

DIAGNOSIS	**RADIOLOGY**	• Thoracic: ↑ cardiac size, valentine-shaped heart, pleural effusion, pulmonary edema, or pulmonary vein dilation	• Thoracic: abnormalities in heart size and shape, major vessels, and pulmonary vascularity • Specific changes may vary with each defect/type	• Thoracic: pulmonary interstitial, alveolar congestion, pulmonary edema, alveolar edema, LA and LV enlargement, hilar lymphadenomegaly, and anatomic changes in the LA, LV, and mainstem bronchi
	MISCELLANEOUS	• Echocardiogram: dilation of atria, LV, or RV, myocardial fibrosis, myocardial hypertrophy in septum or LV, valvular regurgitation, or altered or prominent papillary muscles • ECG: arrhythmias, sinus tachycardia, APC, atrial fibrillation, ↑ amplitude and duration of P waves, or LA and LV enlargement patterns	• Echocardiogram: anatomic abnormalities, shunting lesion location and severity, and abnormal blood flow • ECG: ± chamber enlargement patterns	• Echocardiogram: anatomic changes, pleural and pericardial effusions, presence and severity of atrioventricular valve insufficiency with regurgitation • ECG: recognition and identification of arrhythmia and ↑ P wave duration
TREATMENT	**GENERAL**	• Symptomatic • Fluid therapy • Oxygen therapy • Thoracocentesis	• Supportive • Symptomatic • Surgery: dependent on defect	• Supportive • Symptomatic • Oxygen therapy
	MEDICATION	• β-Blockers: propanolol or atenolol • ACE inhibitor: enalapril • Aspirin • Ca channel blocker: diltiazem • Diuretic: furosemide • Positive inotropes: digoxin • Vasodilator: nitroglycerin ointment • Warfarin	• β-Blockers: propanolol • Antiarrhythmic: lidocaine or procainamide • Ca channel blocker: diltiazem • Diuretic: furosemide • Positive inotropes: digoxin • Vasodilators: enalapril	• ACE inhibitor: enalapril • Adrenergic blocking agent: prazosin • Arterial dilators: hydralazine • Ca channel blocker: diltiazem • Diuretic: furosemide • Positive inotropes: digoxin • Vasodilator: nitroglycerin ointment
	PATIENT CARE	• Heat support • Low stress environment	• Treated as outpatient until complications with chronic heart failure • Standard postoperative care	• Low stress environment

Table 6-1   Cardiopulmonary (Continued)

DISEASE	Cardiomyopathy, Restrictive (feline diastolic dysfunction)	Congenital Heart Disease	Endocardiosis (Chronic Valvular Heart Disease, Chronic Mitral Valve Insufficiency)
PATIENT CARE	• Reradiograph within 12–24 hours to monitor pleural effusion • Monitor electrolytes daily for 3–5 days • Reevaluate patients every 2–4 months • Sodium-restricted diet	• Monitor for clinical signs • Monitor PCV every 1–3 months • Monitor radiographs and echocardiograms at regular intervals • Restrict activity • Sodium-restricted diet	• Monitor BUN and creatinine when using diuretics and ACE inhibitors • Recheck 1 week after initiation of therapy for changes on PE, ECG, or radiographs • Monitor cardiomegaly through radiographs every 6–12 months • Sodium-restricted diet • Restrict activity
PREVENTION/ AVOIDANCE	• Avoid stressful situations	• N/A	• N/A
COMPLICATIONS	• Thromboembolism	• Chronic heart failure • Arrhythmias • Death	• Right-sided heart failure • Tachyarrhythmia • Atrial fibrillation • LA rupture • Tamponade • Death
PROGNOSIS	• Poor	• Guarded without surgery	• Dependent on severity of disease
NOTES	• **Caution:** aggressive fluid therapy must be monitored closely for overload and worsening disease • Pain may indicate thromboembolism to terminal aorta and its branches		• Poodle, Yorkshire terrier, Cavalier King Charles spaniel, Schnauzer, Cocker spaniel

FOLLOW-UP

DISEASE	Congestive Heart Failure		Heartworm Disease
	Left-Sided	**Right-Sided**	
DEFINITION	Heart failure is the failure of the left or right side of the heart to adequately pump blood through the body or through the pulmonary circulation. The causes of congestive heart failure may be mechanical failure (valve insufficiency, aortic regurgitation, or hypertension), myocardial failure (myocarditis, dilated cardiomyopathy, or neoplasia), interference with cardiac filling (severe arrhythmia, hypertrophic cardiomyopathy, or tamponade), or increased requirement for cardiac output (anemia, overexercise, pregnancy, or hyperthyroidism).		Heartworm disease is a problem in dogs throughout most of the United States. It is an infection of *Dirofilaria immitis* transmitted by many species of mosquitoes. The worms reside in the pulmonary arteries and can extend into the right atrium and ventricle.
CLINICAL SIGNS	• Anorexia, muscle wasting, exertional weakness, tiring, pallor and syncope • Arrhythmias, ↑ CRT, murmur, gallop, and weak femoral pulses • Pulmonary edema, tachypnea, dyspnea, crackles, wheezes, cough, hemoptosis, and cyanosis	• Anorexia and muscle wasting, exertional weakness, tiring, pallor, and syncope • Systemic venous congestion • Fluid accumulation: pericardial effusion, pleural effusion, ascites, and subcutaneous edema • Murmur, gallop, arrhythmia, muffled heart sounds, and jugular venous distention • Hepatomegaly and splenomegaly	• Weight loss and muscle wasting • Dyspnea, cough, exercise intolerance, syncope, crackles, and abnormal lung sounds • Ascites • Hypertension • Intermittent vomiting (cats) or hemoptysis • Hepatomegaly
GENERAL	• History • Clinical signs • Cardiac auscultation		• History • Clinical signs • Cardiac auscultation
CBC	• Normal	• Eosinophilia (variable)	• Eosinophilia and basophilia (variable)
BIOCHEMISTRY	• ↑↓ ALT, AST, alkaline phosphatase, BUN, and creatinine • ↑↓ Sodium, potassium, and protein		• ↑↓ Hepatic enzymes and bile acids • ↑ Albumin and globulin • ↓ Azotemia
URINALYSIS	• Normal		• ↑ Protein and globulin
RADIOLOGY	• Thoracic: ↑ cardiac size, systemic or pulmonary venous dilation, pulmonary edema, or hilar lymphadenomegaly	• Thoracic: ↑ cardiac size, distended vena cava, pleural effusion, or ascites	• Thoracic: enlarged, truncated or tortuous arteries, RV enlargement, pneumonitis, or localized or generalized interstitial and/or alveolar infiltrates

DIAGNOSIS

Table 6-1 Cardiopulmonary (Continued)

DISEASE	Congestive Heart Failure — Left-Sided	Congestive Heart Failure — Right-Sided	Heartworm Disease
DIAGNOSIS			
MISCELLANEOUS	• ECG: arrhythmias, wide (and tall if R-sided) P waves, tall and wide QRS complexes, and left axis orientation • Echocardiogram: cause and extent of disease, pericardial or pleural effusion, neoplasia, or heartworm disease • Heartworm tests: microfilaria and adult antigen		• Echocardiogram: RA, RV, and pulmonary artery enlargement, worm burden, and severity of disease • ECG: arrhythmia, RV hypertrophy pattern, or tall P waves • ELISA: adult female worm antigens • Direct blood smear, Knott test or millipore filter test: microfilaria • Immunodiagnostic screens: microfilaria antigen
TREATMENT			
GENERAL	• Symptomatic • Fluid therapy • Oxygen therapy • Thoracocentesis/pericardiocentesis/abdominocentesis, as needed • Dependent on underlying condition		• Supportive
MEDICATION	• β-Blockers: propranolol, atenolol, or metoprolol • ACE inhibitors: enalapril or captopril • Arterial dilators: hydralazine • Ca channel blockers: diltiazem • Diuretic: furosemide • Positive inotropes: digoxin, dobutamine, or dopamine • Sedation: morphine sulfate or acepromazine maleate • Sodium nitroprusside • Venodilators: nitroglycerin ointment	• ACE inhibitors: enalapril or captopril • Diuretic: furosemide • Positive inotropes: digoxin	• Adulticide: thiacetarsamide sodium or melarsamine • Corticosteroids: prednisone or prednisolone (cats) • Larvacide: ivermectin or milbemycin

TREATMENT

PATIENT CARE
- Restrict stress: handling only for extremely necessary procedures
  - Feed patient ½ hour before injection to observe for anorexia
  - Monitor for jaundice, fever, depression, dyspnea, or other signs of thromboembolism
  - Close monitoring after administering injection for signs of toxicity (inflammation at injection site, vomiting, anorexia, lethargy, icterus, and ↑ BUN, ALT, or bilirubin)

PATIENT CARE
- Restrict activity and ↓ anxiety
- Monitor ECG, serum chemistries, and serum digoxin concentrations regularly
- Sodium-restricted diet
  - Monitor for jaundice, fever, depression, dyspnea, or other signs of thromboembolism
  - Strict confinement for 4–6 weeks
  - Start larvacide treatment 4 weeks after adulticidal treatment
  - Retest for microfilaria 7 weeks after adulticidal treatment

FOLLOW-UP

PREVENTION/ AVOIDANCE
- Minimize stress and exercise
  - Prophylactic therapy: milbemycin oxide
  - Heartworm surveillance testing: 6–12 months after initiating preventative and then at regular intervals

COMPLICATIONS
- Aortic thromboembolism (cats)
- Arrhythmias
- Electrolyte imbalances
- Digoxin toxicity
- Renal failure
- Hypertension
- Muscle wasting
  - DIC
  - Thrombocytopenia
  - Heart failure
  - Acute pulmonary thromboembolism
  - Thiacetarsamide sodium toxicity

PROGNOSIS
- Dependent on underlying disease
  - Good when subclinical or mild disease
  - Fair with moderate to severe disease
  - Guarded if untreated or very high worm burden

Table 6-1 Cardiopulmonary (Continued)

DISEASE	Congestive Heart Failure		Heartworm Disease
	Left-Sided	Right-Sided	
NOTES		• **Caution:** Aggressive fluid therapy must be monitored closely for overload and worsening disease	• **Caution:** Very high mortality in cats when thiacetarsamide therapy is used • **Caution:** IM injection can cause pain and sterile abscesses with melarsamine • Each injection is given in a peripheral vein at a different location as distal as possible with thiacetarsamide sodium • Indwelling catheters are not recommended for administration

DISEASE	Hypertension	Myocarditis	Pneumonia
DEFINITION	Hypertension is an increase in pulmonary arterial or systemic blood pressure. It may be either a primary or a secondary condition. Systemic hypertension is diagnosed through a Doppler, whereas pulmonary arterial hypertension is found through cardiac catheterization.	Myocarditis is an inflammation of the heart muscle. Causes are infectious, viral, protozoan, ischemic injury, trauma, or toxicity. Primary infection is rare: typically it is secondary to another disease process.	Pneumonia is an inflammatory response of the lungs. It is most commonly caused by bacteria but also can be caused by aspiration of ingesta, fungi, allergic, foreign body, viral, neoplasia, lung parasites, or contusions. It has a high rate of mortality and morbidity, especially in hospitalized animals.
CLINICAL SIGNS	• Dependent on primary condition • Polyuria/polydipsia (PU/PD), vomiting, diarrhea, anorexia, ascites, or edema • Tachypnea, dyspnea, exercise intolerance, abnormal lung sounds, crackles, cyanosis, and hypoxemia • Abnormal heart sounds, systolic murmur and atrial gallop • Blindness, retinal detachment, dilated pupils, and hemorrhage • Seizures, ataxia, circling, disorientation, and hindleg paresis	• Fever, weakness, exercise intolerance, syncope, and cough • Arrhythmias, murmur, gallop, VPCs, and ventricular tachycardia	• Fever, anorexia, depression, weakness, and lethargy • Tachypnea, exercise intolerance, respiratory distress, cyanosis, productive cough, crackles, wheezes, loud or asymmetric bronchial sounds • Mucopurulent nasal discharge

DIAGNOSIS			
GENERAL	• History • Clinical signs • Doppler reading	• History (e.g., parvovirus, Chagas disease) • Clinical signs • Cardiac auscultation	• History • Clinical signs • Pulmonary auscultation
CBC	• Neutrophilia and lymphopenia (variable) • Thrombocytopenia • ↓ Leukopenia • ↑ PCV	• ↑ CK, LDH, and AST	• Neutrophilic leukocytosis with or without a left shift • Monocytosis
BIOCHEMISTRY	• ↑ Phosphorus, ALT, cholesterol, BUN, creatinine, glucose, and alkaline phosphatase • ↑↓ Albumin • Electrolyte imbalances	• Normal or may reflect underlying condition	• Normal
URINALYSIS	• ↑ Protein, blood, and glucose • ↑↓ Specific gravity with renal dysfunction	• Normal or may reflect underlying condition	• Normal
TREATMENT			
RADIOLOGY	• Thoracic: ↑ cardiac size, ↑ density, pulmonary artery dilation, ascites, and neoplasia • Abdominal: hepatomegaly or abnormal kidneys	• Thoracic: pulmonary edema, congestion, pleural effusion, ↑ cardiac silhouette, or rounded heart shape	• Thoracic: ↑ lung density, lung consolidation, pulmonary artery enlargement, or interstitial pattern with air bronchograms • Contrast study: swallowing disorders
MISCELLANEOUS	• Doppler or oscillmetric technique: systemic hypertension • Echocardiogram: pulmonary hypertension • Ultrasound: adrenal enlargement	• Echocardiogram: pericardial effusion, thickened pericardium or mottled and patchy areas on myocardium • Angiogram: specific chamber involvement or pleural effusion • ECG: arrhythmias and enlargement patterns • Serology: parvovirus, toxoplasmosis, trypanosomiasis, etc.	• Tracheal wash: ↑ neutrophils and bacteria • Bronchoscopy: foreign body or neutrophilic inflammation • Culture: bacteria recognition and identification

Table 6-1 Cardiopulmonary (Continued)

DISEASE	Hypertension	Myocarditis	Pneumonia
TREATMENT			
GENERAL	*Only for complicated disease* • Supportive • Fluid therapy • Oxygen therapy	• Supportive • Pericardiocentesis	• Supportive • Fluid therapy • Oxygen therapy • Surgery: lung lobectomy (rare)
MEDICATION	• α-Adrenergic blocker: prazosin • β-Adrenergic blocker: propranolol • ACE inhibitor: enalapril • Ca channel blocker: diltiazem or amlodipine (cats) • Diuretic: furosemide • Hydralazine	• Dependent on underlying condition • ACE inhibitor: enalapril • Antiarrhythmics: quinidine • Diuretic: furosemide • Positive inotropes: digoxin	• Antibiotics: dependent on type of bacteria isolated and penetration ability into lung tissue (e.g., enrofloxacin) • Bronchodilators: theophylline or terbutaline
PATIENT CARE	• Treat as outpatient if possible to decrease overall stress	• Restrict activity	• Nebulization with bland aerosols • Chest wall coupage • Tracheal manipulation • Restrict activity • Alter patient's position at least every 2 hours • Nutritional support
FOLLOW-UP			
PATIENT CARE	• Sodium-restricted diet • Monitor for signs of hypotension • Monitor blood pressure every 1–2 weeks then every 1–3 months	• Sodium-restricted diet • Monitor ECG and auscultation • Reradiograph	• Airway humidification • Mild exercise • Reradiograph in 48–72 hours, then after 2–6 weeks
PREVENTION/ AVOIDANCE	• Maintain proper weight control • Measure blood pressure (BP) in all renal failure patients	• Vaccinate • Monitor ECG and echocardiogram with patients using doxorubicin • Avoid endemic areas (e.g., Gulf Coast)	• Vaccinate
COMPLICATIONS	• Renal failure • Chronic heart failure • Glomerulonephropathy • Retinopathy/blindness • CNS signs	• Cardiomyopathy • Chronic heart failure	• Chronic bronchitis • Secondary infection/sepsis

PROGNOSIS	• Good if underlying cause can be determined and treated

NOTES	• Canine abnormal systemic values:
	  • Systolic >180 mm Hg
	  • Diastolic >100 mm Hg
	• Feline abnormal systemic values:
	  • Systolic >170–180 mm Hg
	  • Diastolic >120 mm Hg
	• An average of three readings should be done to adequately evaluate a patient's blood pressure
	• Avoid use of phenylpropanalamine (PPA)
	• Maintain low stress before and during the BP measurement

• Dependent on extent and severity of disease
• Good

DISEASE	Pleural Effusion	Rhinitis/Sinusitis	Tracheal Collapse
DEFINITION	Pleural effusion is an accumulation of fluid in the pleural cavity. It may be seen unilaterally or bilaterally. This is an abnormal process that has many causes, typically indicating a more severe underlying condition.	Infection of the nasal sinuses is a common veterinary problem. Acute rhinitis is self-limiting, and chronic sinusitis may require constant treatment. Causes may include bacterial, viral, fungi, foreign body, dental disease, infectious agents, or neoplasia.	A collapsing trachea is a trachea with a range of dynamic variations resulting in collapse somewhere along its length. It also may involve the mainstem bronchi, causing them to collapse also. It can be an acquired weakness or congenital defect. It is most commonly seen in older toy breed dogs.
CLINICAL SIGNS	• Fever, anorexia, depression, pallor, and pleuritis • Tachypnea, dyspnea, open-mouth breathing, exercise intolerance, cyanosis, and cough • Muffled heart and lung sounds • Preference for sternal recumbency	• Sneezing, cough, nasal discharge, gagging, and retching • Fever, lymphadenopathy, bony swelling, oral ulceration, ocular or neurologic changes	• Stertor, stridor, intermittent "honking" cough, change in voice, and gagging • Decreased exercise tolerance • Cyanosis, dyspnea, and syncope • Enlarged tonsils

Table 6-1 Cardiopulmonary (Continued)

DISEASE	Pleural Effusion	Rhinitis/Sinusitis	Tracheal Collapse
GENERAL	• History • Clinical signs • Cardiac auscultation • Pulmonary auscultation • Thoracic palpation and percussion	• History • Clinical signs • Nasal examination	• History • Clinical signs • Airway examination
CBC	• Leukocytosis • Anemia	• Normal or may reflect underlying condition	• Normal
BIOCHEMISTRY	• ↑ Globulin ↓ Albumin: <1g/dL	• Normal or may reflect underlying condition	• Normal
URINALYSIS	• Normal	• Normal or may reflect underlying condition	• Normal
RADIOLOGY	• Thoracic: tumor, lung lobe torsion, diaphragmatic hernia, widening of mediastinum, rounded lung lobe edges, obscured cardiac borders and diaphragm, ascites, and pleural fissure lines • Contrast study: tumor, diaphragmatic hernia, and cardiac disease	• Skull: ↑ fluid and bony changes (e.g., loss of bone detail and deviated septum)	• Thoracic: narrowing or ballooning of tracheal diameter and ↑ R-sided cardiac size • Cervical/pharyngeal: narrowing or ballooning of tracheal diameter
MISCELLANEOUS	• Fluid analysis: color, clarity, viscosity, specific gravity, TP, and nucleated cell count, neutrophils, macrophages, mesothelial cells, lymphocytes, eosinophils, or neoplastic cells • Serology: feline leukemia virus (FeLV), feline infectious peritonitis (FIP), feline immunodeficiency virus (FIV) or heartworm	• Rhinoscopy: foreign body and bony changes • Biopsy: bacteria or fungi • Cytology and culture: bacteria recognition and identification	• Bronchoscopy: severity and small airway disease • Fluoroscopy: narrowing of tracheal diameter may be dynamic

DIAGNOSIS

		Column 1	Column 2	Column 3
TREATMENT	**GENERAL**	• Symptomatic • Fluid therapy • Thoracocentesis • Chest tube placement • Surgery: thoracotomy	• Supportive • Fluid therapy • Radiotherapy • Surgery: nasal exploratory, rhinotomy, or turbinectomy	• Symptomatic • Surgery: application of extraluminal prostheses
	MEDICATION	• Antibiotics: depending on type of bacteria isolated • Analgesics: bupivacaine, nonsteroidal anti-inflammatory drugs (NSAIDs), morphine, or meperidine	• Antibiotics: cephalexin, trimethoprim sulfa, and chloramphenicol • Corticosteroids: prednisone • Fungicides: eniliconazole, itraconazole, thiabendazole, or ketoconazole	• Antitussives: hydrocodone • Bronchodilators: aminophylline, theophylline, or terbutaline • Corticosteroids: prednisone
	PATIENT CARE	• Monitor temperature, respiratory rate and effort, and pulse • Nutritional support • Check chest tube bandage daily	• Airway humidification	• Intensive monitoring during and postoperatively for signs of hypoxia
FOLLOW-UP	**PATIENT CARE**	• Monitor radiographs	• Monitor for relapse of clinical signs	• Limit activity to reduce exercise intolerance
	PREVENTION/ AVOIDANCE	• N/A	• Vaccinate • Maintain good oral hygiene • Prevent exposure to bird feces (aspergillosis and cryptococcosis)	• Maintain proper weight control • Avoid extreme temperature and humidity changes
	COMPLICATIONS	• Death	• Brain infection • Epistaxis	• Death from hypoxia (rare)
	PROGNOSIS	• Guarded to poor	• Fair to good	• Good with surgery • Guarded with symptomatic treatment

	NOTES	• Classification of fluids:
		  • colorless to pale yellow: transudate
		  • yellow to pink: modified transudate or nonseptic exudate
		  • yellow to red-brown: septic exudate
		  • milky white: chylous
		  • red: hemorrhage
		• Pain medication may be injected directly through the chest tube to give pleural analgesia
			• Serous nasal discharge is indicative of acute or allergic disease
			• Mucopurulent discharge suggests bacterial or fungal infection (infection may be only secondary to underlying neoplasia)
				• Obtain both inspiratory and expiratory radiographs: tracheal collapse may be seen at any point during breathing

Electrocardiography

Electrocardiography (ECG) is an essential tool in evaluating the heart's electrical activity. Used along with physical examination, baseline blood work, and radiographs, a complete picture of the heart can be seen. The procedure has become simplified for use in every clinic with affordable equipment, minimal patient stress, and ease of performing the procedure.

Table 6-2 General Electrocardiography

PROCEDURE	Electrocardiography (ECG)
DEFINITION	• The study of the variations in voltage produced by a mass of associated cardiac muscle fibers or bundle of muscle fibers • Evaluates the functional status of the heart, not the mechanical status
TECHNIQUE	See Skill Box 6-1
INDICATIONS	• Cardiac arrhythmias and the status of the myocardium • Tachycardia, bradycardia, extra beats, murmurs, cardiomegaly, and electrolyte disturbances • Exercise intolerance, panting, dyspnea, cyanosis, fainting, seizures and shock
EQUIPMENT	• Electrocardiograph machine
PRECAUTIONS	↑ Stress can exacerbate already critical conditions
NOTES	• ECG activity may continue to appear normal even after mechanical activity has ceased and the patient has no palpable pulse (electromechanical dissociation) • Variations in the body conformations of many dog breeds alters standard measurements

A lead is a pair of electrodes at different angles that have at least one positive charge and one negative charge. Leads are connected in different combinations to obtain varying measurements of the electrical activity of the heart. Correctly placing the leads and the direction of electrical flow measurement allows understanding of many heart deficits.

Table 6-3   ECG Leads

Lead	Measurement	Movement and Electrode Position	Use
Bipolar Standard Leads			
I	Measurement between two limbs	R arm (−) → L arm (+)	• Abnormalities in P-QRS-T deflections and cardiac arrhythmias • Determining mean electrical axis
II		R arm (−) → L leg (+)	
III		L arm (−) → L leg (+)	
Augmented Unipolar Limb Leads			
aVR	Measurement from one limb to a point halfway in between the other two limbs	L arm and leg (−) → R arm (+)	• Determining mean electrical axis and heart position • Confirming information gained from other leads
aVL		R arm and L leg (−) → L arm (+)	
aVF		L arm and R arm (−) → L leg (+)	
Unipolar Precordial Chest Leads			
CV_5RL (rV_2)	• Measurement from the dorsal and ventral surfaces of the heart • The limb leads form a potential equal to that in the center of the heart, allowing voltage to be measured from the center of the heart to the selected location of the chest lead	• R and L arm and L leg (−) → 5th R intercostal space near edge of sternum (+)	• R and L ventricular enlargement, myocardial infarction, bundle branch block, and cardiac arrhythmias • Confirming information gained from other leads
CV_6LL (V_2)		• R and L arm and L leg (−) → 6th L intercostal space near edge of sternum (+)	
CV_6LU (V_4)		• R and L arm and L leg (−) → 6th L intercostal space at costochondral junction (+)	
V_{10}		• R and L arm and L leg (−) → over spinous process of the 7th thoracic vertebra (+)	
Invasive Leads			
Esophageal	• Measurement from limb and base of the heart • The electrocardiograph is run on and compared with lead I	• L arm → base of heart	• Rhythm monitoring and accurate identification of P waves
Intracardiac	• Measurement is based on the position of the exploring catheter tip placed through a jugular venipuncture and attached to an outside electrode	• Dependent on the position of the exploring catheter tip within the heart	• Cardiac arrhythmias (accurate identification of P waves), differentiation between ventricular and supraventricular tachycardia, and for pacing the heart

Skill Box 6-1 / ECG Technique

Position:

Right lateral recumbency

The patient may be placed in a natural position (standing, sitting, or resting) in critical cases or for routine monitoring

Restraint:

Place the animal on a nonconductive table (e.g., Formica or metal covered with a blanket or pad)

Legs should be held parallel to each other and not touching

Forelimbs should be perpendicular to the long axis of the body

**Caution: Chemical restraint should not be used, because it may alter different aspects of the recording

Electrodes:

a. Attach the clips to the animal's skin that has been moistened with conductive gel, paste, or creams, or alcohol

   RA/LA: proximal to the olecranon and on the caudal aspect

   RL/LL: patellar ligament on the anterior aspect

   Cardiac: L intercostal space at costochondral junction and variable, depending on desired unipolar precordial chest lead

b. Apply small metal plates covered with conductive gel, paste, or creams on the pads of the feet

c. Shave the fur and adhere electrode pads (Holter apparatus) for long-term monitoring

The teeth of the alligator clips may be bent out, flattened, or filed to improve patient comfort

Conductive gel, paste, and creams are better at lowering the electrical resistance than alcohol and do not evaporate

Alcohol-soaked pads may be used between the clip and skin

RA/LA electrodes may have to be moved halfway between the olecranon and carpus if cardiac interference is seen

Recording:

1. Turn on the machine
2. Position the stylus in the center of the paper and maintain that position throughout the recording
3. Turn the sensitivity switch to 1 to allow 1 mV input to move the stylus 1 cm (2 large boxes)

   Turn the sensitivity switch to 2 if the tracing is small and unclear or turn it to $\frac{1}{2}$ if the tracing is large and extending to the top and bottom of the paper

4. Turn the record switch to a paper speed of 50 mm/sec and push the standardization button to record the reference size of 1 mV
5. Record the desired leads

   a. Turn the lead selector to 1 and record 2 sets (30 large boxes)

   b. Without turning off machine or changing any other parameters, turn the lead selector to 2 and continue through to aVF and CV_6LU (V_4)

   c. Turn the lead selector to 2 and record 2–4 feet of lead II rhythm strip at 25 mm/sec

   d. If precordial chest leads are desired, stop recording and reposition chest lead for each reading

   e. Return the lead selector to STD and push the standardized button

   When recording an ECG strip, it is best to 'drive' with both hands. The left hand is placed on the stylus position knob to help maintain a centered tracing, because they tend to wander during long readings or when switching leads. The right hand is placed on the lead selector switch to change through the various leads smoothly.

6. Stop recording and remove clips from the patient
7. Fold up ECG strip and record the patient's information (e.g., name, position, excitement level, etc.) on the strip

   **Caution: If the machine does not have a modern 3-prong plug, attach the ground lead wire to a water pipe or object with a common ground

Alterations seen in a recording of a heart rhythm are often remedied by changing technique, position, etc. After trying multiple attempts to remedy an alteration, verify the machine is in proper working condition and not in need of repair.

Table 6-4 ECG Problems and Artifacts

Alteration	Problem	Solution
Baseline is not well defined	• Poorly defined baseline	• The stylus heat and verify whether it is clean • ↕ Sensitivity to ½ to ↕ the amplitude of the wave

Flat line	• An electrode has fallen off	• Replace electrode that has fallen off:
		  • Lead I works and Leads II and III do not—replace L leg
		  • Lead II works and Leads I and III do not—replace L arm
		  • Lead III works and Leads I and II do not—replace R arm

Negative R wave	• True abnormality • Misplaced electrode	• Verify that the electrodes are placed in the correct position
QRS complex off the paper	• Excessive amplitude of QRS complex	• ↓ Sensitivity to ½ to ↓ the amplitude of the wave
Rapid and irregular vibrations of the baseline	• Muscle tremors • Body movements • Purring	• Verify the patient is in a comfortable position and electrodes are comfortably placed • Place a hand over the chest wall with moderate pressure to → body tremors • Blowing in a cat's face or gentle manipulation of the larynx to stop purring • ↓ Sensitivity to ½ to ↓ the amplitude of the wave
Regular sequence of 60 sharp up and down waves	• Electrical interference	• Verify the machine is properly grounded • Verify the electrode clips are clean, securely attached to skin, and moistened (not saturated) with gel or alcohol • Verify that the legs are held apart and the clips are not touching each other, and the animal is not touching anything metal (e.g., table) • Verify that the table is not touching electrical cords and is positioned away from electrical wiring • Verify that the cords are not tangled or coiled up on one another
Up and down movement of baseline	• Respiratory movements (e.g., panting and coughing)	• Verify that the patient is in a comfortable position • Hold the animal's mouth shut for short periods to obtain each lead

Skill Box 6-2 / Heart rate calculation

ECG Paper and Grid Lines: (refer to Figures 6-1, 6-2, 6-3, and 6-4)

25 mm/sec

    Small box = 0.04 sec

    Large box (5 small boxes) = 0.20 sec

    Set (15 large boxes) = 3 sec

50 mm/sec

    Small box = 0.02 sec

    Large box (5 small boxes) = 0.10 sec

    Set (15 large boxes) = 1.5 sec

Rhythm	Paper Speed	
	25 mm/sec	**50 mm/sec**
Regular Rhythm	*Method 1:* the number of small boxes in one cycle / 1,500 = HR/min	*Method 1:* the number of small boxes in one cycle / 3,000 = HR/min
	Method 2: the number of large boxes in one cycle / 300 = HR/min	*Method 2:* the number of large boxes in one cycle / 600 = HR/min
	Method 3: heart rate calculator used according to provided directions	
Irregular Rhythm • The fraction of the last cycle should be estimated in tenths	The number of cycles in two sets (30 large squares-6 sec) × 10 = HR/min	*Method 1:* the number of cycles in two sets (30 large squares—3 sec) × 20 = HR/min
		Method 2: the number of cycles in four sets (60 large squares—6 sec) × 10 = HR/min • Greater accuracy with slower rates

The following description of the movement and image of electrical current are for the standard lead II positioning. Understanding the placement of the positive and negative leads will enable one to decipher movement and image for each lead position.

Waves are recorded as positive waves (movement above the baseline) when most of the electrical current is moving from the negative electrode to the positive electrode. Negative waves (movement below the baseline) occur when most of the electrical current is moving from the positive electrode to the negative electrode.

Table 6-5 ECG Interpretation

Cycle Segment	P wave	P-R Interval	QRS	S-T Interval	T wave	Q-T Interval
Movement*	• SA node → R atrium → L atrium → AV node	• SA Node → ventricle	• R bundle branch and L bundle branch → apex and ventricular free walls → basal regions of free walls and septum	• Basal regions of free walls and septum → apex and ventricular free walls	• Apex and ventricular free walls	• R bundle branch and L bundle branch → apex and ventricular free walls → basal regions of free walls and septum → apex ventricular free walls
Image	• Positive wave	• P wave and ending straight line	• Negative wave (Q) followed by a tall positive wave (R) and ended with a short negative wave (S)	• Straight line with no deviations	• Positive wave	• Negative wave (Q), tall positive wave (R), short negative wave (S) ending with a straight line (S-T segment)
Measurement	• Width: 0.04 sec (2 boxes) • Height: 0.4 mV (4 boxes)	• Start of the P wave to start of Q wave (R wave if no Q wave) • 0.06–0.13 sec (3–6.5 boxes)	• Start of Q wave to the end of the S wave • Width: 0.05–0.06 sec (2.5 boxes) • Height: 2.5–3.0 mV (25–30 boxes)	• End of the QRS complex to the start of the T wave • Width: 0.2 mV (2 boxes) • Height: 0.15 mV (1.5 boxes)	• Height: ≤ ¼ of the amplitude of the R wave	• Start of the Q wave to the end of the T wave
Action	• Depolarization of the R and L atrium	• Time delay to allow filling of ventricles	• Depolarization of the ventricles	• Early phase of ventricular repolarization	• Repolarization of the ventricles	• Summation of depolarization and repolarization of the ventricles

*Electrical impulse movement through the heart
**Measurement taken at a paper speed of 50 mm/sec

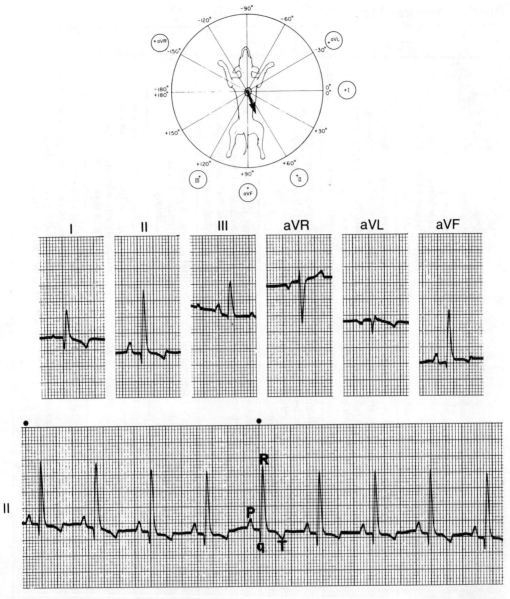

Figure 6-1 Normal canine electrocardiogram.

Rhythm Abnormalities

Table 6-6 Common Rhythm Abnormalities

Rhythm Pattern	Cause	Image	Associated Conditions
Atrial Fibrillation	• Rapid and disorganized depolarization pattern in the atria • ↓ Cardiac output	• Nondistinguishable P waves are replaced by numerous f waves • QRS complexes may be normal or wide and varying amplitude	• Atrial enlargement, congenital heart defects, drug reactions, anesthesia, heartworm disease, trauma, and hypertrophic cardiomyopathy
Atrial Premature Contraction/ Complexes (APC)	• Premature atrial beats originating outside the SA node	• Premature P wave • QRS complexes are normal unless the P wave is so premature they overlap with varying results See Figure 6-2	• Congenital heart disease, cardiomyopathy, electrolyte imbalances, neoplasia, hyperthyroidism, drug reactions, toxemias, atrial myocarditis, and normal variations in aged animals
Respiratory Sinus Arrhythmias	• Irregular sinus rhythm originating in the SA node • Respiratory rate ↑ during inspiration and ↓ during expiration	• Normal sinus rhythm • ↑ Number of cycles during inspiration and ↓ number of cycles during expiration	• Normal finding (brachycephalic), vagal stimulation, and chronic respiratory diseases
S-T Segment Depression	• Net electrical event of myocardial cell repolarization	• Depression of the S-T segment of the QRS complex	• Normal finding, myocardial ischemia (inadequate circulation), hyperkalemia and hypokalemia, cardiac trauma, and acute myocardial infarction
S-T Segment Elevation	• Net electrical event of myocardial cell repolarization	• Elevation of the S-T segment of the QRS complex See Figure 6-3	• Normal finding, myocardial hypoxia (oxygen deficiency), myocardial infarction, and pericarditis
Ventricular Fibrillation	• Weak and uncoordinated ventricular contractions • ↓ To zero cardiac output	• Completely irregular, chaotic, and deformed reflections of varying width, amplitude, and shape	• Shock, anoxia, trauma, electrolyte imbalances, drug reactions, aortic stenosis, cardiac surgery, electric shock, myocarditis, and hypothermia
Ventricular Premature Contraction/ Complexes (VPC)	• An impulse originating in the ventricles instead of the SA node	• P wave is dissociated from the QRS complex • Widened and bizarre QRS complex See Figure 6-4	• Cardiomyopathy, congenital defects, GDV, drug reactions, myocarditis, cardiac neoplasia, hyperthyroidism, and chronic valvular disease

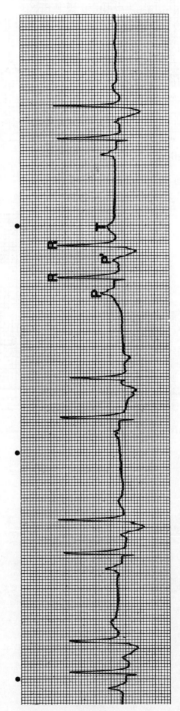

Figure 6-2 Atrial premature contraction/complex.

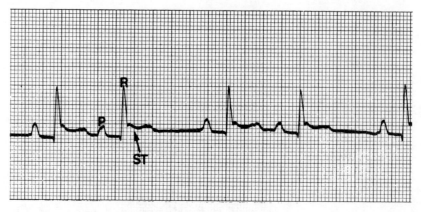

Figure 6-3 S-T Elevation.

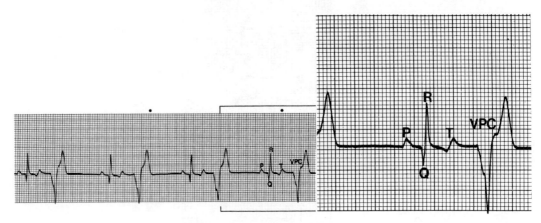

Figure 6-4 Ventricular premature contraction/complex.

DERMATOLOGY

Table 6-7   Dermatology

DISEASE	Acne	
	Canine	Feline
DEFINITION	Chronic inflammatory disorder most often seen in short-coated breeds. It is often associated with superficial and deep pyoderma. It is typically found on the chin and lips of young animals.	Feline acne if often associated with the chin and lower lip. They may have a single episode or a lifelong problem. Poor grooming is thought to be one cause for this condition.
DIAGNOSIS		
CLINICAL SIGNS	• Erythematous papules, swelling, exudate, and scarring	• Comedones, erythema papules, serous crusts, swelling, and alopecia
GENERAL	• Clinical signs	• Clinical signs
CBC	• N/A	• N/A
BIOCHEMISTRY	• N/A	• N/A
URINALYSIS	• N/A	• N/A
RADIOLOGY	• N/A	• N/A
MISCELLANEOUS	• Bacterial culture: bacteria recognition and identification • Biopsy: to confirm diagnosis	• Biopsy: to confirm diagnosis
TREATMENT		
GENERAL	• Symptomatic	• Symptomatic
MEDICATION	• Antibiotics: cephalexin • Antibiotics (topical): mupirocin • Corticosteroids: prednisone or prednisolone • Medicated gels: pyoben • Medicated shampoo: benzoyl peroxide • Retinoids (topical): retin-A gel and tretinoin	• Antibiotics: clavamox or enrofloxacin • Antibiotics (topical): mupirocin • Medicated shampoo: benzoyl peroxide or sulfur-salicylic acid • Retinoids (topical): retin-A gel and tretinoin
PATIENT CARE	• Treated as outpatient	• Treated as outpatient

Table 6-7 Dermatology (Continued)

DISEASE	Acne	
	Canine	Feline
PATIENT CARE	• Prevent self-trauma: (e.g., rubbing of chin, chewing on bones that increase salivation) • Frequent cleaning/shampooing of chin • Warm compresses	• Shampoo 1–2 times weekly and then taper over a 2–3-week period
PREVENTION/ AVOIDANCE	• Lifelong treatment may be necessary	• Lifelong treatment may be necessary
COMPLICATIONS	• Deep pyoderma	• Deep pyoderma
PROGNOSIS	• Excellent	• Excellent
NOTES	• English bulldogs, Boxers, Doberman pinscher, and Great Dane • Discourage owners from expressing the lesions: it can lead to massive inflammation	• Discourage owners from expressing the lesions: it can lead to massive inflammation

FOLLOW-UP

DISEASE	Acral Lick Dermatitis (Lick Granuloma)	Atopy	Flea Allergy Dermatitis (FAD)
DEFINITION	Acral lick dermatitis is an area of a firm, raised, ulcerative, or thickened area that is usually located on the dorsal aspect of the carpus, metacarpus, tarsus, or metatarsus. The area may have a history of trauma, foreign body reaction, neoplasia, allergy, endocrinology, or others. The problem is typically made worse by the constant licking and chewing of the patient.	Animals that have formed allergies to normally innocuous inhaled substances such as pollen, grass, fleas, molds, and mites. This disease is the cause of most dermatologic problems.	The antigens in the saliva of fleas is the cause of a hypersensitivity reaction called flea allergy dermatitis. It is the most common skin disease in most geographic areas, especially during the summer months. Ctenocephalides felis is the type of flea that usually infests both dogs and cats.

DIAGNOSIS

CLINICAL SIGNS	• Excessive licking and chewing, alopecia, ulcerative and thickened	• Pruritis and skin lesions *Dogs* • Face rubbing, foot chewing, alopecia, edema, and hyperpigmentation • Otitis externa, recurrent pyoderma, and seborrheic dermatitis *Cats* • Alopecia, dermatitis, and miliary eczema	• Pruritis: licking, chewing, rubbing, rolling, and scratching • Papules, erythema, broken hairs, dry hair, scaling, hyperpigmentation, and miliary eczema (cats) • Alopecia: tail base, dorsal lumbar region, caudal thighs, groin, abdomen, head, and neck (cats) • Lymphadenopathy (cats)
GENERAL	• History • Clinical signs	• History: seasonal • Clinical signs	• History • Clinical signs • Presence of fleas or flea dirt
CBC	• Normal or may reflect underlying cause	• Eosinophilia (occasional)	• Hypereosinophilia (cats—variable)
BIOCHEMISTRY	• Normal or may reflect underlying cause	• Normal or may reflect underlying cause	• Normal
URINALYSIS	• N/A	• N/A	• N/A
RADIOLOGY	• Lower limb: neoplasia, radiopaque foreign body, bony proliferation, and some forms of trauma	• N/A	• N/A
MISCELLANEOUS	• Skin scraping: bacteria, demodex, dermatophytosis • Bacterial culture: bacteria recognition and identification • Hypoallergenic test diet: food hypersensitivity • Intradermal skin test: atopy • Biopsy: neoplasia	• Intradermal skin test: most reliable specific test • Enzyme-linked immunosorbent assay (ELISA) and radioallergosorbent test (RAST): ↑ values (nonspecific)	• Intradermal skin test: + results (reliable) • Flea combing

Table 6-7 Dermatology (Continued)

	DISEASE	Acral Lick Dermatitis (Lick Granuloma)	Atopy	Flea Allergy Dermatitis (FAD)
TREATMENT	GENERAL	• Symptomatic	• Symptomatic	• Symptomatic
	MEDICATION	• Antihistamines: chlorpheniramine and hydroxyzine HCl • Antibiotics: variable • Psychotropic drugs: clomipramine HCl, amitriptyline, or fluoxetine HCl	• Antihistamines: (e.g., chlorpheniramine, hydroxyzine, and diphenhydramine) • Corticosteroids: prednisone or methylprednisolone • Immunotherapy: SC injection of increasing doses of offending allergen • Medicated shampoos	• Antihistamines: diphenhydramine or chlorpheniramine • Antiparasitic: fipronil • Corticosteroids: triamcinolone • Fatty acid supplements • Insecticide: imidacloprid and selamectin • Lufenuron
	PATIENT CARE	• Treated as outpatient	• Treated as outpatient	• Treated as outpatient
FOLLOW-UP	PATIENT CARE	• Monitor closely for licking and chewing • Check CBC, biochemistry, and ECG every 1–2 months for those receiving tricyclic antidepressants	• Fatty acid supplementation • Frequent bathing to reduce pruritis • Examine patients every 2–8 weeks after treatment, then every 3–12 months	• Flea comb regularly
	PREVENTION/ AVOIDANCE	• Determine underlying disease when possible	• Avoid offending allergen	• Maintain year-round flea control: flea comb, monthly oral medication, and/or spot-ons medication
	COMPLICATIONS	• Deep pyoderma	• Superficial pyoderma • Flea allergy dermatitis • Surface pyoderma	• Superficial or deep pyoderma • Acute moist dermatitis • Acral lick dermatitis
	PROGNOSIS	• Guarded if no underlying disease is found and psychogenic causes are suspected	• Good if allergen is determined	• Excellent

NOTES

- E-Collars, foul-tasting medications and sprays, and bandages may be used to prevent licking and chewing
- Additional attention and exercise may help if psychogenic causes are suspected

- Do not use penicillins or tetracyclines for treatment of superficial pyoderma
- Some type of treatment is usually needed for life
- It may take 3 months to 1 year before results from immunotherapy are seen

- A complete flea control plan includes treating the pet, other pets in household, and indoor and outdoor environment
- Control may take 4–8 weeks to achieve
- With many new alternatives to flea control, dips, sprays, and flea collars should be the last choice for control
- Extra care should be taken when using insecticides to avoid overdose to animals and humans
- Flea-infested animals should also be checked for *Dipylidium caninum*

DISEASE	Food Hypersensitivity	Otitis externa
DEFINITION	Food hypersensitivities show symptoms induced by food ingestion in which there are demonstrable or highly suspected immunologic reactions.	Otitis externa is the inflammation of the soft tissue of the external ear canal. Its causes are often multifactorial, signifying a generalized dermatologic problem. It can be either a primary or a secondary disease, making it very frustrating and difficult to treat.
CLINICAL SIGNS	• Pruritis: feet, ears, face, axillae, and others • Vomiting and diarrhea (variable) • Neurologic signs: seizures and malaise (rare)	• Head shaking, tilting, pain, foul odor, scratching and rubbing at ears • Behavioral changes: irritable or aggressive • Loss of hearing
GENERAL	• History • Clinical signs • Nonseasonal occurrence and partial or incomplete response to corticosteroids	• History • Clinical signs • Otoscopic examination
CBC	• Normal	• Normal or may reflect underlying cause
BIOCHEMISTRY	• Normal	• Normal or may reflect underlying cause
URINALYSIS	• N/A	• N/A

DIAGNOSIS

Table 6-7   Dermatology (Continued)

	DISEASE	Food Hypersensitivity	Otitis externa
DIAGNOSIS	RADIOLOGY	• N/A	• Skull: only used in chronic cases to determine patency of ear canal and rule out otitis media
	MISCELLANEOUS	• Intradermal skin testing: inconsistent findings • Hypoallergenic test diet or novel elimination diet trial	• Cytology: parasites, cells, bacteria, yeast, and fungi • Culture: bacteria recognition and identification • Intradermal skin tests: + results
TREATMENT	GENERAL	• Symptomatic	• Symptomatic • Flush and dry ear canals
	MEDICATION	• If any, dependent on clinical signs	• Antibiotics: cephalexin, trimethoprimsulfa, enrofloxacin, or clindamycin • Antifungals: ketoconazole • Corticosteroids: prednisone • Parasiticides: ivermectin
	PATIENT CARE	• Treated as outpatient	• Treated as outpatient
FOLLOW-UP	PATIENT CARE	• Feed the restricted diet exclusively for 6 weeks • Avoid flavored chew toys, bones, treats, vitamins, and chewable medications	• Recheck ears 1 week after beginning treatment: do not treat before examination, for better visibility
	PREVENTION/ AVOIDANCE	• Restrict the feeding of hypersensitive foods	• Clean ears regularly • Thoroughly dry ears after swimming and bathing • Lateral ear resection surgery
	COMPLICATIONS	• Pruritis: by other sources	• Ruptured ear drum • Otitis media • Permanent ear canal changes: stenosis and calcification
	PROGNOSIS	• Good if offending food is determined	• Excellent if treated early

NOTES

- The diet should consist of foods that the animal has not been previously exposed to (e.g., rice, potatoes, lamb) and without additives or preservatives. (See Table 3-12)
- If no improvement, review other food sources and other forms of allergens (e.g., fleas and inhalant)
- Corticosteroids should only be used with severe pruritis: otherwise, they may alter the results of the hypoallergenic diet test

DISEASE	Pyoderma		Surface (Acute Moist Dermatitis—hot spots, Skin Fold Dermatitis)
	Deep	Superficial	
DEFINITION	Deep pyoderma extends into the dermis and in severe cases into the subcutaneous tissue. This bacterial skin infection has many different forms, two of the most common being folliculitis and furunculosis. It is almost always secondary to another disease process.	The epidermis is the target of a bacterial infection with superficial pyoderma. It can manifest itself in 2 ways: penetrating the stratum corneum (impetigo) or invading the hair follicles (folliculitis).	Self-trauma and deep skin folds are the most common causes of surface pyoderma. A colony of bacteria live on the surface of the epidermis only, without invading the stratum corneum or hair follicles. Acute moist dermatitis (hot spots) and skin fold dermatitis are the two distinct forms of surface pyoderma.
CLINICAL SIGNS	• Anorexia, depression, peripheral lymphadenopathy, and fever • Pustules: inguinal, ventral, abdominal, and axillary areas extending to the whole body • Erythemaous, painful and pruritic skin • Exudate and crust formation, drainage tracts, and hemorrhagic bullae	*Impetigo* • Pustules: inguinal and ventral abdominal area (especially young animals) *Folliculitis* • Pustules: inguinal, ventral abdominal, and axillary areas • Erythema and pruritic skin • Epidermal collarettes: "bull's-eye" lesions	• Biting, licking, and rubbing *Acute moist dermatitis* • Alopecia, thin exudate layer, erythema, surrounded by matted hairs and thickened skin with abrasion *Skin fold pyoderma* • Inflammation, exudate, fetid, alopecia, and erythema

- Possible reasons for certain exudates:
  - Dark, dry, and granular = ear mite infection
  - Moist, yellow, and odiferous = bacterial infection
  - Brown and waxy = yeast infection
  - Yellow and waxy to oily = keratinization disorders
- Use only warmed 0.9% saline to flush an ear canal with a ruptured tympanic membrane
- Plucking hair from within the ear canal may cause irritation and predisposes the animal to otitis externa

Table 6-7 Dermatology (Continued)

DISEASE	Pyoderma		Surface (Acute Moist Dermatitis—hot spots, Skin Fold Dermatitis)
	Deep	Superficial	
DIAGNOSIS			
GENERAL	• History • Clinical signs	• History • Clinical signs	• History • Clinical signs • Self-trauma, environmental irritant, or any pruritic skin
CBC	• Leukocytosis with a left shift (variable)	• Normal or may reflect underlying cause	• Normal or may reflect underlying cause
BIOCHEMISTRY	• ↑ Globulin (variable)	• Normal or may reflect underlying cause	• Normal or may reflect underlying cause
URINALYSIS	• N/A	• N/A	• N/A
RADIOLOGY	• N/A	• N/A	• N/A
MISCELLANEOUS	• Cytology: neutrophils, macrophages, and bacteria • Skin scrapings: ectoparasites • Blood culture: bacteria • Culture: bacteria recognition and identification • Skin biopsy: to confirm folliculitis, perifolliculitis, or furunculosis	• Cytology: neutrophils and bacteria • Skin scrapings: ectoparasites • Culture: bacteria recognition and identification • Skin biopsy: to confirm folliculitis	• N/A
TREATMENT			
GENERAL	• Symptomatic • Fluid therapy (severe cases)	• Symptomatic	• Symptomatic • Wound management
MEDICATION	• Antibiotics: variable • Medicated shampoos	• Antibiotics: variable • Medicated shampoos: antiseptic	• Antibiotics (oral and/or topical): variable • Corticosteroids (topical): panalog cream and neopredef powder
PATIENT CARE	• Clip haircoat on long-coated breeds	• Treated as outpatient	• Treated as outpatient

FOLLOW-UP			
PATIENT CARE	• Bathe twice daily for 1–2 weeks then 1–2 times weekly • Whirlpool baths • Provide a high-quality diet • Supplementation of essential fatty acids • Padded bedding to ease pressure point pyoderma	• Bathe 2–3 times weekly for 2–3 weeks • Prevent self-trauma • Provide a high-quality diet • Supplement with essential fatty acids	• Maintain a clean and dry wound • Prevent self-trauma: restraint, collars, etc.
PREVENTION/ AVOIDANCE	• Determine the underlying cause • Bathe regularly with appropriate shampoo	• Determine the underlying cause • Bathe with appropriate shampoo, especially after swimming	• Determine the underlying cause • Clean and dry the skin folds routinely with astringents
COMPLICATIONS	• Bacteremia or septicemia • Scarring	• Deep pyoderma • Recurrence	• Superficial or deep pyoderma
PROGNOSIS	• Excellent if underlying cause is determined	• Excellent	• Excellent
NOTES	• German shepards		• Cocker spaniel, Springer spaniel, Saint Bernard, Irish setter, Shar pei, Basset hound, Bulldog, Boston terrier, and Pug • Corrective surgery may be performed on chronically infected skin folds

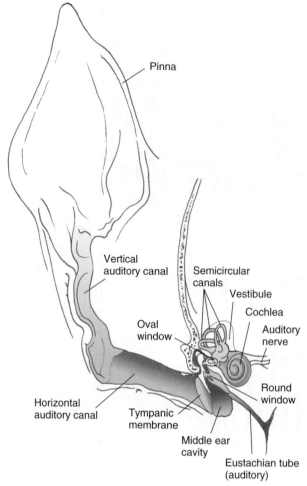

Figure 6-5 Ear.

Skill Box 6-3 / Ear Cleaning and Flushing

1. Prepare solution to clean ears: e.g., chlorhexidine, povidone iodine, Oti-clens, Epi-Otic

2. Using either a bulb syringe or syringe without the needle, fill the ear canal with cleaning solution. Be careful not to form a seal between the instrument and the ear canal, and do not use a direct stream on the tympanic membrane.

3. Put a towel or piece of roll cotton at the entrance of the ear canal and begin gently massaging the ear canal from the bottom up. This will work the solution from the bottom of the ear canal to the opening.

4. Repeat steps 2 and 3 until the ear canal and solution on the towel comes out clean (5–10 times).

5. To dry the ear canal, use either a flushing solution or suction via an infant feeding tube attached to a syringe.

Skill Box 6-4 / Bathing

1. Location: a safe place for both owner and animal to stand, a mixture of hot and cold water available and an area able to withstand water (e.g., shaking wet dog).

   Place a towel or mat in the bottom of the tub to supply traction for the animal.

   Have a leash hook fastened to the wall so the animal can be secured without having to always have a hand on the animal.

2. Supplies: multiple towels, appropriate shampoo, plastic apron, gloves (depending on type of shampoo) and protective eyewear.
3. Comb out and demat the animal before bathing.
4. Wet down the animal completely, making sure to get water down to the skin.
5. Apply the shampoo and lather the entire animal, including face.
6. Leave shampoo on for the amount of time indicated on the bottle or by the veterinarian.

   Use a timer to ensure that the shampoo is on for the correct time: do not guess.

7. Rinse the animal completely, making sure to remove all soapy residue.
8. Dry the animal's haircoat and ear canals with a combination of shaking (removes 95% of the water) and towels.

   Blow in the animal's ear to get it to shake.

   Dry the ear canals, using either a vinegar rinse or with cotton balls.

   **Caution: Keep the animal in a warm place until completely dry to avoid the animal becoming chilled.

9. Comb and brush out the animal after the bath to remove all the hair that was loosened.

   **Caution:
   Do not use lubricants in the eyes, it may trap the shampoo in the eye instead of protecting the eye.
   Do not place an animal in a heater/dryer cage without direct supervision to prevent overheating and death of the animal.
   If drying an animal with a blow dryer, be sure to keep the dryer on the lowest setting and continuously moving to prevent burns to the animals.

ENDOCRINOLOGY/REPRODUCTION

Table 6-8 Endocrinology/Reproduction

DISEASE	Abortion	Diabetes Insipidus	Diabetes Mellitus
DEFINITION	An abortion is the termination of a pregnancy. It may be the result of difficulties with the mother, fetus, or placenta. Exposure to toxins or infections in the dam are well documented.	Diabetes insipidus is a disorder of water metabolism caused by a deficiency of antidiuretic hormone (ADH) caused by either a lack of release of ADH or renal tubular insensitivity to ADH.	A chronic disorder of carbohydrate metabolism, characterized by hyperglycemia and glucosuria and resulting from inadequate production or utilization of insulin. *Type I:* insulin-dependent (low to absent secretory ability) *Type II:* non-insulin-dependent (inadequate or delayed insulin secretion or peripheral tissue insensitivity to insulin)
CLINICAL SIGNS	• Anorexia, lethargy, vomiting, and diarrhea *Early gestation* • Vaginal discharge: fetid and purulent *Late gestation* • Restlessness and abdominal contractions	• PU/PD, nocturia, incontinence • Weight loss and dehydration • Neurologic signs: seizures, disorientation, and blindness	• PU/PD, polyphagia, and weight loss • Later stages: anorexia, lethargy, oily hair coat, dorsal muscle wasting, depression, and vomiting
GENERAL	• History • Clinical signs • Observe for any systemic signs of illness	• Clinical signs	• History • Clinical signs
CBC	• Normal or may reflect underlying cause	• Normal	• Eosinophilia and lymphocytosis (variable) ↑ PCV and TP • Mild nonregenerative anemia • Heinz bodies
BIOCHEMISTRY	• Normal or may reflect underlying cause	• Normal	• ↑ Glucose (>200 mg/dL in dogs; >250 mg/dL in cats), cholesterol, sodium, phosphate, alkaline phosphate, ALT and AST ↓ Potassium • Metabolic acidosis

DIAGNOSIS

DIAGNOSIS			
URINALYSIS	• N/A	• ± ↑ Protein • ⊟ ↓ Specific gravity: <1.010	• ↑↓ Glucose, ketones, and UTI • ↓ Specific gravity: <1.030 µg/dL
RADIOLOGY	• N/A	• N/A	• Thoracic: microcardia and hypoperfusion of lungs
MISCELLANEOUS	• Ultrasound: uterine pathology and retained fetuses • Bacterial culture: bacteria recognition and identification • Necropsy of dead fetuses • RAST or agar gel immunodiffusion (AGID): *B. canis*	• Nuclear imaging and computer tomography (CT): identify pituitary or hypothalamic lesion • Abrupt or Gradual Water Deprivation Test: UA specific gravity of <1.025 ug/dL • ADH Response Test: failure to concentrate urine after exogenous ADH administration	• Ultrasound: pancreatic and liver pathology
TREATMENT			
GENERAL	• Symptomatic • Fluid therapy • Surgery for retained fetuses	• Symptomatic	• Supportive • Fluid therapy
MEDICATION	• Antibiotics: variable • Prostaglandin	• ADH supplement: vasopressin	• Longer-Acting Insulin: long-term treatment (e.g., Lente, Ultralente, or PZI) • Short-Acting Insulin: initial management (e.g., Regular or Semi-lente)
PATIENT CARE	• Postparturition or postoperative nursing care	• Free access to water	• Free access to water • Try to mimic the same feeding schedule used at home

Table 6-8 Endocrinology/Reproduction (Continued)

DISEASE	Abortion	Diabetes Insipidus	Diabetes Mellitus
PATIENT CARE	• Physical examination 7–14 days after treatment	• Free access to water	• Maintain a regimented feeding and medication schedule (see Skill Box 6-5) • Monitor for signs of iatrogenic hypoglycemia, PU/PD, appetite, and body weight (see Skill Box 6-6) • Provide consistent amount of exercise every day to prevent fluctuations in insulin requirements • Serial BGs: initially every few weeks and then, once regulated, every few months • Serum fructosamine or glycosylated hemoglobin: ↑ value
PREVENTION/ AVOIDANCE	• OVH	• Avoid circumstances that might markedly increase water loss	• Prevent or correct obesity • Avoid unnecessary use of corticosteroids or megesterol acetate
COMPLICATIONS	• Pyometra • Sepsis • Shock • Uterine rupture • Infertility • Peritonitis • Death	• Primary disease	• Cataracts (dogs) and diabetic neuropathy (cats) • Seizures or coma • Anemia and hemoglobinemia with severe hypophosphatemia • Secondary infections
PROGNOSIS	• Excellent if treated early	• Very good prognosis with lack of release of ADH • Guarded prognosis with renal insensitivity to ADH	• Cats may recover but may relapse later • Dogs have permanent disease • Normal life span is expected with treatment

FOLLOW-UP

NOTES

- In the first trimester, it is very difficult to determine whether an animal is having infertility problems or experiencing abortions
- Aborted fetuses or placenta may be infectious: isolate animal from all other dogs, pups, and humans

- Meals should coincide with the administration of insulin
- Feed diets of increased fiber and complex carbohydrates to reduce postprandial fluctuations in blood glucose levels
- Patients scheduled for surgery: NPO after 12 AM, give half the normal dose of insulin the morning of surgery, monitor blood glucose levels, and administer R insulin if needed: after the surgery, maintain the patient on a 5% Dextrose IV drip until food intake has resumed
- Keeshond, Puli, Miniature Pinscher, and Cairn terriers

- Water deprivation test is contraindicated in dehydrated animals

DISEASE	Dystocia	Eclampsia (Puerperal tetany)	Hyperadrenocorticism (HAC, Canine Cushing's Syndrome)
DEFINITION	Dystocia results from abnormalities associated with parturition. They are due to either primary or secondary uterine inertia. Primary uterine inertia is the failure of uterine contractions sufficient to deliver. Secondary uterine inertia is fetal obstruction caused by large pups, narrow birth canal, abnormal pup position, etc.	Eclampsia can be a life-threatening condition often seen 1–4 weeks postpartum. It is caused by extremely low serum ionized calcium levels.	Hyperadrenocorticism is most commonly found in dogs in middle to old age. It is caused by the excessive secretion of cortisol by the adrenal glands. The excess glucocorticoid comes from (1) excessive secretion of adrenocorticotropic hormone (ACTH) from a pituitary microadenoma or (2) an adrenocortical tumor. Excessive administration of corticosteroids can also result in iatrogenic HAC, a separate syndrome.

Table 6-8 Endocrinology/Reproduction (Continued)

DISEASE	Dystocia	Eclampsia (Puerperal tetany)	Hyperadrenocorticism (HAC, Canine Cushing's Syndrome)
CLINICAL SIGNS	• Vaginal stenosis • Active straining for >45 minutes, resting phase for >4–6 hours without straining or intermittent weak contractions for >2 hours • Signs of pain or licking or biting of vulva • Purulent or hemorrhagic vaginal discharge	• Restlessness, nervousness, panting, tachypnea, drooling, and whining • Ataxia, stiff gait, muscle tremors, tetany, and convulsions • Hyperthermia and seizures • Dilated pupils and ↓ pupillary light response	• Pendulous, distended or pot-bellied abdomen • Bilaterally symmetric alopecia with a dull, dry haircoat and recurrent skin infections • Thin skin with hyperpigmentation and ↑ fragility (especially cats) • Muscle and testicular atrophy • PU/PD and lower urinary tract disease (LUTD) • Excessive panting and severe respiratory distress • Behavior change, circling, and seizures • Infertility • Polyphagia
GENERAL	• History • Clinical signs • Prolonged gestation: >72 days from the first mating	• History • Clinical signs	• History: exogenous glucocorticoid use
CBC	• ↑↓ PCV and TP • ↓ Glucose and calcium	• Normal	• Steroid leukogram • Mild erythrocytosis (variable)
BIOCHEMISTRY	• Normal	• ↓ Calcium (≤7 mg/dL) and glucose (rare)	• ↑ Alkaline Phosphatase, cholesterol, ALT, and glucose (variable)
URINALYSIS	• N/A	• N/A	• ↑ Protein, blood, bacteria, white blood cells (WBCs), and cortisol-to-creatinine ratio (>35) • ↓ Specific gravity: <1.020
RADIOLOGY	• Abdominal: fetal death characterized by intrafetal gas patterns, collapsed spinal cord, overlapping of the skull bones, or pup in the birth canal	• N/A	• Thoracic: mineralization of bronchial walls • Abdominal: adrenal tumors and hepatomegaly

DIAGNOSIS

	Column A	Column B	Column C
DIAGNOSIS — MISCELLANEOUS	Ultrasound: uterine pathology and fetal viability	ECG: prolonged QT interval, bradycardia, tachycardia, or VPCs	• ACTH Stimulation Test: to diagnose type->20 µg/dL with endogenous HAC, blunted or no response iatrogenic HAC • Low-Dose Dexamethasone Test: to confirm diagnosis—>1 µg/dL during 8-hour test • High-Dose Dexamethasone Suppression Test: to differentiate type—<1.5 µg/dL with pituitary-dependent HAC and >1.5 µg/dL with adrenocortical neoplasia • Endogenous Plasma ACTH Concentration: to differentiate type—>40 pg/mL with pituitary dependent HAC and <20 pg/mL with adrenocortical tumors • Ultrasound: ↑ liver and adrenal glands • CT: visualization of pituitary tumors and possibly pituitary microadenomas (radiographs and ultrasounds can be used, but are not as accurate)
TREATMENT — GENERAL	• Symptomatic • Fluid therapy • Manual manipulation via vagina • Surgery: emergency cesarean section	• Symptomatic	• Symptomatic • Radiation therapy: pituitary macroadenoma or macrocarcinoma • Surgical removal of adrenal tumor
TREATMENT — MEDICATION	• Anesthesia: isoflurane or reversible induction agents • Ecbolic agents: oxytocin, calcium gluconate, ergonovine maleate, or dextrose • Tranquilizer: acepromazine	• Calcium gluconate • Tranquilizers: diazepam	• Corticosteroids: prednisone or prednisolone • Ketoconazole • l-Deprenyl • Mitotane (e.g., Lysodren)
TREATMENT — PATIENT CARE	• Postparturition or standard postoperative care	• Cold water baths and enemas • Hand-raise puppies until crisis is over	• Treated as outpatient

Table 6-8 Endocrinology/Reproduction (Continued)

DISEASE	Dystocia	Eclampsia (Puerperal tetany)	Hyperadrenocorticism (HAC, Canine Cushing's Syndrome)
FOLLOW-UP			
PATIENT CARE	• Postparturition care • Monitor growth and nursing habits of the neonates	• Monitor calcium levels	• Monitor for reoccurrence of previous clinical signs • Perform an ACTH Response Test 5—10 days after initiation of medication (except l-deprenyl) then every 3—6 months • Monitor for inappetance, severely decreased water consumption, attitude, activity, vomiting, or diarrhea relating to the medication
PREVENTION/ AVOIDANCE	• Ovariohysterectomy (OVH) • Scheduled cesarean section	• Do not supplement with calcium during gestation • OVH	• N/A
COMPLICATIONS	• Maternal or fetal death • Increased risk in future pregnancies • Neonate stuck in birth canal	• Cerebral edema • Death	• Thromboembolism • Congestive heart failure • Hypertension • Recurrence of clinical signs • Progression of CNS signs • Infection: skin and urinary • Diabetes mellitus
PROGNOSIS	• Excellent if discovered early	• Good with immediate treatment • Poor with delayed treatment	• Guarded because of the number of complications associated with this disease
NOTES	• Rule out obstructive dystocia before administering ecbolic agents. • Welsh corgis and brachycephalic breeds tend to have a congenitally small pelvis, and the pups tend to have large heads and shoulders	• Response to treatment is rapid: therefore, treat if the diagnosis is suspected while laboratory confirmation is pending • Probable reoccurrence with subsequent litters	• Easy cutaneous bruising is seen in these dogs: venipuncture should be performed with extra care • Poodles, Dachshunds, Boston terriers, and Boxers

DISEASE	Hyperparathyroidism	Hyperthyroidism (feline)	Hypoadrenocorticism (Addison's Disease)
DEFINITION	The disease results from excessive secretion of the parathyroid hormone (PTH). This can be caused by an adenoma, carcinoma, or hyperplasia of the parathyroid gland.	A multisystemic metabolic disorder most commonly seen in middle-aged to old cats. It is caused by an excessive amount of circulating thyroid hormone. The disease causes an increased basal metabolic rate, which in turn causes the disease's clinical signs.	Hypoadrenocorticism is a disease of the adrenal gland resulting in a deficiency of glucocorticoid and/or mineralocorticoid secretion from the adrenal cortex. The cause is often thought to be idiopathic or sometimes caused by infection, hemorrhagic infarctions, metastatic neoplasia, trauma, and amyloidosis. Mostly seen in young to middle-aged female dogs.
CLINICAL SIGNS	• Anorexia, lethargy, depression, shivering, constipation, vomiting, and facial swelling • Weakness, twitching, stiff gait, and seizures • PU/PD	• Weight loss, increased appetite, restlessness, hyperexcitability, and weakness • Unkempt haircoat, excessive shedding and matting • Enlargement of 1 or both thyroid glands • PU/PD • Tachycardia, systolic murmurs, gallop rhythm, and other signs associated with secondary hypertrophic cardiomyopathy • Variable: dyspnea, panting, hyperventilation, vomiting, and diarrhea	• Intermittent anorexia, vomiting, diarrhea, lethargy, muscle weakness, collapse, and depression • Vomiting and diarrhea • PU/PD • Progressing to bradycardia, hyperkalemia-associated arrhythmias, and shock
GENERAL	• Clinical signs • Palpation of a parathyroid gland (cats)	• History • Clinical signs • Palpation of thyroid gland(s)	• History • Clinical signs
CBC	• Normal	• Erythrocytosis (occasional) • Mature leukocytosis and eosinopenia • ↑ PCV and MCV	• Normal
BIOCHEMISTRY	• ↑ Calcium, ALT, and alkaline phosphatase • ↓ Phosphorus	• ↑ ALT, AST, alkaline phosphatase, BUN, creatinine, glucose, phosphorus, and bilirubin	• ↑ ALT, AST, cholesterol, calcium, potassium, creatinine, and BUN • ↓ Phosphorus, sodium, and glucose • Sodium to potassium ratio: ≤27

DIAGNOSIS

Table 6-8 Endocrinology/Reproduction (Continued)

	DISEASE	Hyperparathyroidism	Hyperthyroidism (feline)	Hypoadrenocorticism (Addison's Disease)
DIAGNOSIS	URINALYSIS	• ↓ Specific gravity	• N/A	• ↑↓ Ketones and glucose • Specific gravity: <1.030
	RADIOLOGY	• Skeletal: generalized osteopenia, ↑ bone resorption (alveolar bone of the jaw) and cyst-like areas in the bone	• Thoracic: cardiomegaly	• Abdominal: cystic or renal calculi, cholecystitis, and pancreatitis
	MISCELLANEOUS	• Serum ionized calcium: ↑ values • Serum PTH concentration: ↑ values • Ultrasound: visualization of the parathyroid gland, urolithiasis, and renal abnormalities	• Basal serum thyroid hormone concentration: >4 µg/dL • Free T_4 by equilibrium analysis: ↑ value • T_3 suppression test: >1.5 µg/dL • TRH response test: little to no increase in serum T_4 • Ultrasound: underlying renal disease • Blood pressure: ↑ value	• ACTH stimulation test: primary hypoadrenocorticism is <1 µg/dL and secondary hypoadrenocorticism post-ACTH concentrations is >2.5 µg/dL • Plasma concentration of ACTH: primary is >500 pg/mL and secondary is <20 pg/mL • Plasma aldosterone: ↓ value • Sodium:potassium ratio: <27:1 • ECG: peaking of T waves, prolonged P-R waves until P wave ultimately disappears, QRS complex widens, and R-R intervals become irregular
TREATMENT	GENERAL	• Symptomatic • Fluid therapy • Surgical removal of the parathyroid gland adenoma	• Symptomatic • Radioiodine therapy • Surgery: thyroidectomy	• Supportive • Fluid therapy in severe cases
	MEDICATION	• ± Calcium supplementation • Diuretic: furosemide	• β-Adrenergic-blocking drugs • Methimazole	• Corticosteroids: prednisone • Mineralcorticoids: DOCP or florinef
		• Standard postoperative care	• Treated as outpatient	• Treated as outpatient

FOLLOW-UP

PATIENT CARE	• Check serum calcium 1–2 times daily for 1 week postoperatively	• Check CBC, BUN, creatinine, and serum T_4 every 2–4 weeks during first 3 months of methimazole treatment • Check serum T_4 the first week and then every 3–6 months after thyroidectomy • Check T_4 the second week and then every 3–6 months after radioiodine therapy	• Check electrolytes weekly until stabilized in the normal range • Check electrolytes, BUN, and creatinine monthly for 3 months, then every 3–12 months
PREVENTION/ AVOIDANCE	• N/A	• N/A	• N/A
COMPLICATIONS	• Hypocalcemia (iatrogenic)	• Hypothyroidism (iatrogenic) • Congestive heart failure • Renal damage • Retinal detachment • Diarrhea • Dehydration	• PU/PD from medication
PROGNOSIS	• Excellent with proper treatment • Poor with associated renal disease	• Excellent with treatment • Poor with thyroid carcinoma	• Good to excellent with proper diagnosis and treatment • Poor prognosis for those with tumors causing the disease
NOTES	• This is the only condition that causes an ↑ calcium and ↓ phosphorus • Keeshond, German shepherd, Norwegian Elkhounds, and Siamese cat	• Clinical signs are expected to completely resolve with proper treatment • Radioiodine therapy is the best choice of treatment to cure the disease • Renal disease may become apparent once euthyroidism is established	• Most commonly seen in female dogs <7 years old • The dosage of glucocorticoids needs to be increased during times of stress such as travel, hospitalization, and surgery • Great Danes, Rottweilers, Portuguese Water spaniel, West Highland white terriers, Wheaten terriers, and Standard poodles

Table 6-8 Endocrinology/Reproduction (Continued)

DISEASE	Hypoparathyroidism	Hypothyroidism (canine)	Mastitis
DEFINITION	Hypoparathyroidism is a deficiency in the secretion of the parathyroid hormone. This condition is most commonly seen in dogs as naturally occurring and typically following thyroidectomy in cats.	Hypothyroidism is the most commonly diagnosed endocrine disease in the dog; a condition that results from inadequate production and release of T_4. Caused by either destruction of the thyroid gland or impaired secretion of TSH by the pituitary gland.	Mastitis is a bacterial infection of one or more of the lactating glands. Seen in the postpartum dam and queen.
CLINICAL SIGNS	• Anorexia, weight loss, vomiting, diarrhea, depression, and listlessness • Cataracts • Tachycardia, weak pulses, and panting • Neurologic signs: ataxia, nervousness, tremors, twitching, rigid limb extension, muscles spasms, stiff gait, and seizures	• Weight gain, lethargy, mental dullness, muscle weakness, exercise intolerance, and cold intolerance • Bilaterally symmetrical nonpruritic alopecia on ventral and lateral trunk, caudal thighs, dorsal tail, dorsal nose, and ventral neck • Hyperpigmentation, myxedema, and pyodermas • Bradycardia, impaired myocardial contractility • Anestrus, infertility, abortion, testicular atrophy, and hypospermia	• Anorexia, lethargy, fever, and dehydration • Mammary gland(s): firm, swollen, warm, painful and purulent or hemorrhagic discharge • Abscess of mammary gland(s) • Neglect or failure to thrive of neonates
DIAGNOSIS — GENERAL	• Clinical signs	• Clinical signs	• History • Clinical signs
CBC	• Normal	• Normocytic, normochromic, nonregenerative anemia	• Leukocytosis with left shift or leukopenia with sepsis • ↑ PCV (variable)
BIOCHEMISTRY	• ± Phosphate • ↓ Calcium	• ↑ Cholesterol, CK, and triglycerides	• ↑ TP and BUN
URINALYSIS	• Normal	• N/A	• N/A
RADIOLOGY	• N/A	• N/A	• N/A

DIAGNOSIS	**MISCELLANEOUS**	• Serum PTH concentration: ↓ value • ECG: prolongation of QT and ST segments, deep wide T waves, and tachyarrhythmias	• Basal serum thyroid hormone concentrations: <1.0 µg/dL • TSH stimulation test: <15 µg/dL • Serum TSH concentration: ↑ value • Free T4 by equilibrium analysis: ↓ value	• Milk cytology and culture: neutrophils, macrophages, bacteria recognition and identification
TREATMENT	**GENERAL**	• Supportive • Fluid therapy	• Symptomatic	• Supportive • Fluid therapy • Treatment of abscessed glands
	MEDICATION	• Calcium supplementation • Vitamin D supplementation	• L-thyroxine	• Antibiotics: enrofloxacin, amoxicillin, or erythromycin
	PATIENT CARE		• Treated as outpatient	• Hand-raise neonates or find a surrogate dam • Warm compress and manually milk glands several times a day
FOLLOW-UP	**PATIENT CARE**	• Check serum calcium weekly for 1 month, monthly for 6 months, then every 2–4 months	• Check serum T_4 levels after 1 month of therapy, then every 6–12 months	• Same as above • Monitor the growth and feeding habits of the neonates
	PREVENTION/ AVOIDANCE	• N/A	• N/A	• Clean environment • Clip toenails of neonates • Shave hair around mammary glands
	COMPLICATIONS	• Hypercalcemia (iatrogenic) • Renal disease	• Thyrotoxicosis from administration of high does of L-thyroxine	• Abscessed gland • Hand-raising of neonates
	PROGNOSIS	• Excellent with close monitoring of calcium levels	• Excellent with proper treatment • Poor if disease is caused by a tumor of the thyroid gland	• Good with prompt treatment

Table 6-8   Endocrinology/Reproduction (Continued)

DISEASE	Hypoparathyroidism	Hypothyroidism (canine)	Mastitis
NOTES	• Check albumin level, because it is the most common cause for pseudo-hypocalcemia • Cats with transient hypoparathy-roidism postthyroidectomy typically regain normal function by 4–6 months • Toy poodle, Miniature schnauzer, German shepherd, Labrador retriever, and Scottish terrier	• It has been proposed (controversial) that there is relationship between hy-pothyroidism and von Willebrand's disease • Failure of clinical signs to signifi-cantly improve within 3 months may be attributable to an incorrect diag-nosis • Serum T_4 levels should be checked 4–6 hours after administration of L-thyroxine • Treatment is lifelong • Golden retriever, Doberman pin-scher, Irish setter, Great Dane, Airedale terrier, Old English sheep-dog, Miniature Schnauzer, Cocker spaniel, Poodle, and Boxer	• Avoid antibiotics that may be passed in the milk and cause deleterious ef-fects to the neonates

DISEASE	Pregnancy	Pyometra
DEFINITION	Pregnancy is the condition of carrying a developing embryo(s) in the uterus. Parturition consists of 3 stages. Stage 1 is characterized by restlessness, anxiety, nesting behavior, and shivering, and can last 6–12 hours. Stage 2 is the actual delivery of the fetus. There are visible contractions, and the first fetus should be delivered within 1–2 hours from the on-set of stage 2. There may be a resting period for up to 4 hours after the delivery of a fetus. Stage 3 is the expulsion of the placenta, typically following the delivery of each fetus.	Pyometra may be seen in both dogs and cats following estrus or progesterone administration by 1–2 months. It is caused by a hormonal change in the uterus that allows for secondary infections. Seen with either an open cervix or closed cervix.
CLINICAL SIGNS	• Mammary gland development and lactation • Enlarged abdomen • Nesting instinct	• Lethargy, depression, anorexia, vomiting, diarrhea • Abdominal distention and enlarged uterus *Open-cervix pyometra* • Vaginal discharge: purulent, blood and mucus • PU/PD *Closed-cervix pyometra* • Septicemia, shock, hypothermia, and collapse

DIAGNOSIS	**GENERAL**	• History • Clinical signs • Abdominal palpation: 25–36 days after breeding (dogs) and 21–28 days after breeding (cats)	• History • Clinical signs
	CBC	• N/A	• Neutrophilia with a left shift • Mild nonregenerative anemia
	BIOCHEMISTRY	• ↑ Relaxin and progesterone levels	• ↑ Globulin, protein, ALT, and ALP • Azotemia (variable) • Electrolyte imbalances
	URINALYSIS	• N/A	• ↑ Protein • Isothenuric
	RADIOLOGY	Abdominal: fetal skeletal calcification 42 days of gestation	• Abdominal: enlarged or ruptured uterus and peritonitis
	MISCELLANEOUS	Ultrasound: 16 days of gestation	• Ultrasound: differentiate pyometra from pregnancy • Cytology and culture: bacteria recognition and identification • Vaginoscopy: determine site of origin of purulent discharge
TREATMENT	**GENERAL**	• N/A	• Symptomatic • Fluid therapy • OVH with abdominal lavage
	MEDICATION	• N/A	• Antibiotics: cephalothin, ampicillin, or enrofloxacin • Prostaglandin $F_{2\alpha}$ ($PGF_{2\alpha}$)
	PATIENT CARE	• N/A	• Standard postoperative care
FOLLOW-UP	**PATIENT CARE**	• Provide adequate nutrition throughout pregnancy. See Table 3-10 • Provide a quiet safe place for the dam/queen to deliver • Monitor parturition to become aware of any complications	• Reexam medically managed pyometra cases 2 weeks after initiation of treatment • Vaginal discharge may be seen for 4 weeks posttreatment
	PREVENTION/ AVOIDANCE	• OVH • Supervision	• OVH

Table 6-8 Endocrinology/Reproduction (Continued)

DISEASE	Pregnancy	Pyometra
COMPLICATIONS	• Dystocia • Retained fetuses or placenta • Eclampsia • Mastitis	• Uterine rupture • Sepsis and peritonitis • $PGF_{2\alpha}$ side effects • Estrus sooner after treatment
PROGNOSIS	• Excellent with proper prenatal care	• Good with OVH and no abdominal contamination • Guarded with medical management of closed pyometra
NOTES	• The length of gestation is 63 days from ovulation but may extend from 56–72 days • A transient temperature drop occurs within 24 hours of the onset of parturition • A normal fetal heart rate is twice that of the mother	• Do not perform cystocentesis when pyometra is suspected because of friable uterus and possible contamination of abdomen • Diluting $PGE_{2\alpha}$ with 1:1 sterile saline and walking an animal for 30 minutes after giving the injection may decrease side effects

FOLLOW-UP

Skill Box 6-5 / Client Education—Insulin Administration

1. Do not shake the vial; gently roll it between the palm of your hands to mix.

2. Drawing up the medication:

   a. Pull back the plunger of the syringe to the desired dose.

   b. Insert the needle into the vial, and inject the air to prevent a vacuum in the vial.

   c. Pull back on the plunger again to the desired amount and withdraw the needle from the vial.

   d. Check to make sure there are no bubbles in the syringe, if there are, pull back on the plunger and tap the syringe to move the bubbles to the top. Then push the plunger until all the air is out of the syringe. Verify again that you have the correct amount of insulin within the syringe.

3. Giving the injection:

   a. Locate an area anywhere from midneck to the last rib and halfway down on either side.

   b. Place your index finger against the back of the animal and use your thumb and middle finger to pull up skin to form a tent under your index finger.

   c. Insert the needle, bevel side up, into the skin.

   d. Pull back on the plunger to verify no blood fills the syringe.

   e. Depress the plunger to insert the insulin under the skin.

   f. Remove the syringe and immediately recap it.

   g. Properly dispose of the syringe and needle.

Skill Box 6-6 / Client Education—Monitoring for Hypoglycemia

Prevention

1. Feed the animal the same food and amount at the same times every day.

2. Do not feed table scraps or any diet other than the agreed-on diabetic diet.

3. Feed multiple meals each day.

4. Provide fresh clean water at all times.

5. Maintain a consistent exercise program.

6. Do not administer insulin to a patient that is not eating unless directed to do so by the veterinarian.

Signs to Watch for

1. Seizures/comas

2. Lack of appetite

3. Deviations from normal behavior

4. Depression

5. Drunken state

6. Cataracts

Actions to Take

1. Give Karo syrup orally or sugar water.

2. Take the animal to an animal hospital or emergency clinic immediately.

3. Keep the animal warm.

GASTROENTEROLOGY

Table 6-9   Gastroenterology

DISEASE	Anal Sac Disease	Cholangitis/Cholangiohepatitis	Constipation
DEFINITION	This is the most common disease of the anal area in small animals, especially dogs. It is the impaction, inflammation, infection, abscess, and/or rupture of the anal gland(s).	Cholangitis is inflammation confined to the bile ducts. Cholangiohepatitis is the inflammation of the bile ducts and adjacent hepatocytes. The inflammatory infiltrates are either suppurative, most commonly seen in younger cats, or nonsuppurative, mostly seen in older cats.	Constipation is a condition of prolonged fecal transit time, which contributes to increased water absorption, leaving a hard, dry fecal mass. These fecal masses can cause irritation and inflammation of the intestinal mucosa and disrupt normal motility.
CLINICAL SIGNS	• Scooting, tail chasing, and discomfort in sitting • Chewing, biting, licking, or rubbing at perianal area • Swollen anal glands, tenesmus, malodorous perianal discharge, and painful defecation • Change in behavior	• Anorexia, depression, weight loss, fever, vomiting, jaundice, and dehydration • Ascites and hepatomegaly (occasional) • Generalized lymphadenopathy (rare)	• Tenesmus, blood, mucus, hard, dry feces, and lack of fecal output • Vomiting, dehydration, anorexia, depression, and weakness • Unkempt haircoat • Distended and painful abdomen
GENERAL	• Clinical signs • Palpation of the anal glands	• History • Clinical signs	• History • Clinical signs • Abdominal palpation: enlarged colon with large fecal mass and a colon full of hypersegmented fecal balls • Digital rectal examination: fecal impaction and possible detection of underlying condition
CBC	• N/A	• Mild nonregenerative anemia • Neutrophilia with a left shift	• Stress leukogram • ↑ PCV and TP
BIOCHEMISTRY	• N/A	• ↑ Bilirubin, ammonia, ALT, AST, ALP, and gamma-glutamyltransferase (GGT) • ↓ Albumin and BUN	• ↓ Chloride and potassium
URINALYSIS	• N/A	• ↑ Bilirubin	• N/A

DIAGNOSIS

Table 6-9 Gastroenterology (Continued)

DISEASE	Anal Sac Disease	Cholangitis/Cholangiohepatitis	Constipation
DIAGNOSIS			
RADIOLOGY	• N/A	• Abdomen: hepatomegaly and cholelithiasis	• Abdominal: enlarged colon with large fecal mass or a colon full of hypersegmented fecal balls and possible detection of underlying condition

MISCELLANEOUS	• Exudate/secretion cytology: WBCs and bacteria
	• Culture: bacteria recognition and identification
		• Ultrasonography: cholelithiasis, cholecystitis, obstruction, pancreatic abnormalities and ↑ echogenecity of the liver
		• Biopsy:
		  —Suppurative, ↑ neutrophils, intrahepatic cholestasis, and portal fibrosis
		  —Nonsuppurative, lymphocytic portal infiltrates
		• Culture: bile, bacteria recognition and identification
			• Ultrasound: obstructive tumors
			• Colonoscopy: obstructive mass or lesions

TREATMENT			
GENERAL	• Expression of glands (see Skill Box 6-7) • Duct cannulation and irrigation • Surgery: anal sacculectomy	• Supportive • Fluid therapy • Laparotomy to relieve obstruction	• Supportive • Fluid therapy • Manual evacuation of the colon • Surgery: colotomy or colectomy

MEDICATION	• Antibiotics (systemic): chloramphenicol, penicillin, or aminoglycosides
	• Antibiotics (topical): panalog
		• Antibiotics: ampicillin, amoxicillin cephalosporins, and metronidazole
		• Corticosteroids: prednisolone
		• Ursodeoxycholic acid: actigal
			• Laxatives
			  —Bulk-forming: canned pumpkin or psyllium
			  —Emollient: colace, docusate sodium (DSS)
			  —Lubricant: mineral oil, laxatone, or sterile lubricant jelly
			  —Osmotic: lactulose, milk, or glycerin
			  Motility modifier: cisapride

PATIENT CARE	• Treated as outpatient • Standard postoperative if surgery	• Nutritional support • Vitamin supplementation	• Encourage to defecate: clean litter pan, multiple walks

FOLLOW-UP — **PATIENT CARE**	• High-fiber diet • ↑ Exercise • Express anal glands every 3–4 days for 2 weeks until material is normal	• Check liver enzymes and bilirubin every 7–14 days initially, then quarterly	• Encourage activity and exercise after postoperative recovery • Diet with ↑ fiber (e.g., metamucil or pumpkin filler)
PREVENTION/ AVOIDANCE	• High-fiber diet • Routine expression	• Control inflammatory bowel disease	• Same as above
COMPLICATIONS	• Rupture • Septicemia • Fecal incontinence after anal sacculectomy	• Recurrence of nonsuppurative forms • Diabetes mellitus • Hepatic lipidosis • Pancreatitis and triad disease • Death	• Obstipation • Perforation of colon wall during manual evacuation • Peritonitis, diarrhea or stricture formation postsurgery • Megacolon
PROGNOSIS	• Excellent • Guarded to poor, with fecal incontinence	• Good with early treatment of suppurative disease • Variable with nonsuppurative	• Fair with lifelong treatment • Poor with megacolon
NOTES	• Color and consistency of anal gland contents: —Clear or pale yellow-brown = normal —Thick, pasty brown = impaction —Creamy yellow or thin green yellow = inflammation —Red-brown exudate = abscessed	• **Caution:** Drugs used must be selected with care to not further damage the liver through metabolism • **Caution:** Corticosteroids should not be used in suppurative forms • Himalayan, Persian, and Siamese cats	• Typically seen in the transverse and descending colon • Avoid bulk-forming fiber diets, because they will contribute to fecal retention

Table 6-9 Gastroenterology (Continued)

DISEASE	Diarrhea		Exocrine Pancreatic Insufficiency (EPI)
	Acute	Chronic	
DEFINITION	Diarrhea can be acute or chronic (lasting longer than 3–4 weeks) and involve either the small bowel or the large bowel. The causes include dietary indiscretion, toxins, drugs, intestinal parasites, infectious diseases, and systemic or metabolic disturbances.		EPI is the insufficient secretion of digestive enzymes and clinical signs of malabsorption. It occurs with severe progressive loss of acinar tissue from atrophy. Most commonly seen in middle-aged to older dogs.
CLINICAL SIGNS	• Inappetence, lethargy, fever, vomiting, abdominal pain, and dehydration • Clinical signs of an underlying condition *Small Bowel Diarrhea* • Watery, voluminous, and fetid *Large Bowel Diarrhea* • Watery, mucoid, bloody feces with tenemus and ↑ sense of urgency		• Weight loss, ↓ muscle mass, ravenous appetite, ↑ water intake, vomiting, coprophagia, and pica • Diarrhea, malodorous, flatulence, borborygmus, and a large amount of stool • Dull haircoat, unthrifty, excessive shedding, and greasy oily hair around perineum
DIAGNOSIS — GENERAL	• History • Clinical signs • Abdominal palpation: mass lesions, pain, mesenteric lymphadenopathy, thickened or fluid-distended bowel loops • Digital rectal palpation: masses, strictures, or anal diseases		• History • Clinical signs
CBC	• Normal or may reflect underlying disease	• Eosinophilia and macrocytosis • Anemia	• Mild lymphophenia and eosinophilia
BIOCHEMISTRY	• Normal or may reflect underlying disease		• ↓ ALT • ↓ Cholesterol, lipids, and polyunsaturated fatty acids
URINALYSIS	• Normal or may reflect underlying disease		• Normal

DIAGNOSIS	**RADIOLOGY**	• Abdominal: foreign bodies, obstruction, intussusception, and ileus	• Abdominal: obstruction, mass, foreign body, and organomegaly • Contrast study: bowel wall thickening or irregularity, tumor, stricture, or foreign body	• N/A
	MISCELLANEOUS	• Fecal flotation: parasites or bacteria • Fecal or rectal smear cytology: infectious agents or inflammatory cells • ELISA: parvo • Folate and cobalamin: variable, depending on conditions and locations of problems • IFA Giardia/Cryptosporidium: positive	• Fecal flotation: parasites or bacteria • Fecal cytology: infectious agents or inflammatory cells • Folate and cobalamin: variable, depending on conditions • Ultrasonography: bowel wall thickening or irregularity, mass, foreign body, intussusception, ileus, or other disease process • Endoscopy: perform biopsies	• TLI assay: <5 μg/dL (dogs) and <31 μg/dL (cats) • Fecal proteolytic activity: ↓ values • Oral bentiromide digestion test: minimal ↑ PABA • Folate: variable, depending on different conditions • Cobalamin: ↓ value
TREATMENT	**GENERAL**	• Supportive • Fluid therapy • Surgery: laparotomy to remove obstruction	• Supportive • Fluid therapy • Surgery: laparotomy to remove obstruction or mass or obtain full-thickness biopsy specimen	• Symptomatic
	MEDICATION	• Antibiotics • Antisecretory drugs: opiates, anticholinergics, chlorpromazine, loperamide, and salicylates • Anthelmintics: fendendazole and metronidazole	• Anthelmintics: fenbendazole and metronidazole	• Antibiotics: tetracyclines, metronidazole, and tylosin • H$_2$-receptor blocker: cimetidine and ranitidine • Pancreatic enzyme replacement added to each meal
	PATIENT CARE	• NPO for at least 24 hours • Provide a clean litter box or frequent walks	• Provide a clean litter box or frequent walks	• Divide daily food intake into 2–3 meals • Diet should be low in fiber and highly digestible • Multivitamin, especially fat-soluble vitamins, cobalamin, and tocopherol

Table 6-9 Gastroenterology (Continued)

	DISEASE	Diarrhea		Exocrine Pancreatic Insufficiency (EPI)
		Acute	Chronic	
FOLLOW-UP	PATIENT CARE	• Recheck fecal analysis after treatment for parasites • Small, frequent meals • Bland or hypoallergenic diet	• Bland or hypoallergenic diet • Monitor fecal output, consistency, and frequency • Monitor body weight	• Monitor weight gain and fecal consistency • Gradually decrease enzyme replacement as animal returns to normal
FOLLOW-UP	PREVENTION/ AVOIDANCE	• Yearly fecal analysis	• Yearly fecal analysis	• N/A
FOLLOW-UP	COMPLICATIONS	• Intussusception	• Dehydration • Abdominal effusion with intestinal adenocarcinoma • Inflammatory bowel disease	• Small bowel bacterial overgrowth • No response to pancreatic enzyme replacement
	PROGNOSIS	• Excellent in mild cases and with proper treatment of severe cases • Poor with chronic diarrhea unresponsive to treatment		• Good with dietary and enzyme management • Poor when associated with diabetes mellitus
	NOTES	• Most acute diarrhea is self-limiting within 3–4 days		• German shepherds

DISEASE	Hepatic Disease or Failure (Liver Disease)	Hepatic Lipidosis (Fatty Liver Disease)	Inflammatory Bowel Disease (IBD)
DEFINITION	Hepatic failure results from the sudden loss of >75% of functioning hepatic mass. Hepatic disease is the accumulation of inflammatory cells in the liver over an extended period with adequate liver function. Causes include infectious agents, drugs, toxins, immune-mediated, traumatic injury, thermal injury, and hypoxia.	Hepatic lipidosis is seen almost exclusively in cats. It is the result of >50% of cells in the liver accumulating excessive trigylcerides. This disease will lead to death if left untreated. This occurs when there is difference in the rates of deposition and metabolism of fat.	IBD is a group of gastrointestinal diseases that infiltrate the mucosa and submucosa with inflammatory cells. It may involve the stomach, small and large intestines, or a combination. Lymphocytic-plasmacytic is the most common type of IBD, found in both dogs and cats.

DIAGNOSIS

CLINICAL SIGNS	• Jaundice, yellow to orange urine, vomiting, diarrhea, anorexia, depression, lethargy, ascites, and pallor • PU/PD • Bleeding: hemorrhages, melena, and hematuria • Abdominal pain • Neurologic signs: seizures, dementia, ataxia, and circling	• Prolonged anorexia • Lethargy, vomiting, and constipation or diarrhea • Hepatomegaly, jaundice, muscle wasting, weakness, and pallor	• Intermittent vomiting • Diarrhea, flatulence, hematochezia, mucus, and tenesmus • Weight loss and listlessness • Poor haircoat • Thickened bowel loops and mesenteric lymphadenopathy
GENERAL	• History • Clinical signs • Abdominal palpation: hepatomegaly and hepatodynia	• History: obesity • Clinical signs	• Clinical signs
CBC	• Nonregenerative anemia • Thrombocytopenia • ± Nucleated RBCs	• Nonregenerative, normocytic, normochromic anemia with poikilocytosis (if prolonged) • Neutrophilia and lymphopenia (variable)	• Mild, nonregenerative anemia or mild leukocytosis without a left shift (cats) • Neutrophilic leukocytosis with a left shift (dogs)
BIOCHEMISTRY	• ↑ ALT, AST, ALP, GGT, total bilirubin, globulin, ammonia, BUN (acute), glucose (chronic), and cholesterol • ↓ Albumin, BUN (chronic), glucose (acute), and cholesterol	• ↑ ALP, ALT, AST, ammonia, and bilirubin • ↓ Potassium, phosphorus, albumin, and BUN • Azotemia (variable)	• ↑ T_4 (cats) • ↓ Protein (dogs) and albumin (cats)
URINALYSIS	• ↑ Bilirubin, urobilinogen, ammonia, bilirubin crystals, and ammonium biurate crystals • ↓ Specific gravity	• ↑ Lipids and bilirubin	• N/A
RADIOLOGY	• Thoracic: metastasis to lung parenchyma • Abdominal: ↑ or ↓ in liver size, changes in tissue characteristics and contours	• Abdominal: hepatomegaly	• Abdominal: survey films to rule out other diseases • Barium contrast study: mucosal abnormalities and thickened bowel loops

Table 6-9 Gastroenterology (Continued)

	DISEASE	Hepatic Disease or Failure (Liver Disease)	Hepatic Lipidosis (Fatty Liver Disease)	Inflammatory Bowel Disease (IBD)
DIAGNOSIS	MISCELLANEOUS	• Ultrasound: masses, abscesses, cysts, obstructions, and lesions • Biopsy: to determine the nature and severity of hepatic disease • Bile acid concentrations: ↑ values • Fasting bile acids concentrations: >30 μmol/L • Postprandial bile acid concentrations: >30 μmol/L • Blood ammonia concentrations: ↑ values • Ammonia tolerance test: ↑ values	• Ultrasound: hepatomegaly and hyperechoic liver • Biopsy: hepatocellular vacuoles • Coagulation tests: ↑coagulation times for PT, APTT, and ACT (variable)	• Fasting serum trypsinlike immunoreactivity (TLI): to rule out EPI • Cobalamin and folate assays: variable depending on different conditions • Ultrasound: measure stomach and intestinal wall thickness and rule out other diseases • Endoscopy: obtain intestinal biopsies *Cats* • FeLV/FIV: + results
TREATMENT	GENERAL	• Symptomatic • Supportive • Fluid therapy • Paracentesis with respiratory distress	• Supportive • Fluid therapy	• Symptomatic • Fluid therapy if vomiting • Surgery: entertomy biopsies
	MEDICATION	• Antibiotics: penicillin, ampicillin, cephalosporins, metronidazole, and aminoglycosides • Cholchicine • Corticosteroids: prednisolone • GI protectants: sulcralfate • H₂ blocker: ranitidine and cimetidine • Lactulose • Phenobarbital • Ursodeoxycholic acid: actigal • Vitamin K therapy	• Antiemetic: metoclopramide • Antibiotics: metronidazole • Lactulose • Vitamin K therapy	• 5-Aminosalicylic drugs: sulfasalazine, olsalazine, and mesalamine • Antibiotics: metronidazole or tylosin • Antidiarrheal drugs: loperamide and diphenoxylate • Azathioprine • Corticosteroids: prednisone • Chemotherapy: chlorambucil
	PATIENT CARE	• Moderate activity restriction • Nutritional support • Monitor body weight, temperature, pulse, respiration, and mental status • Vigilant monitoring for signs of infection • Vitamin and mineral supplements	• Aggressive nutritional support via syringe, nasogastric tube, esophagostomy tube, or gastrotomy tube • Vitamin supplementation: thiamine, taurine, arginine, ʟ-carnitine, and ʟ-citrulline	• Nutritional support if severely malnourished • Vitamin supplementation: folic acid, cobalamin, and fat-soluble vitamins

FOLLOW-UP			
PATIENT CARE	• Monitor CBC and serum biochemistry frequently, depending on severity of presenting condition • Follow-up biopsies at 6 and 12 months • Dietary modifications	• Continuous feeding via tube by owners for 4–6 weeks or for 10 days post vomiting, eating on their own, and normal biochemical values • Monitor potassium and phosphorus • Monitor body weight and hydration	• Hypoallergenic dietary management • Periodic evaluations until patient stabilizes
PREVENTION/ AVOIDANCE	• Vaccinate against infectious agents • Screen susceptible breeds • Avoid hepatotoxic drugs	• Prevent anorexia (especially obese cats) • Monitor food intake in obese cats during times of stress or other disease processes	• N/A
COMPLICATIONS	• Liver failure and liver encephalopathy • Renal disease or failure • Sepsis • GI ulceration • DIC and bleeding diatheses • Death	• Vomiting • Tube dysfunction • Hepatic failure • Death	• Malnutrition and dehydration • Adverse drug reactions • Anemia • Protein-losing enteropathy • Small intestinal bacterial overgrowth
PROGNOSIS	• Dependent on the amount of viable liver mass left after treatment • ↑ Prognosis with determination of underlying cause	• Grave if left untreated • 65% of patients recover with proper treatment*	• Good with continuous maintenance of remission and control of relapses • Course of disease tends to be progressive in prone breeds.
NOTES	• **Caution:** Drugs used must be selected with care to not further damage the liver through metabolism • **Caution:** Avoid alkalinizing agents (e.g., lactate, sodium bicarbonate) with patients with hepatic encephalopathy • Bedlington terriers, Doberman pinschers, Cocker spaniels, Labrador retrievers, Standard poodles, Skye terriers, and West Highland white terriers	• **Caution:** Avoid dextrose supplementation, because it interferes with fat oxidation • Most cats are obese before this disease process starts • Vitamin K should be given IM at least 12 hours before biopsies • Biopsy samples typically float when placed in formalin	• Basenjis, soft-coated Wheaten terriers, and Shar peis

*Saunders Manual of Small Animal Practice, S. Birchard & R. Sherding

Table 6-9   Gastroenterology (Continued)

DISEASE	Megaesophagus (Esophageal Hypomotility)	Pancreatitis	Peritonitis
DEFINITION	Megaesophagus is a segmental or diffuse hypomotility and dilation of the esophagus. There are three main causes: congenital, acquired idiopathic, or secondary to another condition such as myasthenia gravis.	Pancreatitis is inflammation of the pancreas that can be either acute or chronic. Chronic pancreatitis is often seen with morphologic changes in the pancreas. It can be caused by obesity, ingestion of excessive fat, or multiple other disease processes.	A life-threatening condition that requires progressive medical management for resolution. Peritonitis is an inflammatory process involving all or part of the peritoneal cavity.
CLINICAL SIGNS	• Regurgitation, salivation, halitosis, weight loss, and emaciation • Dyspnea, raspy breath sounds, pulmonary crackles, mucopurulent nasal discharge, cough, and fever • Neurologic deficits • Generalized muscle weakness or atrophy	• Vomiting, diarrhea, anorexia, depression, dehydration, fever, and weakness • Cranial abdominal pain: panting, hunched-up, praying position, restlessness, or trembling	• Abdominal pain, reluctance to move, tucked up abdomen, and praying posture • Tachycardia and tachypnea • Fever, vomiting, diarrhea, and dehydration • Shock
GENERAL	• History • Clinical signs • Palpation of dilated esophagus	• History • Clinical signs • Abdominal palpation: enlarged and painful pancreas	• History • Clinical signs • Abdominal palpation: pain or organomegaly
CBC	• Neutrophilia and left shift	• Neutrophilia with or without a left shift • Leukocytosis • ↑ PCV	• Neutrophilia with or without a left shift • Leukocytosis • Anemia
BIOCHEMISTRY	• Normal or may reflect underlying disease	• ↑ Amylase, lipase, ALP, ALT, bilirubin, BUN, creatinine, cholesterol, lipids, and glucose • Calcium (variable) • ↓ Azotemia (acute type)	• ↑ Amylase, lipase, ALT, AST, and bilirubin • ↓ Protein, glucose, and potassium • Electrolyte imbalances • Azotemia
URINALYSIS	• Normal or may reflect underlying disease	• Normal	• N/A

DIAGNOSIS

DIAGNOSIS	**RADIOLOGY**	• Thoracic: distention of esophagus with air, fluid, or food • Contrast study: ↓movement and pooling of fluid	• Thoracic: pulmonary edema or pleural effusion (rare) • Abdominal: displacement of stomach and duodenum, ↑ density, ↓ contrast gastric distention, static gas pattern, thickened and corrugated walls of the duodenum	• Abdominal: free fluid or air, ↓ detail, ileus, distention of loops of bowel with fluid or gas • Iodinated contrast studies: GI to locate perforation
	MISCELLANEOUS	• Acetylcholine receptor antibody titer: screen for myasthenia gravis • Fluoroscopy: ↓ strength and coordination or peristaltic contractions • Endoscopy: dilated esophagus, foreign body, neoplasia, and esophagitis	• Canine pancreatic-like immunoreactivity (cPLI): ↑ value • TLI: ↑ value • Ultrasound: irregular enlargement and abscesses of the pancreas and hypoechoic changes • CT: identification and management of abscesses	• Ultrasound: free fluid, abscesses, masses, and cause of peritonitis • Abdominocentesis cytology: bacterial recognition and identification and ↑ WBCs • ± Culture
TREATMENT	**GENERAL**	• Symptomatic • Supportive	• Symptomatic • Supportive • Fluid therapy • Surgery: laparotomy	• Supportive • Fluid therapy • Peritoneal lavage • Surgery: laparotomy, correct primary cause, lavage and drainage
	MEDICATION	• Antibiotics for aspiration pneumonia: variable • H_2 blockers: sulcralfate • Metoclopramide	• Analgesics: meperidine HCl and butorphanol • Antibiotics: ampicillin, cephalosporins, trimethoprim-sulfa, and enrofloxacin • Antiemetics: chlorpromazine • Corticosteroids (shock): prednisone • Glucagon • Somatostatin • Vasopression	• Analgesics: variable • Antibiotics: penicillin, cephalosporins, or aminoglycosides
	PATIENT CARE	• Nutritional support to ensure passage of food past dilated esophagus • ↑ Caloric density diet	• NPO • Potassium supplementation • Complete rest and confinement	• Standard postoperative care • Limit activity • Nutritional support

Table 6-9 Gastroenterology (Continued)

FOLLOW-UP

DISEASE	Megaesophagus (Esophageal Hypomotility)	Pancreatitis	Peritonitis
PATIENT CARE	• Offer small frequent meals with patient in upright position for 10–15 minutes after meal	• After vomiting has stopped for 1–2 days, slowly reintroduce water followed by a gradual reintroduction of a high-carbohydrate diet	• Check CBC, chemistry profile, and urinalysis every 1–2 days even in patients who are responding
PREVENTION/ AVOIDANCE	• Diligent feeding rituals will increase life span • Early detection of recurrent pneumonias	• Avoid fatty foods and dietary indiscretion • Maintain optimum weight control • Avoid corticosteroid treatment	• N/A
COMPLICATIONS	• Weight loss • Aspiration pneumonia	• Septic shock → Protein and oncotic pressure • Peritonitis • Worsening pancreatitis	• Herniation of abdominal contents • Adhesions
PROGNOSIS	• Fair with diligent supportive care	• Fatal without treatment • Poor with complications	• Poor even with adequate treatment
NOTES	• Feeding small "meat balls" of canned food to a patient in an upright position often gives the least regurgitation	• Patients with recurrent pancreatitis may try a trial period of enzyme therapy	• **Caution:** Do not use povidone-iodine solution for lavage, because it may be absorbed and produce toxic effects • Use a contrast medium with minimal abdominal effects in case of leakage (e.g., iohexol)

DISEASE	Protein-Losing Enteropathy	Vomiting
DEFINITION	Protein-losing enteropathy is a disease of excessive loss of serum protein into the intestinal tract. It can be a primary GI tract disease or the result of a generalized condition such as congestive heart failure, nephrotic syndrome, or metastatic neoplasia.	Vomiting is the forceful, reflex expulsion of gastric or proximal small bowel contents from the oral cavity. Its duration can be acute or chronic (>7 days).
CLINICAL SIGNS	• Diarrhea • Thickened bowel loops • Ascites, edema, pleural effusion, and dyspnea	• Nausea: hypersalivation, repeated swallowing, and licking of lips • Others, depending on underlying disease

DIAGNOSIS

GENERAL
- History
- Clinical signs
- Abdominal palpation: intestines

- History
- Examination of vomitus

CBC
- ± Anemia
- ± Lymphopenia

- Normal or may reflect underlying disease

BIOCHEMISTRY
- ↓ Albumin, globulin, calcium, and cholesterol

- Normal or may reflect underlying disease

URINALYSIS
- Normal

- Normal or may reflect underlying disease

RADIOLOGY
- Thoracic: rule out cardiac disease or fungal disease
- Abdominal: rule out fungal disease, tumors, or intestinal obstruction
- Contrast: tumor or bowel disease

- Thoracic: heartworm disease
- Abdominal: foreign body, pancreatitis, or pyometra

MISCELLANEOUS
- Fecal examinations: rule out parasites and bacterial overgrowth
- TLI and folate: results dependent on disease process
- Cobalamin: ↓ values
- Serum bile acids: assess hepatic function
- Ultrasound: abdominal abnormalities or tumors
- Endoscopy: mucosal visualization and biopsy
- T_4: ↑ values (cats)

- Depending on underlying disease

TREATMENT

GENERAL
- Symptomatic
- Supportive
- Blood transfusions
- Surgery: laparotomy for full-thickness biopsies

- Symptomatic
- Fluid therapy
- Surgery: exploratory laparotomy

MEDICATION
- Antibiotics: metronidazole, tylosin, or sulfasalazine
- Chemotherapy: chlorambucil
- Corticosteroids: prednisone
- Diuretics: furosemide

- Antiemetic: metoclopramide, diphenhydramine, prochlorperazine, and chlorpromazine
- Antisecretory: cimetidine, famotidine, and rantidine
- GI protectants: sucralfate

PATIENT CARE
- Treated as outpatient
- Standard postoperative care

- NPO

Table 6-9 Gastroenterology (Continued)

DISEASE	Protein-Losing Enteropathy	Vomiting
PATIENT CARE	• Dietary modifications, depending on underlying cause • Recheck body weight and protein concentrations every 7–14 days • Monitor for recurrence of clinical signs	• After vomiting has stopped for $1/2$–1 day, slowly reintroduce water followed by a gradual reintroduction of a single-protein and carbohydrate diet • Wean back to regular diet over 4–5 days
PREVENTION/ AVOIDANCE	• Control inflammatory bowel disease	• Avoid dietary indiscretion
COMPLICATIONS	• Respiratory difficulty • Malnutrition, severe • Diarrhea, severe • Slow wound healing	• Dehydration • Electrolyte imbalances • Aspiration pneumonia
PROGNOSIS	• Guarded	• Excellent in mild cases and with proper treatment of severe cases
NOTES	• ↑ Risk of morbidity postoperatively because of slow wound healing because of ↓ albumin	• Types of vomiting: —Undigested or partially digested food >12–16 hours old = delayed gastric emptying —Projectile vomiting = gastric or upper small bowel obstruction —blood flecks, clots = ulcer disease

FOLLOW-UP

Skill Box 6-7 / Anal Sac Expression

1. Supplies: gloves, lubricant (e.g., K-Y Jelly), alcohol, absorbent material (e.g., rolled cotton, paper towels, baby wipes) and deodorizer.
2. Put alcohol-soaked absorbent material into the gloved hand doing the expression to catch the expressed material, insert the forefinger into the rectum, and immobilize the sac between the forefinger and the thumb on the outside of the rectum.
3. Gently apply pressure to the sac with thumb and forefinger, milking from the bottom of the sac upward toward the duct opening,
4. Note the amount and character of the material expressed. Normal secretions are a dark, foul-smelling substance that is a liquid to a paste in consistency. Material that is very thick or purulent should be brought to the attention of the veterinarian.
5. Clean the perianal area of the animal with alcohol-soaked material and then spray with a deodorizer.

If using powdered gloves, put 2 gloves on the hand doing the expression, then remove one glove after each sac is expressed.

If having difficulty expressing a gland, try rolling the skin outward with the finger outside the rectum to better expose the duct.

If having trouble with positioning, switch and use the thumb on the inside and the forefinger on the outside or teach yourself to be ambidextrous and express the right gland with the left hand and vice versa.

HEMATOLOGY

Table 6-10 Hematology

DISEASE	Anemia		Disseminated Intravascular Coagulation (DIC)
	Nonregenerative	Regenerative	
DEFINITION	Anemia is a decreased number of necessary red blood cells (RBC) and is a primary bone marrow dysfunction. It can be caused by RBC loss, destruction, or depression of production. Anemia is typically broken down into two types: regenerative (loss and destruction) and nonregenerative (depression of production). Regenerative anemia can be immune-mediated, causing the destruction of RBCs, ending in immune-mediated hemolytic anemia (IMHA).		Disseminated intravascular coagulation is a complex condition that is always secondary to another disease process. It is defined as an excessive activation of the clotting mechanism with complete consumption of clotting factors.
CLINICAL SIGNS	• Weakness, exercise intolerance, collapse, fever, lymphadenopathy, depression, and anorexia • Tachypnea or dyspnea, tachycardia, and soft systolic heart murmur • Mucous membranes: pallor, petechial hemorrhages, or icteric • Retinal hemorrhages • Melena • Splenomegaly • Flea infestation		• Clinical signs of underlying disease • Petechiae and spontaneous hemorrhage from orifices
GENERAL	• History • Clinical signs		• History • Clinical signs
CBC	• ↑ MCV • PCV, mean cell hemoglobin concentration (MCHC), and TP • Leukopenia and thrombocytopenia	• ↑ MCHC • ↓ PCV, MCV, and TP • Reticulocytosis, neutrophilia and thrombocytosis • Nucleated RBCs • Basophilic stippling (cats)	• Thrombocytopenia • Schistocytes • ↓ Platelet count and fibrinogen levels • Presence of fibrin degradation products
BIOCHEMISTRY	• Normal or may reflect underlying disease	• ↑ Bilirubin	• Normal or may reflect underlying disease
URINALYSIS	• Hematuria • ± Bilirubinuria		• Hematuria
RADIOLOGY	• Abdominal: splenomegaly	• Thoracic: fluid • Abdominal: fluid	• Normal or may reflect underlying disease

DIAGNOSIS

DIAGNOSIS

MISCELLANEOUS

- Fecal analysis: hookworms and coccidia
- Bone marrow biopsy: ↓ erythroid precursors
- ELISA: FeLV in-house screening

- Fecal analysis: hookworms and coccidia
- Bone marrow biopsy: ↑ erythroid precursors
- COOMBS test and anti-nuclear antibody (ANA) serology: + results
- Slide agglutination test: + results indicates anemia is immune-mediated

- FDP assay: ↑ times
- Coagulation tests: prothrombin time, activated clotting time, activated partial thromboplastin time: ↑ times
- Latex agglutination test: ↑ value

TREATMENT

GENERAL

- Supportive
- Blood transfusions
- Fluid therapy

- Symptomatic
- Aggressive fluid therapy
- Blood transfusions

MEDICATION

- Cyclosporine
- Erythropoietin
- Ferrous sulfate

- Antibiotics: tetracyclines
- Corticosteroids: prednisone
- Chemotherapy: azathioprine and cyclophosphamide
- Ferrous sulfate

- Antibiotics
- Corticosteroids (endotoxic shock)
- Heparin
- Mannitol
- Aspirin

PATIENT CARE

- Monitor for adverse reactions to drugs and transfusions
- Monitor heart rate, respiratory rate, and temperature
- Heat support
- Restrict activity
- Nutritional support

- Avoid IM injections and neck leads
- Strict confinement
- Feed soft foods
- Use peripheral blood vessels from blood draws and catheter placement

FOLLOW-UP

PATIENT CARE

- Check CBC every 3–5 days until normal
- Monitor blood pressure

- Check PCV weekly until normal, then every 2 weeks for 2 months, then monthly
- Check CBC monthly during treatment

- Related to underlying disease

PREVENTION/ AVOIDANCE

- Neuter cryptorchid males
- Monitor CBCs of patients receiving cancer drugs

- N/A

- Related to underlying disease

Table 6-10   Hematology (Continued)

DISEASE	Anemia		Disseminated Intravascular Coagulation (DIC)
	Nonregenerative	Regenerative	
COMPLICATIONS	• Sepsis • Hemorrhage • Erythropoietin related • Blood transfusion related	• DIC • Embolisms • Infections • Cardiac arrhythmias • Hypoxia	• Related to underlying disease
PROGNOSIS	• Guarded to poor unless underlying disease can be diagnosed and treated • Recovery may take weeks to months	• Poor to good prognosis with appropriate treatment • Guarded to poor prognosis with IMHA	• Grave
NOTES		• IMHA: Old English sheepdog, Cocker spaniel, Poodles, Irish setters, English Springer spaniels, and Collies	• **Caution:** Venipuncture sites can lead to excessive hematomas, place pressure wraps after procedure

FOLLOW-UP

DISEASE	Thrombocytopenia, Immune-Mediated (IMT, Idiopathic Thrombocytopenic Purpura, ITP, Autoimmune Thrombocytopenia)	Von Willebrand's Disease
DEFINITION	Thrombocytopenia is a deficiency of platelets. Primary immune-mediated is the destruction of platelets with no identifiable cause. It may occur as a single entity or as a combination of other immune-mediated diseases.	Von Willebrand's disease is a bleeding disorder caused by a deficiency or dysfunction of the plasma protein (von Willebrand's factor, vWf) used for normal platelet functions. This is the most common inherited bleeding disorder in dogs.
CLINICAL SIGNS	• Fever, anorexia, lethargy, pallor, and weakness • Epistaxis, hematochezia, and cutaneous, retinal, and mucosal hemorrhages • Melena	• Spontaneous hemorrhage from mucosal surfaces of oral and nasal cavities, GIT, and genitourinary tract • ↑ Hemorrhage from wounds and surgery sites

		(Column 1)	(Column 2)
DIAGNOSIS	GENERAL	• History • Clinical signs • Patient response to treatment	• History • Clinical signs
	CBC	• Thrombocytopenia <50,000/µL • Microthrombocytosis • Neutrophilia or neutropenia • Schistocytes • Autoagglutination • Anemia: type dependent on when bleeding occurred	• Anemia • Neutrophilia and a mild left shift • Reticulocytosis after acute bleeding
	BIOCHEMISTRY	• Mild ↑ ALT and ALP (variable) • ↓ Protein	• Normal
	URINALYSIS	• ↑ Protein and blood (rare)	• Normal
	RADIOLOGY	• Thoracic: tumors • Abdominal: tumors	• N/A
	MISCELLANEOUS	• Serology: ehrlichiosis, Rocky Mountain spotted fever, dirofilariasis, and leptospirosis • ANA titer: + results • Coagulation profiles: ↓ clotting times • Bone marrow cytology: ↑ megakaryocytes	• Buccal mucosa bleeding time: ↑ time • Toenail bleeding time: ↑ time • Von Willebrand's factor assay: ↓ values
TREATMENT	GENERAL	• Supportive • Fluid therapy • Blood transfusion • Surgery: splenectomy	• Supportive • Fluid therapy • Hormonal therapy
	MEDICATION	• Corticosteroids: prednisone, prednisolone or dexamethasone • Chemotherapy: vincristine, cyclophosphamide, azathioprine, danazol, or cyclosporine	• Cryoprecipitate: a concentrated form of vWF and factor VIII • Desmopressin acetate: ↑ vWF and ↓ bleeding time
	PATIENT CARE	• Treated as outpatient • Standard postoperative care • Strict confinement	• Avoid IM injections, neck leads, trauma, etc. • Strict confinement • Feed soft foods • Use peripheral blood vessels from blood draws and catheter placement

Table 6-10 Hematology (Continued)

DISEASE	Thrombocytopenia, Immune-Mediated (IMT, Idiopathic Thrombocytopenic Purpura, ITP, Autoimmune Thrombocytopenia)	Von Willebrand's Disease
PATIENT CARE	• Strict confinement until normal platelet counts return • Monitor platelet counts periodically after recovery	• Monitor for hemorrhages for 48 hours after surgery
PREVENTION/ AVOIDANCE	• Avoid unnecessary vaccinations • Minimize stress • Avoid medications that are suspected of having caused initial ITP • OVH for intact females to prevent hormonal imbalances	• Neuter affected dogs
COMPLICATIONS	• GI ulceration • CNS hemorrhage • Hemorrhagic shock	• Hemorrhage
PROGNOSIS	• Good with corticosteroid treatment	• Depends on the concentration of the von Willebrand factor
NOTES		• Thyroid supplementation: evidence exists that it may ↑ vWF concentration and ↓ bleeding tendency • Doberman pinscher, Scottish terrier, Shetland sheepdog, Golden retriever, Pembroke Welsh corgi, and Standard poodle

FOLLOW-UP

INFECTIOUS DISEASE

Table 6-11   Infectious Disease

DISEASE	Brucellosis ZOONOTIC	Ehrlichiosis	Feline Immunodeficiency Virus (FIV, Feline AIDS)
DEFINITION	A disease caused by *Brucella canis*. This bacteria can be found in the lymphatic system, genital tract, eye, kidney, and intervertebral discs.	The most common rickettsial disease of dogs caused by *Ehrlichia spp.* Mostly found on the Gulf coast, Eastern seaboard, Midwest, and California.	An immunodeficiency syndrome characterized by chronic and recurrent infection. Gradually selecting and destroying T-lymphocytes.
CLINCAL SIGNS	• Generalized lymphadenopathy, splenomegaly, paresis/paralysis, and spinal hyperesthesia *Male* • Scrotal swelling or dermatitis, enlarged epididymis, or testicular atrophy *Female* • Abortion, infertility, and vaginal discharge for 1–6 weeks post-abortion	*Acute* • Fever, organomegaly, lymphadenopathy, dyspnea, exercise intolerance, oculonasal discharge, and neurologic signs (e.g., ataxia, vestibular dysfunction) *Chronic* • Weight loss, fever, epistaxis, spontaneous bleeding, pallor, organomegaly, uveitis, arthritis, neurologic signs, and intermittent limb edema	*Stage 1* • Usually subclinical: fever, neutropenia, and lymphadenopathy *Stage 2* • Latent phase: could last for years *Stage 3* • Terminal phase: stomatitis, gingivitis, periodontitis, pneumonia, rhinitis, conjunctivitis, abscesses, skin infections, otitis, and urinary tract infections
GENERAL	• Clinical signs	• History • Clinical signs	• History of exposure • Clinical signs
CBC	• Normal	*Acute* • Thrombocytopenia • Anemia (variable) • Leukopenia *Chronic* • Nonregenerative anemia • Lymphocytosis • Pancytopenia • Leukopenia or leukocytosis	*Stage 3* • Anemia • Lymphopenia • Neutropenia

DIAGNOSIS

Table 6-11 Infectious Disease (Continued)

DISEASE	Brucellosis ZOONOTIC	Ehrlichiosis	Feline Immunodeficiency Virus (FIV, Feline AIDS)
BIOCHEMISTRY	• ↕ Globulin • ↓ Albumin	*Acute* • ↑ Globulin • Mild ↑ ALT, ALP, BUN, and creatinine • ↓ Albumin *Chronic* • ↕ Globulin, BUN, and creatinine • ↓ Albumin	• ↑ Protein and globulins
URINALYSIS	• Normal	*Acute* • ↑ Protein	• ↑ Protein
RADIOLOGY	• Diskospondylitis: if found, check for Brucellosis	• N/A	• N/A
MISCELLANEOUS	• Lymph node cytology: nonspecific reactive hyperplasia • Semen cytology: >80% of sperm are morphologically abnormal, inflammatory cells • RSAT: accurate for negative dogs, detects infected dogs 3–4 weeks after infection • AGID: highly sensitive, detects infected dogs 4–12 weeks after infections • Cultures: blood, urine, semen, vaginal discharge, and aborted fetuses	• IFA: titers > 1:10 (2–3 weeks after exposure) *Acute* • Bone marrow cytology: hypercellular or megakaryocytic *Chronic* • Bone marrow cytology: erythroid hyperplasia and ↑ mast cells	• ELISA: in-house screening kits • Western Blot: confirms + results of ELISA

DIAGNOSIS

			TREATMENT / FOLLOW-UP	
TREATMENT	**GENERAL**	• Symptomatic • Fluid therapy • Dental care	• Supportive • Blood transfusion • Fluid therapy	• Supportive
	MEDICATION	• Antibiotics for secondary infection: metronidazole • Appetite stimulants: cyproheptadine and diazepam • Corticosteroids: prednisone • Immune stimulants: interferon	• Antibiotics: tetracycline or doxycycline • Corticosteroids: prednisone or prednisolone	• Antibiotics: minocycline and dihydrostreptomycin
	PATIENT CARE	• Nutritional support	• Restrict activity	• Treated as outpatient
FOLLOW-UP	**PATIENT CARE**	• Maintain current vaccines to prevent infection of respiratory disease	• Restrict activity • Platelet count every 3 days until normal • Repeat serologic testing in 9 months: should be undetectable in 12 months	• Multiple antibiotic courses of treatment • Serologic titers monthly for 3 months, then at 6 months • Restrict activity in working dogs
	PREVENTION/ AVOIDANCE	• Isolate affected cats • Neuter males • Quarantine and test incoming cats • Retest high-risk cats regularly	• Tick control and avoidance through sprays, collars, and spot-ons • Avoid tick-infested areas	• Neuter infected intact animals • Quarantine and test all new dogs and breeding individuals
	COMPLICATIONS	• N/A	• N/A	• Infertility • Sexual transmission
	PROGNOSIS	• Poor prognosis in terminal phase: ≤ 1-year survival	• Excellent • Poor if bone marrow is severely hypoplastic	• Early detection ↑ response to therapy • Guarded if late detection
	NOTES	• Transmitted through bite wounds, in utero, and transfusions • Theroretically transmitted through intimate contact or fomites • Shed in the saliva • Most commonly seen in unneutered roaming males • A kitten may test + when <6 months old because of maternal antibodies: retest at 8–12 months after all maternal antibodies are gone	• Transmitted by the brown dog tick and transfusions • Incubation period is 7–21 days • German Shepherds and Doberman pinschers	• Transmission is after breeding or abortion, or after contact with semen, vaginal discharge, and urine by penetration of oronasal, conjunctival, or genital mucous membranes • Lasts for 6–64 months • Low risk of human infection: mild and easily treated

Table 6-11 Infectious Disease (Continued)

DISEASE	Rocky Mountain Spotted Fever ZOONOTIC	Salmon Poisoning
DEFINITION	This is a tick-borne disease caused by *Rickettsia rickettsii*. It is the most important rickettsial disease in humans. Found on the east coast, midwest, and plains region.	A rickettsial disease caused by *Neorikettsia helminthoeca*, found in the Pacific Northwest. Attacks the tissue of the small intestinal epithelium and associated lymph system.
CLINICAL SIGNS	• Anorexia, fever, lethargy, vomiting, diarrhea, depression, myalgia, lymphadenopathy, dyspnea, and cough • DIC • Edema of face and limbs • Ocular pain, anterior uveitis, scleral injection, and conjunctivitis • Vasculitis, petechial hemorrhages, epistaxis, and spontaneous bleeding into urine, feces, etc. • Neurologic signs: altered mental states and vestibular signs	• Pyrexia, diarrhea, vomiting, hypothermia, profound weight loss, naso-ocular discharge, and lymphadenopathy
GENERAL	• History • Clinical signs • Ticks recently removed from the dog	• History of ingesting raw salmonoid fish meat • Clinical signs
CBC	• Leukocytosis with a left shift ± Toxic neutrophils • Monocytosis • Mild anemia • Thrombocytopenia	• N/A
BIOCHEMISTRY	↑ ALT, ALP, BUN, creatinine, cholesterol, and albumin ↓ Sodium and chloride • Metabolic acidosis	• N/A
URINALYSIS	• ↑ Protein and blood	• N/A
RADIOLOGY	• N/A	• N/A
MISCELLANEOUS	• Micro-IFA: titers >1:128 • Direct immunofluoresence with skin biopsies: rickettsial antigens as early as 3–4 days postinfection	• Direct fecal smear: operculated fluke eggs (*Nanophyetus salmincola*) • Giemsa-stained fine-needle aspiration (FNA) of lymph nodes: hyperplasia with intracytoplasmic rickettsial bodies in macrophages

DIAGNOSIS

TREATMENT GENERAL	• Supportive • Blood transfusions • Fluid therapy	• Supportive
MEDICATION	• Antibiotics: tetracyclines or doxycycline	• Antibiotics: tetracyclines or doxycycline • Anticestodal: praziquantel
PATIENT CARE	• Restrict activity	• Restrict activity
FOLLOW-UP PATIENT CARE	• Monitor platelet count every 3 days until normal • Micro-IFA titers 2–4 weeks after initial titer: 2–4-fold rise in titer • Restrict activity	• Monitor temperature, hydration, electrolytes, and acid–base balances
PREVENTION/ AVOIDANCE	• Tick and rodent control • Using gloves or instruments to check daily for ticks, and remove entire tick if found	• Prevent eating of raw fish (salmonoid type) • Thoroughly cook or freeze fish
COMPLICATIONS	• N/A	• N/A
PROGNOSIS	• Good if early diagnosis and treatment • Poor if in later stages with CNS disease	• Good with treatment
NOTES	• **Caution:** handling of an infected tick may result in transmission of the disease even without attachment • Transmitted by the American deer tick, wood tick, lone star tick, and transfusions • The tick must be attached for 5–20 hours to infect dogs • Primary host is rodents and rabbits • Incubation time is 2 days to 2 weeks • High titers can be seen for 1 year after successful treatment	• Transmitted through eating raw salmon or related fish carrying encysted forms of the fluke *Nanophyetus salminicola* • Incubation of 5–21 days

Table 6-11 Infectious Disease (Continued)

DISEASE	Tetanus	Toxoplasmosis ZOONOTIC
DEFINITION	Disease caused by *Clostridium tetani*, which is found in the soil and as part of the normal bacterial flora of the intestinal tract of mammals.	This disease, caused by the protozoan parasite, *Toxoplasma gondii*, can invade and multiply in any cell in the body.
CLINICAL SIGNS	• Stiffness, tetanic spasms, localized muscle rigidity then involving entire nervous system, trismus, ears erect, and ↑ salivation • Altered heart and respiratory rates, laryngeal spasms, and dyspnea	• Subclinical most of the time • Anorexia, depression, fever, lethargy, weight loss, diarrhea, and vomiting • Anterior and posterior uveitis • Pneumonia and dyspnea • Myocarditis, pancreatitis, icterus, and abdominal effusion • Neurologic signs: seizures, ataxia, tremors, paresis, paralysis, stiff gait, and CNS disease
GENERAL	• Clinical signs • Recent wound (especially with high levels of necrosis and anaerobic conditions)	• Clinical signs
CBC	• N/A	• Leukopenia with degenerative left shift or neutrophilic leukocytosis • Nonregenerative anemia
BIOCHEMISTRY	• N/A	• ↑ Bilirubin, bile acids, AST, ALT, ALP, creatinine, amylase and lipase • ↓ Albumin
URINALYSIS	• N/A	• ↑ Protein and bilirubin
RADIOLOGY	• N/A	• Abdominal: hepatomegaly and effusion • Thoracic: effusion, patchy alveolar and interstitial pulmonary infiltrates
MISCELLANEOUS	• N/A	• IgM: elevated 2 weeks postinfection, <1:16 = negative • IgG: elevated 2–4 weeks postinfection, >1:512 = active infection or 2–4-fold rising titer 2 weeks apart • Antigen serum titers: + 1–4 weeks postinfection

DIAGNOSIS

TREATMENT

GENERAL
- Supportive
- Fluid therapy
- Wound debridement and cleansing
- Monitor blood pressure and ECG

- Supportive
- Fluid therapy

MEDICATION
- Antibiotics: penicillin G or metronidazole
- Anticonvulsants/Muscle relaxants: diazepam or chlorpromazine
- Tetanus antitoxin

- Antibiotics: clindamycin
- Ophthalmic drops: 1% prednisone

PATIENT CARE
- Keep patient in a dark quiet area and do not disturb
- Provide soft bedding to prevent decubital sores
- Prevent urinary and fecal retention with urinary catheterization and enemas
- Nutritional support: force feeding and stomach tube not advised because it may cause tetanic state

- Typically treat as outpatient
- Confine patients that have neurologic signs

FOLLOW-UP

PATIENT CARE
- Monitor blood pressure and ECG

- Examine 2 days and 14 days after initiation of treatment for improvement

PREVENTION/ AVOIDANCE
- Prevent skin wounds: maintain clean and safe runs and yards
- Give proper wound care management
- Aseptic surgical technique

- Prevent ingestion of raw meat, bones, viscera, or unpasteurized milk
- Prevent free roaming to hunt prey or access to the housing of food-producing animals

COMPLICATIONS
- N/A

- N/A

PROGNOSIS
- Extremely guarded when severely affected

- Guarded: can be become carriers and relapse clinically if immunocompromised

NOTES
- Clinical signs show up 5 days to 3 weeks later
- Death is of respiratory dysfunction
- Animals can be pretested for anaphalytic reaction to the antitoxin by giving an intradermal injection first and monitoring for 30 minutes

- **Caution:** disease can be transmitted to an unborn fetus by an infected human mother
- Transmitted by ingesting infected animal tissues, cat feces, and transplacental infection
- Excrete eggs 3–10 days after infection for 1–2 weeks: can shed again if stressed
- Oocysts must first sporulate to become infectious
- Oocysts can last in the soil for >1 year

MUSCULOSKELETAL

Table 6-12   Musculoskeletal

DISEASE	Arthritis		Cruciate Disease
	Acute	Degenerative Joint Disease (DJD, Osteoarthritis)	
DEFINITION	There are two types of clinically diagnosed arthritis, degenerative and acute inflammatory. Acute arthritis is a pathogenic organism within the closed space of a joint and is broken down into 3 types: septic, traumatic, and immune-mediated. DJD is a progressive deterioration, characterized by a loss of hyaline cartilage matrix and death of chondrocytes. There is no cure for DJD: treatment is based on alleviating clinical signs and slowing progression.		Cruciate disease results in a partial or complete instability of the stifle joint. The tearing of the anterior cruciate ligament can be done acutely or as a degenerative process.
CLINICAL SIGNS	• Stiff gait, lameness, ↓ range of motion (ROM), crepitus, and joint swelling • Reluctance to jump or climb stairs, pain or instability	• Episodic lameness, pain, swelling, crepitus, and laxity • ↑ Lameness following moderate to heavy exercise • Stiff on rising after recumbency	• Acute or intermittent lameness and muscle atrophy of hind limb musculature
GENERAL	• History • Clinical signs • Joint palpation and manipulation	• History • Clinical signs • Joint palpation	• History • Clinical signs • Joint palpation: + anterior drawer sign
CBC	• Leukocytosis	• N/A	• N/A
BIOCHEMISTRY	• N/A	• N/A	• N/A
URINALYSIS	• ↑ Protein	• N/A	• N/A
RADIOLOGY	• Affected joint: joint capsular distension, soft tissue thickening, joint effusion, and bone lysis	• Affected joint: osteophytes, subchondral sclerosis, narrowed joint space and remodeling of subchondral bone/epiphyses	• Affected joint: joint effusion with capsular distention, periarticular osteophytes, compression of infrapatellar fat pad, and calcification of cruciate ligament

DIAGNOSIS

		Condition 1	Condition 2	Condition 3
DIAGNOSIS	MISCELLANEOUS	• Synovial fluid analysis: ↑WBCs and bacteria • Synovial tissue biopsy: neoplasia • Joint fluid culture: ↑WBCs, bacteria, and turbidity • ANA test: + results • Tick-borne agent serology: + results	• N/A	• Arthrocentesis: rule out sepsis and immune-mediated disease • Arthroscopy: confirmation and severity of disease • Magnetic resonance imaging (MRI): confirmation and severity of disease
TREATMENT	GENERAL	• Supportive • Arthrocentesis • Surgery: arthrotomy and reconstructive procedures	• Supportive • Surgery: resection arthroplasty, joint replacement, and arthrodesis	• Symptomatic • Cage rest • Surgery: tibial plateau leveling osteotomy (TPLO), patellar tendon procedure, fascial strip "over-the-top" procedure, imbrication procedure, or extracapsular suture stabilizing technique
	MEDICATION	• Chondroprotective agents: adequan or glucosamine with chondroitin sulfate • Corticosteroids: prednisone or triamcinolone hexacetonide • Methylsulfonyl methane • NSAIDS: carprofen or etodolac	• NSAIDs: buffered aspirin, carprofen, or etodolac • Corticosteroids: prednisone • Chondroprotective agents: glucosamine with chondroitin sulfate	• Chondroprotective drugs: glucosamine with chondroitan sulfate or polysulfated glycosaminoglycans • NSAIDs
FOLLOW-UP	PATIENT CARE	• Physical therapy: hot/cold treatment, swimming, range of motion (ROM) exercises and massage	• Treated as outpatient	• Placement of Robert Jones bandage
	PATIENT CARE	• Moderate activity, but restricted to a level that minimizes discomfort • Strict confinement with acutely painful episodes • Obesity control • Physical therapy: swimming	• Weight control • Encourage moderate and consistent exercise (e.g., swimming—low impact)	• Cryotherapy • Physical therapy: ROM exercises and massage • Restricted activity: leash-only exercise and no use of stairs for 3 months postoperatively • Full exercise by 6–9 months postoperatively • Control obesity

Table 6-12 Musculoskeletal (Continued)

FOLLOW-UP

DISEASE	Arthritis		
	Acute	Degenerative Joint Disease (DJD, Osteoarthritis)	Cruciate Disease
PREVENTION/ AVOIDANCE	• Maintain appropriate weight control • Early recognition to prevent proceeding to secondary condition	• Maintain proper weight control • Early use of glucosamine with chondroitin sulfate to slow progression	• Selective breeding • Maintain proper weight control
COMPLICATIONS	• Nonambulatory • DJD	• Nonambulatory	• Osteoarthritis
PROGNOSIS	• Good with septic form • Fair to guarded with immune-mediated form	• Progressive	• Excellent with surgery
NOTES			• Joint is palpated for drawer motion, movement of tibia relative to femur during the tibial compression test, and thickening of joint capsule • 20%–40% of dogs rupture the opposite cranial cruciate ligament within 17 months • Rottweilers and Labrador retrievers

DISEASE	Hip Dysplasia	Osteochondrosis or Ostchondritis Dessicans (OCD)	Osteomyelitis
DEFINITION	Hip dysplasia is the most common condition of the hip joint and cause of osteoarthritis in that joint. Hip dysplasia is a faulty development of the hip joint contributing to joint laxity and subluxation early in life. Joint instability occurs as muscle development and maturation lag behind the rate of skeletal growth.	Osteochondrosis is a defect in endochondral ossification leading to an excessive retention of cartilage. This defect may occur in any limb joint. Un-united anconeal process and fragmented coronoid process also may be seen along with osteochondrosis or separately. It is often seen in animals between 5 and 10 months of age.	Osteomyelitis is an infection of the bone and its soft tissue elements and membranes. Infectious organisms often complicate an existing condition, leading to a very difficult, sometimes impossible, infection to treat.

DIAGNOSIS

CLINICAL SIGNS	• Lameness of hindleg(s), pain, crepitus, joint laxity, and ↓ range of motion (ROM) • Gait abnormalities: hopping or swaying • Muscle atrophy from disuse	• Varying degrees of lameness, crepitus, pain, muscle atrophy, and hyperextension pain	• Anorexia, lethargy, fever, and depression • Lameness, pain, inflammation, and intermittent draining tracts
GENERAL	• History • Clinical signs • Joint palpation	• History • Clinical signs • Joint palpation	• History • Clinical signs • Skeletal palpation • Neurologic examination
CBC	• N/A	• N/A	• Neutrophilic leukocytosis
BIOCHEMISTRY	• N/A	• N/A	• Normal or may reflect underlying disease
URINALYSIS	• N/A	• N/A	• Normal or may reflect underlying disease
RADIOLOGY	• Joint: subluxation of femoral head, flattening of femoral head, shallow acetabulum, periarticular osteophytes, or widening of joint space between femoral head and cranial acetabulum	• Skeletal: joint abnormalities, bone lengths, arthritis, sclerosis of underlying bone or bone flap/fragments ("joint mice")	• Skeletal: soft tissue swelling, bone resorption, sclerosis, bone sequestra, fracture nonunion, cortical thinning, widening of fracture gap, reactive periosteal new bone, foreign bodies, or fungal lesions • Contrast: sinus location and severity and foreign bodies
MISCELLANEOUS	• N/A	• CT/MRI: location and severity of lesion • Joint tap and fluid analysis: confirms involvement and mononucleated cells • Arthroscopy: confirming OCD lesion	• Radionuclide imaging: detecting osteomyelitis • Cytology: toxic neutrophils, phagocytized bacteria or fungal organisms • Culture and sensitivity

Table 6-12   Musculoskeletal (Continued)

	DISEASE	Hip Dysplasia	Osteochondrosis or Ostchondritis Dessicans (OCD)	Osteomyelitis
TREATMENT	**GENERAL**	• Surgery: triple pelvic osteotomy (TPO), femoral head and neck excision arthroplasty, pectineal myectomy, intertrochanteric osteotomy or total hip replacement	• Symptomatic • Surgery: arthrotomy or arthroscopy	• Symptomatic • Wound management: debridement, drainage and irrigation • Surgery: sequestrectomy, amputation, bone grafts, or biopsy
	MEDICATION	• Analgesics: variable • Chondroprotective agents: adequan or glucosamine with chondroitin sulfate • NSAIDS	• NSAIDs	• Antibiotics: variable
	PATIENT CARE	• Postoperative radiographs to evaluate surgery • Physical therapy • Restrict activity	• Cryotherapy postoperatively • Place modified Robert Jones bandage	• Sterile dressing applied to surgical wounds left to close by secondary intention • Irrigate daily with sterile saline
FOLLOW-UP	**PATIENT CARE**	• Restrict activity postoperatively • Monitor radiographs to assess degeneration	• Cryotherapy for 15–20 minutes three times daily for 3–5 days if no bandage placed • Physical therapy: ROM exercises • Restrict activity for 4 weeks then gradually increase to normal activity over the next 4 weeks • Reradiograph 4–6 weeks postoperatively • Obesity control	• Monitor radiographs for fracture healing
	PREVENTION/ AVOIDANCE	• Selective breeding • Nutritional manipulation for large-breed dogs during growth and development • Avoid excessive exercise	• Selective breeding • Maintain proper weight control	• Proper wound and fracture management

	(continued from previous page)	Panosteitis (Enostosis)	Patellar Luxation, Medial
FOLLOW-UP			
COMPLICATIONS	• Osteoarthritis • Disuse atrophy	• Recurrence and relapse • Limb deformity or impaired function • Neurologic disease	• Osteoarthritis • Nonambulatory
PROGNOSIS		• Good with acute disease • Poor with chronic disease	• Good, depending on severity of disease and joint affected
NOTES		• Great Danes, Labrador retrievers, Newfoundlands, Rottweilers, Bernese mountain dogs, English setters, and Old English sheepdogs	• St. Bernards, German shepherds, Labrador retrievers, Golden retrievers, and Rottweilers
DIAGNOSIS			
DISEASE		Panosteitis (Enostosis)	Patellar Luxation, Medial
DEFINITION		Panosteitis is a disease of young large-breed dogs that begins in the medullary bone marrow in the region of the nutrient foramen. Its cause is unknown. It gives intermittent lameness of one or multiple limbs. The disease is self-limiting, but its clinical signs will remain for months.	Medial patellar luxation is generally a condition of small-breed dogs. It is typically a congenital or developmental malformation of the stifle joint, causing the patella to displace from the femoral trochlea.
CLINICAL SIGNS		• Anorexia, lethargy, and fever • Lameness to nonweightbearing, shifting from one limb to the other, and pain	• Intermittent lameness of hindlimb, "skipping" and pain
GENERAL		• History • Clinical signs • Bone palpation	• History • Clinical signs • Patella palpation: laxity
CBC		• Eosinophilia (variable)	• N/A
BIOCHEMISTRY		• Normal	• N/A
URINALYSIS		• Normal	• N/A
RADIOLOGY		• Skeletal: ↑ density, progressive mottling and radiopacity within the medullary cavity, new bone formation, and thickened bone cortices	• Hindlimb: bowing or torsion of tibia or femur and shape of femoral trochlea
MISCELLANEOUS		• N/A	• N/A

Table 6-12 Musculoskeletal (Continued)

	DISEASE	Patellar Luxation, Medial	Panosteitis (Enostosis)
TREATMENT	GENERAL	• Supportive • Symptomatic • Surgical: trochleoplasty, trochlear sulcoplasty, recession sulcoplasty, trochlear chondroplasty, chondroplasty, wedge recession, patelloplasty, or tibial tuberosity translocation	• Supportive
	MEDICATION	• NSAIDs: carprofen, etodolac, or aspirin	• Corticosteroids: prednisone • NSAIDS
	PATIENT CARE	• Cryotherapy immediately postoperatively then 15–20 minutes daily for 3–5 days if no bandage • Placement of Robert Jones bandage • Physical therapy: ROM exercises if no bandage	• Treated as outpatient
FOLLOW-UP	PATIENT CARE	• Restricted activity: leash only exercise and no use of stairs for 3 months postoperatively • Full exercise by 6–9 months postoperatively • Correct obesity	• Restrict activity • Recheck lameness every 2–4 weeks for more serious orthopedic problems
	PREVENTION/ AVOIDANCE	• Selective breeding • Maintain proper weight control	• N/A
	COMPLICATIONS	• Recurrence after surgery • DJD	• N/A
	PROGNOSIS	• Excellent with surgery	• Excellent
	NOTES	• Miniature and Toy poodles, Yorkshire terriers, Pomeranians, Pekingese, Chihuahuas, and Boston terriers	• German shepherd, Irish setter, Saint Bernard, Doberman pinscher, Airedale, Basset hound, and Miniature Schnauzer

Skill Box 6-8 / Physical Therapy

Skill	Effect	Cause	Technique
1. Superficial heat	Relieving pain and improving blood supply	Smooth muscle tone decreases and blood vessel diameter increases	1. Whirlpool baths/ hydrotherapy 2. Hot packs for 20 minutes using towels soaked in water as hot as the owner can tolerate laid over the affected area 3. Infrared lamps 4. Circulating hot water blankets
2. Cold	Reduce swelling and muscle spasm	Local vessel constriction and reduction in local tissue metabolism	1. Ice packs with early application for 15–20 minutes using an ice-soaked towel laid over the affected area with evenly applied compression **Fill a Styrofoam cup with water and freeze to use as a cold treatment** ****Caution:** Ice packs containing crushed ice are less effective because of the uneven application • Ice should be applied immediately after an injury. Heat is used once the bleeding and swelling have stopped, usually after 72 hours. Using heat too soon greatly increases swelling and bleeding into tissues, exacerbating the injury.
3. Massage	Reducing muscle spasms and relieving excess fluid in interstitial or joint spaces, increase circulation to paralyzed musculature and mobilize tissue that is abnormally adhered to adjacent structures	Increase circulation, release scar tissue, balance muscle function, and relax the animal	1. Gently stroke or lightly knead the area, moving toward the heart with even pressure and longitudinally along the muscle

Skill Box 6-8 / Physical Therapy (Continued)

Skill	Effect	Cause	Technique
4. Passive exercise	Improve synovial fluid production in the joints, reduce tissue adhesion, and increase joint mobility	Reducing dense connective tissues and enhancing venous and lymphatic drainage	1. Manual ROM exercises: at least 3 times a day, perform 10 flexions and extensions on each joint and then cycle the entire limb through its full range of motion 10 times **Caution:** ROM exercises should never exceed the pain-free range: they should be stopped at normal range or until physical limitations are established to prevent further damage and inflammation **Caution:** Avoid passive exercises when acute inflammation is present 2. Hydrotherapy: passive or active exercises in a whirlpool with a water temperature of 96°–104° F
5. Active exercise	Increasing strength, endurance, and flexibility	Contraction of the muscle crossing the joint	1. Active ROM exercises: at least 3 times a day, encourage the animal to move its leg or foot and then apply gentle resistance to the animal's movement **Apply a warm compress to the joints before active ROM exercises to aid in joint movement** 2. Swimming 3. Hydrotherapy: passive or active exercise in a whirlpool with a water temperature of 65°–75° F **Caution:** Do not start until after skin sutures have been removed 4. Walking with support

Skill Box 6-8 / Physical Therapy (Continued)

Skill	Effect	Cause	Technique
6. Electrical stimulation	Pain relief, disuse atrophy, blood and lymph circulation, and wound repair	Stimulation of sensory and motor nerves	1. High-voltage or low-voltage devices are attached by electrodes to specific areas of interest
7. Ultrasound	Increases extensibility	Heating fibrous structures	1. An ultrasound head is applied directly to the skin of the affected area for 5 minutes, moving in slow sweeps with varying frequencies, depending on the injury

NEUROLOGY

Table 6-13 Neurology

DISEASE	Encephalitis	Epilepsy	Intervertebral Disk Disease
DEFINITION	Encephalitis is an inflammatory disease of the brain with random progression. The causes of this condition are wide ranging, from breed predilections, infectious diseases, viral, protozoa, fungal, and bacterial infections. The clinical signs, diagnosis, and treatment are all dependent on determining the underlying disease.	Epilepsy is a condition of recurring seizures regardless of their cause. Primary epilepsy has no known cause: it may be genetic/hereditary. Secondary epilepsy is acquired through brain injury or inflammation.	Intervertebral disk disease is an age-related condition affecting an individual disk or disks. This condition may lead to protrusion or extrusion of the disk, leading to compression of the spinal cord, nerve roots, or meninges. The process can be either a degenerative or an infectious process (diskospondylitis).
CLINICAL SIGNS	• Dependent on underlying disease • Fever, hyperthermic, depression, vomiting, and photophobia • Lung disease, abnormal heart and respiratory rates • GI upset • Corneal changes • Seizures, circling, head tilt, tremors, paralysis, nystagmus, pacing, and behavioral changes	*3 Stages of Seizures* • Aura—immediately preceding seizure—restlessness, crying, and hiding • Ictus—actual seizure—lasting <2–5 minutes, stiff, muscle spasms, jaw chomping, salivating profusely, urinates, defecates, vocalizes, and paddles with all four paws • Postictus—immediately following seizure—lasting <30 minutes, behavioral changes, weakness, blindness, hungry, thirsty, depressed, pacing or tired	• Paresis and paralysis of some or all limbs • Pain or crying when touched • Reluctance to move or jump • Stiff or hunched stance/appearance
GENERAL	• History • Clinical signs • Neurologic examination	• History • Clinical signs • Neurologic examination	• History • Clinical signs • Spine palpation
CBC	• Dependent on underlying disease • Leukocytosis	• Normal	• Normal
BIOCHEMISTRY	• Dependent on underlying disease • ↑ Protein and creatine kinase	• Normal	• Normal

DIAGNOSIS

DIAGNOSIS

	Column 1	Column 2	Column 3
URINALYSIS	• Normal or may reflect underlying disease	• Normal	• Leukocytes • ↑ Protein and bacteria
RADIOLOGY	• Thoracic: lung abnormalities • Skull: sinusitis or rhinitis (cryptococcosis)	• Thoracic: tumors • Abdominal: tumors • Skull: hydrocephalus, trauma, or tumor	• Spine: narrowed, wedge-shaped disk space, small intervertebral foramen, collapsed articular facets or mineralized disk material in the spinal cord, intervertebral foramen or vetebral endplate lysis or sclerosis
MISCELLANEOUS	• CSF analysis: ↑ WBCs and protein, fungi, or bacteria • CSF titers: + results • Serology: Antibody recognition and identification • EEG: diffuse multifocal cerebral involvement • CT/MRI: tumor • Ophthalmoscopy: retinitis, chorioditis, uveitis, or vasculitis of retinal vessels	• Electroencephalography: tumor, inflammation, or metabolic disease • CT: tumor, inflammation or granulomas • MRI: tumor and inflammation • Ophthalmoscopy: retinitis, chorioditis, uveitis, or vasculitis of retinal vessels • CSF analysis	• Myelography: location and severity of disk lesion • CT/MRI: location and severity of disk lesion • CSF analysis: inflammatory cells and infectious agents

TREATMENT

	Column 1	Column 2	Column 3
GENERAL	• Symptomatic • Supportive • Radiation therapy	• Symptomatic	• Symptomatic • Cage rest for 2 weeks • Acupuncture • Surgery: laminectomy, hemilaminectomy, or decompression
MEDICATION	• Dependent on underlying disease • Antibiotics: enrofloxacin or clavamox • Corticosteroids: dexamethasone • Fungal: itraconazole or fluconazole	*Acute (IV)* • Diazepam • Phenobarbital • Sodium pentobarbital *Chronic (oral)* • Phenobarbital • Potassium bromide	• Corticosteroids: prednisone, prednisolone, or methyl prednisolone succinate

Table 6-13 Neurology (Continued)

	DISEASE	Encephalitis	Epilepsy	Intervertebral Disk Disease
TREATMENT	PATIENT CARE	• Dependent on underlying disease • Monitor neurologic functions • Frequent turning to prevent decubital sores and pulmonary edema • Cold water or alcohol baths or ice packs for hyperthermia	• Constant monitoring for seizures • Cold water or alcohol baths or ice packs for hyperthermia	• Careful handling of patients to prevent further trauma: protect the spine during any movement • Nutritional support • Monitor for worsening neurologic signs • Monitor urine output and defecation • Turn recumbent patients at least every 4 hours and keep well padded
FOLLOW-UP	PATIENT CARE	• Monitor neurologic functions • Monitor blood work dependent on underlying disease	• Avoid swimming	• Restrict activity • Physical therapy: range of motion exercises or hydrotherapy, start 2 weeks postoperatively • Monitor urinalysis in nonambulatory patients • Use harnesses to keep pressure off cervical disks • Control obesity
	PREVENTION/ AVOIDANCE	• Tick control • Vaccinations • Proper wound management	• Castrate affected animals • Maintain antiseizure medication	• Maintain proper weight control • Avoid strenuous exercise with prone breeds
	COMPLICATIONS	• Dependent on underlying disease • Death	• Phenobarbital complications • Status epillepticus	• Recurrence of neck pain
	PROGNOSIS	• Variable, dependent on underlying disease • Many forms are lethal	• Proper treatment gives ↓ seizure frequency	• Excellent with surgery

NOTES		
• **Caution:** Chosen drugs must be able to cross the blood–brain barrier • Determining the underlying disease that is causing this condition is critical to the patient's survival	• Most seizures occur while sleeping or at rest, often at night or in early morning • German shepherds, Irish setters, Miniature poodles, Siberian huskies, Beagles, Cocker spaniels, Labrador retrievers, Keeshonds, and miniature Schnauzers	• **Caution:** Corticosteroids should not be used with diskospondylitis • **Caution:** Do not use corticosteroids and NSAIDs together because of GI hemorrhage • For confinement to work, it must be strict, with only leash walks to eliminate • Beagles, Toy poodles, Dachshunds, Doberman pinschers, and all chondrodystrophic breeds

DISEASE	Meningitis	Myasthenia Gravis	Myelopathy
DEFINITION	Bacterial infection of the meninges is the cause of meningitis. It can be the result of septicemia, local invasion, or bite wounds. Secondary inflammation of the brain or spinal cord also may be seen with meningitis.	Myasthenia gravis is associated with autoantibodies directed at nicotinic acetylcholine receptors. This leads to a loss of acetylcholine receptors (AChRs), which impairs neuromuscular transmission and causes muscle weakness and episodic collapsing.	Myelopathy is a degenerative process affecting the myelin and axons of the spinal cords. This slow, progressive problem has no known cause but is limited to the hind limbs. There is no known treatment: only supportive therapy.
CLINICAL SIGNS	• Depression and fever • Hyperesthesia and neck pain • Nasal, sinus, and inner ear infection • Ataxia, tremors, and mild paresis in all four limbs	• Muscle weakness, body trembling, gait abnormalities, paresis/paralysis • Dysphagia, regurgitation, excessive drooling, masticatory dysfunction, and voice change • Dysphonia and dyspnea • Ventroflexion of head	• Abnormal gait and worn toenails • Knuckling and scuffing of hind limbs, muscle atrophy, crossing over of hind limbs, and swaying when turning
DIAGNOSIS — GENERAL	• History • Clinical signs • Neurologic examination	• History • Clinical signs (episodic) • Neurological examination	• History • Clinical signs • Neurologic examination
DIAGNOSIS — CBC	• Neutrophilic leukocytes • Leukopenia	• Normal or may reflect underlying disease	• Normal

Table 6-13 Neurology (Continued)

DISEASE	Meningitis	Myasthenia Gravis	Myelopathy
DIAGNOSIS			
BIOCHEMISTRY	• ↑ Globulin	• Normal or may reflect underlying disease • ↑ CK	• Normal
URINALYSIS	• Pyuria and bacteriuria	• Normal or may reflect underlying disease	• Normal
RADIOLOGY	• Spine: bony infection • Skull: sinus, nasal cavity or ear infection	• Thoracic: megaesophagus or cranial mediastinal mass	• Thoracic: metastasis and tumors • Abdominal: same as above • Spine: ossification, spondylosis, or narrowed intervertebral disk space
MISCELLANEOUS	• Cytology of the skin, eyes, nasal discharge, and sputum: bacteria, fungal, protozoa, rickettsial or viral • Cerebrospinal fluid (CSF) analysis: bacteria or neutrophilic pleocytosis	• Thyroid and adrenal function tests • ANA Assay: + result • Serum antibodies against nicotinic AChRs: + result • Edrophonium chloride challenge test: ↑ muscle strength after injection • Electrodiagnostic evaluation: location and severity of disease • Fluoroscopy: dysfunction of swallowing	• CSF analysis: ↑ protein
TREATMENT			
GENERAL	• Symptomatic • Supportive • Fluid therapy	• Supportive • Fluid therapy • Oxygen therapy • Surgery: feeding tube placement or tumor removal	• Supportive
MEDICATION	• Antibiotics: chloramphenical, trimethoprim, sulfonamides, or metronidazole • Anticonvulsants: diazepam or phenobarbital • Corticosteroids: dexamethasone	• Anticholinesterase drugs: pyridostigmine bromide or neostigmine • Corticosteroids: prednisone	• Aminocaproic acid (variable)
PATIENT CARE	• Intensive care monitoring • Restricted activity	• Nutritional support	• Treated as outpatient

FOLLOW-UP

PATIENT CARE	• Monitor for neurologic signs, fever, systemic signs, and leukocytosis	• Feed animal in an upright position and ensure the animal remains upright for at least 10 minutes after eating • Feed different consistencies of food to determine which works best • Radiograph every 4–6 weeks to monitor megaesophagus • Recheck AChR antibody titers every 6–8 weeks until normal	• Keep as active as possible to delay onset of nonambulatory state *Nonambulatory* • Cart for mobility • Avoid decubital sores • Urinary catheter • Vitamin supplementation
PREVENTION/ AVOIDANCE	• Treat local infections early and thoroughly to prevent spread of infection to the CNS	• N/A	• N/A
COMPLICATIONS	• Irreversible damage to the brain and spinal cord • DIC	• Aspirate pneumonia • Tertiary heart block • Respiratory arrest	• Decubital sores • Fecal and urine incontinence
PROGNOSIS	• Variable, depending on degree of infection and inflammation	• Good • Guarded with cranial mediastinal mass	• Guarded to poor • Patients eventually lose function of both hind and front limbs
NOTES		• Jack Russel terriers, Springer spaniel, Smooth Fox terriers, Golden retrievers, German shepherds, Labrador retrievers, Dachshunds and Scottish terriers	• There have been no controlled studies to show the efficacy of aminocaproic acid • German shepherds, Collies, Labrador retriever, Chesapeake Bay retrievers, and Kerry blue terriers

Table 6-13 Neurology (Continued)

DISEASE	Vestibular Disease of Older Dogs, Acute	Wobbler Syndrome (Caudal Cervical Spondylomyelopathy, Cervical Vertebral Instability)
DEFINITION	Vestibular disease is an acute condition affecting geriatric dogs. It is the disturbance of the peripheral vestibular system. Otitis media is a common cause of the disease in younger dogs.	Wobbler syndrome is caused by pressure placed on the spinal cord by malformation of bone or spinal ligaments. It leads to instability or chronic disk disease. It is thought that overnutrition and rapid growth may be a contributing factor to this condition.
CLINICAL SIGNS	• Head tilt, loss of balance, circling, falling, rolling, disorientation, ataxia, and nystagmus • Facial paresis/paralysis or Horner's syndrome • Nausea and vomiting	• Abnormal gait, knuckling or dragging of toes, rigid flexion of neck, and ataxia • Pain, paraparesis, and ambulatory or nonambulatory tetraparesis
DIAGNOSIS — GENERAL	• Clinical signs • Neurologic examination	• History • Clinical signs
CBC	• Normal	• Normal
BIOCHEMISTRY	• Normal	• Normal
URINALYSIS	• Normal	• Normal
RADIOLOGY	• Normal	• Spine: bony changes, herniation, subluxation, or narrowing of intervertebral disk space • Myelogram: site and type of cord compression
MISCELLANEOUS	• N/A	• CSF analysis: ↑ protein • Thyrotropin stimulation test: minimal to no response
TREATMENT — GENERAL	• Supportive • Fluid therapy	• Surgery: ventral spondylectomy, dorsal laminectomy, fenestration, stabilization or fusion of involved vertebrae
MEDICATION	• Antibiotics: trimethoprim-sulfa • Antiemetics: dimenhydrinate • Tranquilizers: diazepam	• Corticosteroids: prednisone
PATIENT CARE	• Treated as outpatient	• Urinary catheter • Avoid decubital sores • Physical therapy of all limbs to prevent ankylosis • Restrict activity of ambulatory patients or use a neck brace

PATIENT CARE	• Restrict activity as needed for disorientation • Reexamine 2–3 days after discharge to verify continued improvement • Monitor neurologic functions
PREVENTION/ AVOIDANCE	• Prompt recognition and treatment of ear infections if present • Limit running and jumping • Use harness instead of a neck collar
COMPLICATIONS	• Dehydration • Electrolyte imbalances • Renal insufficiencies • Failure of surgical repair • Degenerative changes of surrounding disk spaces • Decubital sores • Urinary tract infection or urine scalding
PROGNOSIS	• Excellent • Most patients return to normal in 2–3 weeks • Good when presented ambulatory • Poor when nonambulatory with tetraparesis
NOTES	• **Caution:** Flexion and tension stress during radiographs can make clinical signs worse • Great Dane and Doberman pinscher

FOLLOW-UP

ONCOLOGY

Table 6-14 Oncology

DISEASE	Neoplasia
DEFINITION	Neoplasia is the development of a new and abnormal formation of tissue, as a tumor or growth. The new tissue serves no useful function but grows at the expense of the healthy organism.
CLINICAL SIGNS	• Presence of a tumor or two effects attributable to adjacent organ/tissue injury (e.g., halitosis, swelling, pain) • Anorexia, vomiting, diarrhea, lethargy, depression, inappetance, and weight loss

DIAGNOSIS

GENERAL	• History • Clinical signs • Physical examination: tumor and lymph node palpation
CBC	• Variable: see specific tumor type • Anemia: normocytic and normochromic
BIOCHEMISTRY	• Variable: see specific tumor type
URINALYSIS	• Variable: see specific tumor type
RADIOLOGY	• Thoracic (ventrodorsal [VD] and left and right laterals): tumor identification, metastases, lymphadenopathy or pleural effusion • Abdominal: tumor identification, metastases, lymphadenopathy, or organomegaly
MISCELLANEOUS	• Ultrasound: tumor identification, lymphadenopathy, or guided biopsy • CT or MRI: tumor identification, metastases, lymphadenopathy, tumor margins, and tissue of origin • Fine-needle aspirate, core biopsy, or surgical biopsy of tumor or enlarged lymph node(s) • Cytology: cells fulfilling the criteria for malignancy • Histopathology: clean margins and tumor grade

TREATMENT

GENERAL	• Symptomatic • Radiation therapy • Surgery: excision with 2–3-cm clean margins
MEDICATION	• Variable: see specific tumor type • Chemotherapy agents • Corticosteroids • Analgesics
PATIENT CARE	• Standard postoperative care after surgical excision

FOLLOW-UP

PATIENT CARE	• Variable: see specific tumor type • Monitor specific blood values • Monitor response to treatment, chemotherapy (see box 6-10) appetite, elimination, and energy level
PREVENTION/ AVOIDANCE	• N/A
COMPLICATIONS	• Variable: see specific tumor type
PROGNOSIS	• Dependent on tumor type, size, location, time of discovery, and completeness of excision
NOTES	

DISEASE	Histiocytoma (Button Tumor)	Mammary Gland Neoplasia	Mast Cell Tumor
DEFINITION	A histiocytoma is a benign skin tumor often found on the head, ear pinna, and limbs. They are most commonly seen in dogs younger than 2 years of age.	Mammary gland neoplasia is very prevalent among female intact dogs and very rare in male dogs. The tumors show malignancy 50% of the time. If the tumors are malignant, they have usually metastasized by the time of diagnosis.	Mast cell tumors are malignant tumors that arise from mast cells. They are a very unpredictable tumor in their appearance, growth rate, and response to treatment.
CLINICAL SIGNS	• Firm, small, dome- or button-shaped mass • Fast-growing, solitary, nonpainful, and might be ulcerated	• Firm nodular mass, ± ulceration • Nipples: red, swollen, and tan or red exudate • Fever	*Dogs* • Lymphadenopathy, erythema, and edema • Tumor: solitary skin or SC mass, present for days to months, recent rapid growth *Cats* • Anorexia and vomiting (cats) • Tumor; found in SC tissue or dermis, papular or nodular, solitary or multiple, hairy or alopecic or ulcerated

Table 6-14 Oncology (Continued)

DISEASE	Histiocytoma (Button Tumor)	Mammary Gland Neoplasia	Mast Cell Tumor
GENERAL	• Clinical signs	• Clinical signs • Mammary gland palpation	• History • Clinical signs
CBC	• N/A	• Anemia • Leukocytosis	• Eosinophilia and basophilia (variable) • Anemia and mastocythemia (rare)
BIOCHEMISTRY	• N/A	• Normal	• Normal
URINALYSIS	• N/A	• Normal	• Normal
RADIOLOGY	• N/A	• Thoracic: pleural effusion and lung metastases • Abdominal: ascites and ↑ size of sublumbar lymph nodes	• Abdominal: ↑ spleen, liver and lymph nodes
MISCELLANEOUS	• Cytology: pleomorphic round cells, variably sized and shaped nuclei, appearance of hepatocytes, variable amounts of pale blue cytoplasm resembling monocytes, ± lymphocyte, plasma cell, and neutrophil infiltrate	• Ultrasound: ascites and size of sublumbar lymph nodes • Cytology: cells with cytoplasmic basophilia, variable nuclear/cytoplasmic ratios, and if malignant have typical carcinoma clumps (e.g., acinar)	• Ultrasound: visceral metastasis • Cytology: round cells with basophilic cytoplasmic granules not forming sheets or clumps and ± eosinophilic infiltrate • Biopsy: confirmation and severity of disease • Histopathology: confirmation of completeness of excision • Buffy coat smear: mast cells • Darier's sign: a tumor that has been manipulated with degranulate, causing erythma and wheal formations.
GENERAL	• Spontaneous regression • Surgery: excision or cyrosurgery	• Symptomatic • Surgery: mastectomy	• Symptomatic • Chemotherapy • Radiotherapy • Surgery: aggressive excision and splenectomy

DIAGNOSIS (rows GENERAL through MISCELLANEOUS)

TREATMENT (row GENERAL at bottom)

		Column 1	Column 2	Column 3
TREATMENT	MEDICATION	• Chemotherapy: doxorubicin, clophosphamide, and mitoxantrone (see Skill Boxes 6-9 and 6-10)	• N/A	• Chemotherapy: L-asparginase, vinblastine, cyclophosphamide, lomustine, and vincristine • Corticosteroids: prednisone • GI protectants: sulcralfate • H_1-blockers: diphenhydramine • H_2-blockers: cimetidine or ranitidine
	PATIENT CARE	• Standard postoperative care	• Standard postoperative care	• Standard postoperative care
	PATIENT CARE	• Monitor its growth and the presence of new tumors	• Reexamine every 2 months for recurrence of mammary tumors	• Monitor CBC before each chemotherapy administration • Monitor for the presence of new tumors • Monitor lymph node enlargement
FOLLOW-UP	PREVENTION/ AVOIDANCE	• N/A	• Early hysterectomy: ≤2nd heat cycle	• N/A
	COMPLICATIONS	• N/A	• Anemia • Osteoporosis • Hypercalcemia • DIC • Ascites • Pleural effusion	• Bleeding • Hemorrhagic gastroenteritis • Chemotherapy toxicity • Radiation reaction • Metastasis to regional lymph nodes, liver, spleen and bone marrow
	PROGNOSIS	• Excellent	• Dependent on size, time of detection and the completeness of excision	• Dependent on the area affected, time of detection and the completeness of excision
	NOTES	• Boxers, Dachshunds, Cocker spaniel, Great Danes and Shetland sheepdog	• Freely movable tumor implies benign and fixed to body wall or skin implies malignant • Removal of all four glands of the affected chain is recommended	• Animals with tumors on the extremities tend to live longer than animals with trunk tumors • Boxers, Boston terriers, Bullmastiffs, English setters and Siamese cats

Table 6-15 Types of Cancer

Type of Cancer	Clinical Signs	Diagnosis	Treatment	Follow-Up	Complications	Prognosis
CARCINOMA *Adenocarcinoma* Anal Sac • Mostly seen in geriatric female dogs, with a very high rate of metastasis	• Dyschezia, tenesmus, PU/PD, pruritis, ulceration, bleeding, weakness, and paresis	• ↑ Calcium • ↓ Phosphorus	• Fluid therapy • Furosemide • Chemotherapy: cisplatin (dogs) (see Skill Boxes 6-9 and 6-10)	• Examination, radiographs, ultrasound, and blood work every 3 months after surgery	• Renal failure, fecal incontinence, sepsis, metastasis, and reoccurrence	• Poor
Nasal • Most tumors begin as unilateral but progress to bilateral	• Epistaxis, epiphora, sneezing, nasal discharge, halitosis, and seizures • Facial deformity: nasal bone swelling	• Skull radiographs: tumor location and extent • CT, MRI, or rhinoscopy: tumor location, extent and effect on surrounding structures and biopsy • Mycotic cultures: fungal rhinitis	• Radiotherapy • Cisplatin (dogs) • Butorphanol	• Survey radiographs, CT, or MRI when clinical signs return	• Brain involvement across cribriform plate	• Fair with radiation • Poor with brain involvement
Pancreas • Liver metastasis is very common	• Fever, icterus, ascites, and maldigestion • Palpable abdominal mass	• Mild anemia and neutrophilia • ↑ Amylase and lipase	• Palliative	• Monitor quality of life	• Diabetes insipidus, pancreatitis, intestinal or biliary obstruction, pancreatic abscess, or peritonitis	• Grave

Prostate • Prostate tumors are always malignant	• Tenesmus, dyschezia, constipation, hematuria, stranguria, dysuria, rear limb lameness, exercise intolerance, cachexia, fever, and dyspnea • Inflammatory leukogram • ↑ Alkaline phosphatase • Azotemia • UA: blood, pyuria and malignant epithelial cells • Contrast cystography: distortion of prostatic urethra	• Castration • Radiotherapy • Analgesics: NSAIDs or opioid drugs • Chemotherapy: cisplatin (dogs), carboplatin, and doxorubicin • Stool softeners	• Monitor ability to urinate and defecate • Monitor pain levels	• Grave
Salivary Gland	• Swelling of upper neck, ear base, upper lip or maxilla, or mucous membrane of lip, dysphagia and pain on opening mouth	• Radiotherapy	• Monitor for tumor growth every 3–6 months	• Unknown
Thyroid • High rate of metastasis • Biopsy and FNA can cause excessive bleeding • Rare in cats	• Dyspnea, dysphagia, dysphonia, regurgitation, and PU/PD • Nonregenerative anemia • See Canine Hypothyroidism signs • Cervical radiographs and ultrasound: displacement of normal structures • Radioiodine study: thyroid hormone production • Thyroid gland scintigraphy: location	• Radiotherapy • β-blockers • Analgesics: butorphanol • Chemotherapy (see Skill Box 6-9): doxorubicin and cisplatin • Methimazole • Thyroxine	• Examine tumor site and radiographs every 3 months	• Anemia, DIC, respiratory distress, hypothyroidism, hypoparathyroidism, and laryngeal paralysis • Depending on size of tumor and lymph node involvement • Larger fixed tumors have a poor prognosis

Table 6-15 Types of Cancer (Continued)

Type of Cancer	Clinical Signs	Diagnosis	Treatment	Follow-Up	Complications	Prognosis
Squamous Cell Carcinoma						
Digit • Often seen in large, black dogs • Arises from subungual epithelium	• Swelling and ulceration • Lameness: chronic and progressive	• Affected foot radiographs: lysis of the 3rd phalanx	• Chemotherapy (see Skill Boxes 6-9 and 6-10): cisplatin (dogs), mitoxantrone, bovine collagen matrix with 5-fluorouracil • Piroxicam • Retinoids	• Limit sun exposure • Use sunscreen or tattoo low-pigmented areas of the paws		• Good
Ear • Areas of low pigmentation and those subjected to solar radiation are more at risk	• Crusty eczematous lesions on edge of pinna and ulceration		• Photodynamic therapy • Radiotherapy • Cryosurgery • Hyperthermia • Bleomycin • Chemotherapy: cisplatin (intralesional injections) • Etretinate • Vitamin E	• Limit sun exposure • Use sunscreen or tattoo low-pigmented areas of the ears		• Good with complete excision
Gingiva	• Excessive salivation, dysphagia, halitosis, bloody oral discharge, loose teeth, and facial deformity • Plaque-like areas that bleed easily	• Skull radiographs: bone involvement and lysis • CT: bone involvement and lysis	• Cryosurgery • Radiotherapy • Chemotherapy (see Skill Boxes 6-9 and 6-10): cisplatin (dogs), mitoxantrone, and carboplatin • Butorphanol	• Feed soft foods or by enteral feeding tube		• Poor because of local invasion (cats) • The more rostral the tumor is located, the better the prognosis (dogs)

Clinical Signs / Characteristics	Diagnosis	Treatment	Monitoring	Complications	Prognosis
Skin • Areas of low pigmentation and those subjected to solar radiation are more at risk • Malignant tumor of squamous epithelium • Crusty, ulceration and pigmentation • Facial skin involvement (cat) • Nail bed involvement (dog)	• Extremity radiographs: bone involvement • Biopsy punch	• Radiotherapy • Cryosurgery • Photodynamic therapy • Chemotherapy: cisplatin (dogs), carboplatin, mitoxantrone, or bovine collagen matrix with 5-fluorouracil (dogs) • Retinoids	• Reexamination and radiographs every 3 months for 1 year then every 6 months for 1 year • Limit sun exposure • Use sunscreen or tattoo low-pigmented areas of the skin	• Good with superficial lesions • Guarded with nail bed or digit involvement	• Good
Transitional Cell Carcinoma _Bladder, Urethra_ • High rate of metastasis • FNA may cause seeding of tumor cells along the needle tract • Recurrent stranguria, pollakiuria, dysuria, hematuria, PU/PD, urinary incontinence, and tenesmus	• Azotemia if at trigone • UA: blood and malignant epithelial cells • Urine culture • Double-contrast cystography: irregularities or mass lesions • IV pyelography, voiding urethrogram or vaginogram	• Radiotherapy • Chemotherapy: cisplatin (dogs) • Piroxicam	• Cystography or ultrasonography every 6–8 weeks • Thoracic radiographs every 2–3 months	• Transplantation of cells during surgery or biopsy • Urinary incontinence, urethral or ureteral obstruction, or renal failure	• Grave
SARCOMA **Chondrosarcoma** Bone • Affects large-breed dogs • Lameness, swelling, pain in affected limb, nasal discharge, and pain at tumor site	• Affected limb radiographs • CT scan: local extent • Nuclear bone scan: staging of disease	• Radiotherapy • Chemotherapy: cisplatin (dogs) and doxorubicin	• Thoracic radiographs monthly for 3 months, then every 3 months	• Brain involvement	• Dependent on tumor grade

Table 6-15 Types of Cancer (Continued)

Type of Cancer	Clinical Signs	Diagnosis	Treatment	Follow-Up	Complications	Prognosis
Nasal and Paranasal Sinus • Affects large-breed dogs	• Epiphoria, sneezing, nasal discharge, halitosis, facial deformity, pain, and seizures	• Skull radiographs: tumor, fluid, and destruction of caudal turbinates • CT or MRI: integrity of cribriform plate and orbital invasion	• Radiotherapy • Chemotherapy: doxorubicin	• Radiographs and CT/MRI may be repeated when clinical signs return		• Fair
Fibrosarcoma Bone • Primarily affects the axial skeleton	• Lameness, swelling, pain, and fracture	• Affected limb radiographs • CT: extent of disease	• Radiotherapy • Chemotherapy: cisplatin (dogs)	• Thoracic radiographs monthly for 3 months, then every 3 months		• Guarded
Gingiva	• Excessive salivation: halitosis, dysphagia, bloody oral discharge, loose teeth and facial deformity	• Skull radiographs: bone involvement • Biopsy: intraoral	• Cryosurgery • Radiotherapy • Chemotherapy: doxorubicin	• Feed soft foods		• Fair
Hemangiosarcoma Bone	• Lameness, swelling, fracture, and pale mucous membranes	• Bone radiographs: lysis • Regenerative anemia, nucleated RBCs, poikilocytosis, and anisocytosis • Thrombocytopenia and leukocytosis • ↓ Protein	• Chemotherapy: doxorubicin and cyclophosphamide	• Examination, thoracic radiographs and ultrasound every 3 months for 1 year then every 6 months	• Pathologic fractures • Rupturing tumors causing hemorrhage	• Unknown

	Clinical signs	Diagnostics	Treatment	Monitoring	Complications	Prognosis
Heart • Pulmonary metastasis very common	• Abdominal and pleural effusion, dyspnea, syncope, arrhythmia, pulse deficits, exercise intolerance, hindlimb paresis, hepatomegaly, and jugular distension	• Fibrin degradation products, PT and PTT: ↑ values • Fibrinogen: →↓ values • CT: extent of disease • Anemia and nucleated RBCs • Azotemia	• Pericardial and pleuralcentesis • Chemotherapy: doxorubicin, vincristine or cyclophosphamide	• Examination, thoracic radiographs, and ultrasound monthly	• Centesis complications	• Grave
Spleen, Liver • Rapid growth and widespread metastatic vascular neoplasia	• Weakness, intermittent collapse, ataxia, lameness, seizures, dementia, and paresis • Pale mucous membranes, tachycardia, enlarged abdomen, and peritoneal fluid	• Regenerative anemia with polychromasia, reticulocytosis, nucleated RBCs, and anisocytosis • Leukocytosis, neutrophilia, and thrombocytopenia • ↑ Liver enzymes • Fibrin degradation products, PT and PTT: ↑ values • ECHO: tumor location and metastasis	• Fluid therapy • Blood transfusions • Chemotherapy: cyclophosphamide, doxorubicin, chlorambucil, methotrexate, and vincristine • Diphenhydramine • Biologic response modifier L-MTP-PE • Surgical: splenectomy	• Restricted activity • Thoracic and abdominal radiographs and abdominal ultrasound every 3 months	• Tumor rupture leading to hemorrhage • Sepsis • Vomiting and diarrhea • Skin sloughs	• Poor

Table 6-15 Types of Cancer (Continued)

Type of Cancer	Clinical Signs	Diagnosis	Treatment	Follow-Up	Complications	Prognosis
Lymphosarcoma/Lymphoma						
Cat • Most common sites are alimentary tract, anterior mediastinum, liver, spleen, and kidneys	• Weight loss • Dependent on form (mediastinal, renal, alimentary, solitary or multicentric) • Open-mouthed breathing, coughing, regurgitation • Renal failure signs • Thickened intestines	• Anemia, leukocytosis, and lymphoblastosis • ↑ Creatinine, BUN, ALT, AST, and calcium • UA: ↑ bilirubin, protein and isothenuria • Serology: + FeLV • Cobalamin and folate: ↓ values	• Chemotherapy: vincristine, cytosine arabinoside, methotrexate, cyclophosphamide, chlorambucil, L-asparginase, doxorubicin, and actinomycin-D • Corticosteroids: prednisone	• Examination, CBC, and platelet count before each weekly cycle of chemotherapy	• Leukopenia • Sepsis	• Dependent on form
Dog • Seen most commonly is solid tissues: lymph nodes, bone marrow and visceral organs • Increased risk with exposure to the herbicide: 2,4 dichlorophenoxyacetic	• Lymphadenopathy, organomegaly and ascites • Coughing, difficulty swallowing, drooling, labored breathing and exercise intolerance • Anterior uveitis or lymphoid infiltrate	• Anemia, lymphocytosis, lymphopenia, neutrophilia, monocytosis, circulating blasts and thrombocytopenia • ↑ ALT, ALP and calcium • ECHO: cardiac contractility	• Radiotherapy • Fluid therapy • Thoraco- and abdominocentesis • Chemotherapy: doxorubicin, vincristine, cyclophosphamide, L-asparginase, methotrexate, and chlorambucil • Corticosteroids: prednisone • Retinoids	• Restrict activity of patients with low WBCs or platelet count • Monitor CBC and platelet count during chemotherapy • Echocardiogram and ECG: cardiotoxicity of doxorubicin	• Leukopenia and neutropenia • Vomiting and diarrhea • Alopecia • Pancreatitis • Sepsis • Tissue sloughing • DIC	• Good

Osteosarcoma • Most common bone tumor in dogs, typically affecting the appendicular skeleton of large to giant breeds	• Swelling, lameness, and pain • Pathologic long-bone fracture	• Affected bone radiograph: bone lysis, proliferation in the metaphyseal region of long bones and soft tissue swelling • Nuclear bone scans: bony or soft tissue metastatic disease	• Radiotherapy • Analgesics: butorphanol, piroxicam, fentanyl, and morphine sulfate • Biologic response modifiers: L-MTP-PE • Chemotherapy: cisplatin (dogs), carboplatin, and doxorubicin	• Restrict activity • Monitor radiographs every 2–3 months • Monitor CBC and platelet count 7–10 days after chemotherapy	• Metastasis (>90% of cases at examination) and hypertrophic osteopathy • Guarded once metastases is present
Vaccine-induced Sarcoma • Typically fibrosarcoma, but may be many other types of sarcoma • Most common with FeLV and rabies	• Firm, painless, SC swelling located at a previous vaccination site	• Tumor site radiograph: bone lysis or extension of the tumor along other tissue planes	• Radiotherapy • Chemotherapy: doxorubicin or cyclophosphamide	• Evaluate monthly for 3 months, then every 3 months • Monitor CBC and platelet count before each chemotherapy treatment	• Poor

Skill Box 6-9 / Chemotherapy Administration

1. Review the patient's record, and recheck the chemotherapy protocol and drug calculations.

   It is best to have a second person confirm the drug calculations.

   **Caution: Chemotherapy drugs differ as to their body weight calculations (e.g., kilograms, pounds, or square meters): be sure to verify the correct form. Also, most drugs are based on lean body weight, not actual body weight.

2. Prepare yourself and assistant with safety gear

   a. Latex gloves, 2 pairs, or a pair of high-risk gloves

   b. Full face shield or protective eyewear

   c. Mask—dust or mist respirator or a mask with a filter (surgical masks do not have a filter and are not sufficient)

   d. Gown—disposable with long sleeves, closed front, and cuffs

3. Prepare all materials needed to prepare and administer the drug

   a. Oral

      1. Drug

      2. Hemostat or pill-gun

   b. SC/IM

      1. Alcohol-soaked gauze sponges

      2. Chemo-pin

      3. Drop cloth

      4. Drug

      5. Gauze sponges

      6. Syringe

   c. IV

      1. Same as above

      2. Catheter

      3. Clippers

      4. Scrub preparation materials

      5. Tape

4. Preparation of the drug

   a. Remove plastic cover of vial, and wipe the top with an alcohol swab

   b. Insert the chemo-pin into the vial

   c. Attach syringe to the chemo-pin while holding the vial upright

   d. If adding a dilutent, add slowly and then mix contents of vial completely, with the luer-lock syringe left in place

   e. Turn vial upside down and aspirate drug into syringe slowly to avoid excess air bubbles

   f. Push any excess air back into the syringe before separating from vial

g. Wrap gauze around the connection between the syringe and vial and gently pull apart

h. Place a covered needle onto the syringe

Note: If not using a chemo-pin, all the above steps are accomplished with a needle attached to the end of the syringe. This greatly increases the risk of aerosolizing the drug, so extreme care should be taken in maintaining equalized pressure in the vial and when attaching and detaching the syringe from the vial.

Do not fill a syringe more than two-thirds full, to prevent the plunger from detaching from the syringe.

If an agent is to be administered via a dripset, fill the dripset with diluent before adding the chemotherapy agent to reduce the risk of contamination when attaching the line to the patient.

5. Preparation of the patient for IV administration

   a. Select vein: peripheral veins are recommended because they provide better visualization of any drug that becomes extravascular.

   b. Aseptically clip and prepare the site.

   c. Place a catheter: butterfly, over-the-needle, or through-the-needle intracatheter

   Caution: Once a vein has been unsuccessfully punctured, a new vein should be used. If this is not possible, it is recommended that time be allowed for the proper clotting to occur before a proximal site is used.

   d. Assure patency of the catheter by flushing at least 12 mL nonheparinized 0.9% sodium chloride.

   Caution: Heparinized saline may cause the drug to form a precipitate.

6. Administration of the drug

   e. With an alcohol-soaked gauze around the end of the catheter, insert the needle into the catheter and administer the drug at the correct rate but at an even pace to avoid leakage around venipuncture site

   f. Flush the catheter with nonheparinized 0.9% sodium chloride after administration to avoid irritation to the vein

   g. Monitor for allergic reactions for up to 1 hour after administration of certain drugs (e.g., L-asparginase)

   Caution: To avoid aerosolization of the drug, an alcohol-soaked gauze sponge should be placed over the injection site whenever inserting or removing the needle or catheter

   Caution: Once the drug has been administered and a flush has been given, do not aspirate the drug back into the catheter because this dilutes the drug and leaves a small amount of diluted drug in the catheter.

   h. Apply a pressure wrap after removing the catheter, and maintain pressure for several minutes

7. Disposal

   a. Place all items in a zip-lock bag to prevent aerosolization

   b. Dispose of the waste into an approved container

c. Clean the preparation and administration surfaces thoroughly

Before removing your gloves, place capped syringes and any other used products that may aerosolize in the waste container into your hands, and pull your gloves off over the materials and then dispose of them.

8. Caring for a patient receiving chemotherapy

a. Wear gloves when handling waste from the patient for the first 48 hours.

b. Do not hose down cages when cleaning because of risk of aerosolization.

c. Closely monitor response to drug (e.g., attitude, appetite, eliminations, and general behavior).

Skill Box 6-10 / Chemotherapy Client Education

1. Monitor appetite, attitude, eliminations and general behavior

Clinical Sign	When to Call	
	Monitor	Call Clinic
Appetite	Picky but still eating treats	Inappetance
Urination	Normal	Bloody urine
Bowel movements	Soft stool	Diarrhea
Vomiting	Single event	Frequent and retching
Attitude	Slightly lethargic	Lethargic and/or reluctant to move
Temperature	≤103° F	>103° F

2. Wear gloves when cleaning up urine, feces, or vomitus from your pet for 48 hours after receiving chemotherapy.

3. Maintain a low-stress environment.

4. Assure proper scheduling of chemotherapy and blood work visits.

OPHTHALMOLOGY

CHAPTER 6 / GENERAL MEDICINE 293

Table 6-16 Ophthalmology

DISEASE	Anterior Uveitis	Cataracts	Conjunctivitis
DEFINITION	Anterior uveitis is inflammation of the iris and ciliary body. Corneal ulceration, trauma, autoimmune, lens-induced, or infections can cause anterior uveitis, but the disease may also be primary.	Cataracts are pathologic changes in the eye that lead to opacity. The changes are in the lens protein composition or disruption of lens fiber arrangement. The general causes are hereditary, inflammatory, metabolic, traumatic, nutritional, or toxic.	Conjunctivitis is a general term for inflammation of the ocular mucous membrane that covers the sclera and lines the inner surface of the eyelids. Its causes can be infectious, foreign body, trauma, tear film deficiency, chemical or environmental irritants, immune-mediated, or caused by other eye diseases.
CLINICAL SIGNS	• Photophobia, blepharospasm and epiphora, hypotony, and aqueous flare • Conjunctival hyperemia, fibrinous exudate, miosis, and corneal edema • Blindness	• Any opacity in the lens of a dilated eye, aqueous flare, and synechia • Visual impairment or blindness	• Hyperemia, discharge, chemosis, pain, or tissue proliferation
DIAGNOSIS GENERAL	• Clinical signs • Ophthalmic examination	• History • Clinical signs • Ophthalmic examination	• History • Clinical signs • Ophthalmic examination
CBC	• Normal	• N/A	• N/A
BIOCHEMISTRY	• ↑ Globulin	• Normal or may reflect underlying disease	• N/A
URINALYSIS	• N/A	• N/A	• N/A
RADIOLOGY	• Thoracic: tumors or evidence of fungal disease • Abdominal: tumors	• N/A	• N/A

Table 6-16 Ophthalmology (Continued)

	DISEASE	Anterior Uveitis	Cataracts	Conjunctivitis
DIAGNOSIS	**MISCELLANEOUS**	• Ocular ultrasound: foreign body and penetrating wounds • Serology: toxoplasmosis, FeLV, FIP, and FIV • Tonometry: ↓ pressure or ↑ pressure when secondary to glaucoma	• Serology: systemic mycoses, rickettsial disease, brucellosis, toxoplasmosis, FeLV, and FIV • Electroretinogram: degree of retinal atrophy • Ocular ultrasound: retinal detachment • Tonometry: ↓ pressure	• Culture and sensitivity: bacteria or fungi recognition and identification • Schirmer tear test: ↓ tear production • Fluorescein stain: ulceration and nasolacrimal duct patency • Tonometry: ↑ pressure • Cytology: inflammation, neoplasia, viral or chlamydial infection • Biopsy: neoplasia or preocular mucin deficiency • Serology: FeLV or FIV
TREATMENT	**GENERAL**	• Symptomatic	• Supportive • Surgery: phacofragmentation, extracapsular extraction, and implantation of an intraocular lens • Laser surgery: capsulotomy	• Symptomatic • Surgery: keratectomy or removal of foreign body, hairs, or mass
	MEDICATION	• Antibiotics: clindamycin • Corticosteroids (systemic) : prednisone • Corticosteroids (topical): 1% prednisolone acetate or 0.1% dexamethasone • Mydriatic-cycloplegic: 1% atropine • NSAIDs: 0.03% flurbiprofen or 1% suprofen	• Corticosteroids: 1% prednisolone acetate	• Antibiotics (systemic): tetracycline, erythromycin, and chloramphenical • Antibiotics (topical): triple antibiotic or pilocarpine • Antiviral: trifluridine • Corticosteroids (systemic): megestrol acetate • Corticosteroids (topical): 1% dexamethasone • Lacrimostimulants • NSAIDs
	PATIENT CARE	• Treated as outpatient	• Treated as outpatient	• Irrigate the eye with an eyewash solution to remove any exudate • Clip the hair surrounding the eye • Apply an Elizabethan collar to prevent self-trauma

FOLLOW-UP

PATIENT CARE	• Reexamine 5–7 days after initiation of treatment then every 2–3 weeks • Monitor intraocular pressure	• Maintain the eyes clear of exudate • Examine 5–7 days after initiation of treatment and then as needed
PREVENTION/ AVOIDANCE	• N/A	• Vaccinate • Isolate patients with infectious conjunctivitis • Minimize stress for patients with herpetic conjunctivitis
COMPLICATIONS	• Blindness • Secondary glaucoma • Cataracts • Endophthalmitis or panophthalmitis • Iris atrophy • Lens luxation	• Corneal sequestration • Symblepharon • Keratoconjunctivitis sicca (KCS)
PROGNOSIS	• Depends on severity of disease on presentation	• Excellent with bacterial conjunctivitis • Fair with feline herpesvirus, immune-mediated diseases, or KCS
NOTES	• **Caution:** Corticosteroids are contraindicated in cases of primary conjunctivitis and corneal ulceration • It takes 2 months for the blood–aqueous barrier to completely heal after an insult; therefore, continue to treat for 2 months	• **Caution:** Differentiate from nuclear sclerosis, which is an increase in the clarity of the nucleus of the lens and is a normal aging process • Miniature poodles, American cocker spaniel, Miniature Schnauzers, Golden retrievers, Boston terriers, Siberian huskies, Persians, Birmans, Himalayans • **Caution:** Corticosteroids are contraindicated in cases of primary conjunctivitis and corneal ulceration

Table 6-16   Ophthalmology (Continued)

DISEASE	Entropion	Cilia Disorders (Distichiasis, Trichiasis, and Ectopic Cilia)	Glaucoma
DEFINITION	Entropion is the inward rolling of the eyelid, causing contact of the eyelashes or eyelid hair with the eye.	Cilia disorders are the abnormal location or positioning of the eyelashes. Trichiasis is cilia arising from normal sites that are directed toward the eye. Distichiasis is the growing of cilia from the meibomian glands and emergence from their ducts. Ectopic cilia are cilia that arise from the meibomian gland and erupt through the palpebral conjunctival surface.	Glaucoma is an increase in intraocular pressure with subsequent damage to the optic nerve. Chronic glaucoma is often caused by retinal and optic nerve degeneration and buphthalmos.
DIAGNOSIS			
CLINICAL SIGNS	• Conjunctivitis with serous discharge to blepharospasm with corneal ulceration and purulent discharge • Visual impairment or blindness • Corneal rupture	• Blepharospasm, epiphora, vascularization, and pigmentation • Hyperemia, discharge, chemosis, pain, or tissue proliferation	• Hyperemia, corneal edema, buphthalmos, dilated pupil, epiphora, and blepharospasm • ↓ Pupillary light response • Impaired vision or blindness • Weak to absent menace response
GENERAL	• History • Clinical signs • Ophthalmic examination	• History • Clinical signs • Ophthalmic examination	• History • Clinical signs • Ophthalmic examination
CBC	• N/A	• N/A	• Normal or may reflect underlying disease
BIOCHEMISTRY	• N/A	• N/A	• Normal or may reflect underlying disease
URINALYSIS	• N/A	• N/A	• Normal or may reflect underlying disease
RADIOLOGY	• N/A	• N/A	• Skull: fungi or neoplastic lesions
MISCELLANEOUS	• N/A	• N/A	• Tonometry: ↑ pressure, >25–30 mm Hg for dogs and >31 mm Hg for cats • Ocular ultrasound: structural abnormalities • Electroretinography: vision loss

TREATMENT			
GENERAL	• Surgery: correction of anatomic entropion or eyelid eversion suture technique	• Surgery: cryoepilation, electroepilation, tarsoconjunctival resection, facial fold resection, or medial canthal closure	• Supportive • Symptomatic • Surgery: cyclocryosurgery, intraocular prosthesis, or enucleation
MEDICATION	• Antibiotic (topical): triple antibiotic	• Antibiotics (topical): triple antibiotic	• Autonomic agents: pilocarpine 2%, epinephrine 1%, dipivefrin HCl 0.1%, or timolol maleate 0.5% • Carbonic anhydrase inhibitors: dichlorphenamide or methazolamide • Diuretics: 20% mannitol or glycerin
PATIENT CARE	• Treated as outpatient	• Treated as outpatient	• Warm, moist compresses twice daily for 5–7 days postoperatively • Monitor every 1–2 days for 1 week for improvement • Treat the other eye prophylactically daily with an autonomic agent
FOLLOW-UP			
PATIENT CARE	• Do not allow rubbing at eyes/sutures		• Treat swelling with topical antibiotics, corticosteroids or hypertonic saline
PREVENTION/ AVOIDANCE	• Selective breeding	• Clip hair on facial folds and around the eyes	• Yearly ophthalmic examination in predisposed breeds • Examinations 2–3 times a year on unaffected eye when one eye already has glaucoma
COMPLICATIONS	• Conjunctivitis • Impaired vision	• Recurrence • Conjunctivitis • Keratitis	• Blindness • Chronic ocular pain
PROGNOSIS	• Good	• Excellent with facial fold resection • Fair to good with hair removal	• Fair with surgery • Poor with medical treatment alone
NOTES	• Chow, Shar pei, and hunting dogs	• Cats do not have cilia, and dogs only normally have them on the upper eyelid	• Normal intraocular pressure is 15–25 mm Hg • 50% of animals develop glaucoma in the second eye within 8 months of the initial diagnosis • 40% of dogs will be blind in affected eye within 1 year, regardless of treatment • May take up to 6 weeks for vision to return

Table 6-16 Ophthalmology (Continued)

DISEASE	Keratitis		Keratoconjunctivitis Sicca (KCS, Dry Eye Syndrome)
	Nonulcerative	Ulcerative (Corneal Ulceration)	
DEFINITION	Keratitis is inflammation of the cornea with possible corneal erosion. It can be caused by trauma, foreign bodies, bacterial infection, irritant, cilia disorders, KCS, feline herpesvirus, or corneal exposure.	Ulceration is the loss of a full-thickness of epithelium with at least some stromal loss. This can be caused by trauma, bacterial infection, pseudomonas, feline herpesvirus, epithelial dystrophy, corneal dryness, neurotrophic keratitis, or complications from other diseases.	KCS is a lack of normal tear production, causing drying and inflammation of the cornea and conjunctiva. It is thought to be an immune-mediated disease against the lacrimal gland. It also can be caused by long-term use of sulfonamides.
CLINICAL SIGNS	• Tearing, squinting, rubbing at eyes, or photophobia • Corneal edema, prolapsed third eyelid, and hyperemia • Serous to mucopurulent discharge, blepharospasm, and neovascularization	• Blepharospasm, photophobia, epiphoria, and rubbing at eyes • Hyperemia, corneal opacity, surface depression, or corneal edema • Serous to mucopurulent discharge • Neovascularization • Miosis, aqueous flare, and hypotony	• Mucoid to mucopurulent discharge • Hyperemia, chemosis, thickened conjunctiva, periocular crust, and puritis • Cornea: dull, opaque, pigmentation, superficial vascularization, and ulceration • Blindness • Blepharospasm, photophobia, and eye rubbing
DIAGNOSIS			
GENERAL	• History • Clinical signs • Ophthalmic examination	• History • Clinical signs • Ophthalmic examination	• History • Clinical signs • Ophthalmic examination
CBC	• N/A	• N/A	• N/A
BIOCHEMISTRY	• N/A	• N/A	• N/A
URINALYSIS	• N/A	• N/A	• N/A
RADIOLOGY	• N/A	• N/A	• N/A
MISCELLANEOUS TREATMENT	• Schirmer tear test: ↓ production • Virus isolation: feline herpesvirus • Cytology: recognition and identification of bacterial • Symptomatic	• Culture and sensitivity: bacteria or fungi recognition and identification • Fluorescein stain: retention of stain • Virus isolation: + feline herpesvirus • Symptomatic	• Schirmer tear test: ↓ production, <10 mm/min • Flourescein stain: ulcer • Cytology: severity of bacterial overgrowth

		Column A	Column B	Column C
TREATMENT	**GENERAL**	• Symptomatic • Contact lenses • Plesiotherapy with strontium-90 generated beta-radiation • Surgery: debridement, laceration repair, keratotomy, keratectomy, superficial keratotomy, or conjunctival flap surgery	• Symptomatic • Debridement of ulcer edges • Surgery: conjunctival flap, tissue adhesion, pedicle flap, keratectomy, linear keratotomy, contact lenses, and collagen shields	• Symptomatic • Surgery: transposition of the parotid salivary duct
	MEDICATION	• 2% Cyclosporine • Antibiotics: chloramphenicol, tobramycin, erythromycin, triple antibiotic, or gentamicin • Antiviral: trifluridine or idoxuridine • Atropine • Mucolytics: acetylcysteine • NSAIDs: aspirin	• Antibiotics (systemic): variable • Antibiotics (topical): gentamicin, tobramycin, and triple antibiotic	• Antibiotics: variable • Artificial tears supplementation • Cyclosporine • Mucolytics: acetylcysteine • Tear stimulants: pilocarpine
	PATIENT CARE	• Treated as outpatient	• Restrict activity with deep ulcer to prevent rupture • Apply an Elizabethan collar to prevent self-trauma	• Clean eyes regularly to keep them clear of discharge
FOLLOW-UP	**PATIENT CARE**	• Examination every 1–2 weeks to monitor progress until resolved	• Monitor healing process with flourescein stain every 1–2 days until improvement is seen	• Monitor Schirmer tear test every 2–4 weeks until normal • Clean eyes regularly to keep them clear of discharge
	PREVENTION/ AVOIDANCE	• N/A	• Lubricant ointment administration in brachycephalic dogs • Continuous treatment with KCS	• N/A
	COMPLICATIONS	• KCS • Keratitis, ulcerative • Blindness	• Desmetocele • Chronic ophthalmitis • Glaucoma • Rupture of globe • Endophthalmitis • Blindness • Phthisis bulbi	• Keratitis, ulcerative
	PROGNOSIS	• Dependent on severity of disease, may require life-long treatment	• Fair to good: may take several weeks to heal	• Good with lifelong treatment

Table 6-16 Ophthalmology (Continued)

DISEASE	Keratitis		Keratoconjunctivitis Sicca (KCS, Dry Eye Syndrome)
	Nonulcerative	Ulcerative (Corneal Ulceration)	
NOTES		• **Caution:** Corticosteroids are contraindicated in cases of primary conjunctivitis and corneal ulceration	• Schirmer tear test: at least 15 mm/min of wetting • Acetylcysteine 5% is mixed 1:1 with artificial tears for ophthalmic use • Cocker spaniels, Bulldogs, West Highland terrier, Lhaso apsos, Miniature Schnauzers, and Shih tzus

DISEASE	Lens Luxation	Prolapsed Gland of the Third Eyelid (Cherry Eye)
DEFINITION	Lens luxation is the actual movement of the lens either anteriorly or posteriorly. Often caused by glaucoma, uveitis, cataracts, trauma, or primary zonular degeneration	Cherry eye is caused by a weak attachment to the nictitating membrane gland, allowing it to protrude/prolapse from the leading edge of the third eyelid.
CLINICAL SIGNS	• Corneal edema, iridonesis, hyperemia, aphakic crescent, and pain	• Conjunctivitis, blepharospasms, epiphora, or hyperemia • Appearance of swelling at medial canthus
GENERAL	• Clinical signs • Ophthalmic examination	• History • Clinical signs
CBC	• Normal or may reflect underlying disease	• N/A
BIOCHEMISTRY	• Normal or may reflect underlying disease	• N/A
URINALYSIS	• Normal or may reflect underlying disease	• N/A
RADIOLOGY	• Thoracic: metastasis from intraocular neoplasia	• N/A
MISCELLANEOUS	• Wood's lamp: fluorescence of a clear lens • Tonometry: glaucoma • Ocular ultrasound: structural abnormalities	• N/A

DIAGNOSIS

TREATMENT	**GENERAL**	• Supportive (posterior luxation) • Surgery (anterior luxation): cyclocryosurgery, evisceration, intrascleral prosthesis, or enucleation	• Surgery: repositioning of the nictitating membrane gland and anchoring securely
	MEDICATION	• 1% Tropicamide • 2% Pilocarpine • Carbonic anhydrase inhibitors: dichlorphenamide • Corticosteroids (topical): 0.1% dexamethasone • Mannitol	• Antibiotics: variable • Corticosteroids (topical): 1% dexamethasone
	PATIENT CARE	• Treated as outpatient	• Standard postoperative care
FOLLOW-UP	**PATIENT CARE**	• Examine within 24 hours and then frequently after that until intraocular pressure stabilizes • Examine every 3 months	• Do not allow rubbing at eyes/sutures
	PREVENTION/ AVOIDANCE	• Selective breeding	• Selective breeding
	COMPLICATIONS	• Uveitis • Corneal edema • Dyscoria • Blindness • Synechia • Glaucoma • Retinal detachment • Vitreous entrapment in the incision	• Reprolapse of the gland • Infection at surgery site
	PROGNOSIS	• Good with surgery	• Excellent with surgery
	NOTES	• **Caution:** Pupil should not be dilated with acute anterior lens luxation • Poodles, Shar peis, Whippet, Norwegian Elkhound, and terriers	• Cocker spaniels, Bulldogs, Pitbull terriers, Beagles, Bloodhounds, Lhasa apsos, Shih tzus, and Shar peis

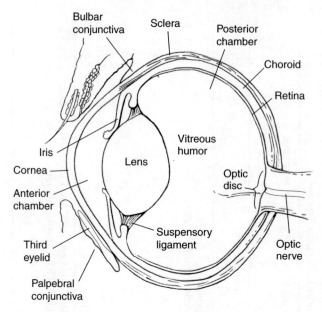

Figure 6-6 Eye

UROLOGY

Table 6-17 Urology

DISEASE	Cystic Calculi (Urocystoliths)	Feline Lower Urinary Tract Disease (FLUTD) (Feline Urologic Syndrome, FUS)	Pyelonephritis (Upper Urinary Tract Infection)
DEFINITION	Any macroscopic concretions found within the urinary bladder are called cystic calculi. They can be found anywhere along the urinary tract but are most commonly seen in the urinary bladder.	FLUTD is inflammation of the lower urinary tract, including the bladder and urethra. It is typically idiopathic. It can also occur secondarily to bacterial infection, crystalluria, or iatrogenic (e.g., urinary catheterization).	Pyelonephritis is inflammation of the renal parenchyma, collecting diverticula, ureters, and its pelves. It is typically used to refer to a "kidney infection." Most commonly secondary to bacterial invasion.
CLINICAL SIGNS	• Dehydration • Dysuria, stranguria, pollakuria, and hematuria • Malodorous or cloudy urine • Abdominal discomfort • Recurrent bacterial UTI	• Licking at perineal area and straining to urinate • Hematuria, polyuria, pollakiuria, periuria, dysuria, or anuria • Thickened, firm, contracted bladder wall	• Lethargy, anorexia, fever, vomiting, and dehydration • PU/PD • Lumbar or abdominal pain • Malodorous or discolored urine • Dysuria, pollakiuria, hematuria, and stranguria
GENERAL	• History • Clinical signs • Bladder palpation (variable)	• History • Clinical signs • Abdominal palpation: bladder • Perineal examination	• History • Clinical signs • Abdominal palpation: kidney
CBC	• Normal or may reflect an underlying disease	• Normal or may reflect an underlying disease	• Neutrophilic leukocytosis with a left shift (variable) • Nonregenerative anemia
BIOCHEMISTRY	• Normal or may reflect an underlying disease • ↑Potassium, BUN, and creatinine • Metabolic acidosis	• Normal or may reflect an underlying disease	• ↑BUN, creatinine, and phosphorus
URINALYSIS	• Bacteria and crystals • Change in pH, depending on type of crystal • Urine culture: recognition and identification of bacteria	• Pyuria, blood, bacteria, and crystals • Urine culture: recognition and identification of bacteria	• Pyuria, bacteria, blood, protein, and leukocyte casts • ↓Specific gravity • Urine culture: recognition and identification of bacteria

DIAGNOSIS (row group label)

Table 6-17 Urology (Continued)

DISEASE	Cystic Calculi (Urocystoliths)	Feline Lower Urinary Tract Disease (FLUTD) (Feline Urologic Syndrome, FUS)	Pyelonephritis (Upper Urinary Tract Infection)
DIAGNOSIS			
RADIOLOGY	• Abdominal: radiopaque calculi • Contrast: radiolucent calculi and vesicourachal diverticula	• Abdominal: anatomic abnormalities, calculi, urethral plugs, tumors, or urachal diverticula • Contrast: urethral strictures, tumors, radiolucent uroliths, or vesicourachal diverticula	• Abdominal: ↑ size of kidneys and contours (variable)
MISCELLANEOUS	• Bile acids or ammonia concentration: ↑ with ammonium urate calculi and portosystemic shunts • Ultrasound: all types of calculi • Stone analysis and bacterial culture: needed for long-term treatment	• Ultrasound: anatomic abnormalities, calculi, tumors, or urachal diverticula	• Ultrasound: dilation of renal pelves and proximal ureter, kidney size, and nephrolithiasis • Pyelocentesis: bacteria and neutrophils
TREATMENT			
GENERAL	• Symptomatic • Medical dissolution (struvite only) • Urohydropulsion • Surgery	• Symptomatic	• Symptomatic • Surgery: nephrotomy • Lithotripsy (rare)
MEDICATION	• Allopurinol (ammonium urate) • Antibiotics: variable • MPG or D-penicillamine (cystine) • Urine alkalinizer: potassium citrate	• Analgesics: butorphanol • Antibiotics: variable • Anticholinergics: propantheline • Glycosaminoglycan: pentosan polysulfate sodium • Phenoxybenzamine • Tranquilizers: diazepam • Tricyclic antidepressant: amitriptyline • Urine acidifier: DL-methionine, ammonium chloride	• Antibiotics: variable
PATIENT CARE	• Access to clean litter box or frequent walks • Monitor for anuria	• Access to clean litter box or frequent walks • Monitor for anuria • Treated as outpatient	• Access to clean litter box or frequent walks • Treated as outpatient

FOLLOW-UP

PATIENT CARE	• Monitor urine pH and specific gravity • Strict diet restrictions, depending on type of calculi* • Monitor dissolution monthly by radiographs, urinalysis, urine culture, and ultrasonography • Monitor radiographs every 3–4 months on patients with surgical removal for recurrence	• ↑ Water consumption by feeding canned food mixed with water, adding sodium chloride to the food or subcutaneous fluids • Monitor males for urethral obstruction	• Perform a urinalysis and urine culture 7–14 days after initiation of antibiotic to verify its efficacy • Perform a urinalysis and urine culture 7 days and 28 days after completing the antibiotics
PREVENTION/ AVOIDANCE	• Strict diet restrictions, depending on type of calculi* • Monitor urine pH	• Acidifying or low-magnesium diet • Avoid stress • Encourage water consumption • Maintain a clean litter box	• Correct ectopic ureters
COMPLICATIONS	• Recurrence • Urethral obstruction • Secondary bacterial UTI	• Urethral obstruction (male cats)** • Recurrence	• Chronic renal failure • Recurrence • Nephrolithiasis • Septicemia or septic shock • Metastatic infection
PROGNOSIS	• Excellent with treatment	• Excellent	• Fair to good: may have irreversible kidney damage

NOTES	• Calculi and urine pH
	  —Struvite: alkaline urine
	  —Ammonium urate and silica: neutral to acid urine
	  —Cystine: acid urine
	  —Calcium oxalate: any urine pH		

*See Table 3-12, Disease and Their Nutritional Requirements
**See Chapter 5, Emergency Care

Table 6-17 Urology (Continued)

DISEASE	Renal Failure		Urinary Tract Infection (Cystitis, Urethrocystitis)
	Acute, (ARF)	Chronic, (CRF)	
DEFINITION	Acute renal failure is a rapid decline in renal function. It is the accumulation of uremic toxins caused by filtration failure, dysregulation of fluids, electrolytes, and acid–base balances. Unlike CRF, this condition may be reversible if diagnosed quickly and treated aggressively.	Chronic renal failure is the progressive decline in the function of the kidneys leading to their shutdown over months to years. The damage is irreversible. The causes may be familial, toxins, infections, neoplasia, or infectious disease.	Urinary tract infection is usually a bacteria-induced inflammation of the lower urinary tract, including the bladder and urethra. The cause is an ascending bacterial infection that is from the urethral orifice or hematogenous.
CLINICAL SIGNS	• Anorexia, lethargy, depression, dehydration, vomiting, and diarrhea • Hypothermia or fever • Oral ulceration and halitosis • Oliguria, polyuria, or anuria • Tachypnea and bradycardia • Enlarged painful kidneys and nonpalpable urinary bladder • Ataxia and seizures	• Lethargy, anorexia, vomiting, diarrhea, constipation, dehydration, weakness, and exercise intolerance • Oral ulceration and halitosis • PU/PD and nocturia • Small, firm nodular kidneys • Subcutaneous edema or ascites • Blindness • Seizures and coma	• Malodorous, cloudy urine and hematuria • Dysuria, pollakiuria, stranguria, periuria, or urinary incontinence • Thickened, firm contracted bladder wall
GENERAL	• History • Clinical signs • Abdominal palpation: kidney	• History • Clinical signs • Abdominal palpation: kidney	• History: recent catheterization or urinary tract surgery • Clinical signs • Abdominal palpation: kidneys and bladder • Digital rectal examination: prostate in males
CBC	• Leukocytosis with or without a left shift (variable) • Lymphopenia • Monocytosis • ↑ PCV • Nonregenerative anemia (variable)	• Nonregenerative anemia	• Normal or may reflect underlying disease

DIAGNOSIS

DIAGNOSIS	**BIOCHEMISTRY**	• ↑ Protein, BUN, creatinine, phosphate, glucose, and potassium • ↓ Calcium and bicarbonate • Metabolic acidosis	• ↑ Protein, BUN, creatinine, amylase, lipase, and phosphate • ↓ Potassium • ± Calcium • Metabolic acidosis	• Normal or may reflect underlying disease
	URINALYSIS	• Pyuria, bacteria, crystals, and casts (e.g., cellular and granular) • ↑ Protein and glucose • ↓ Specific gravity • Urine culture: recognition and identification of bacteria if present	• Protein (variable) • ↑ Specific gravity • Protein:creatinine ratio: to determine severity of proteinuria and glomerular disease • Urine culture: recognition and identification of bacteria	• Pyuria, blood, protein, and bacteria • Urine culture: recognition and identification of bacteria
	RADIOLOGY	• Abdominal: renal size and shape and renal uroliths • Contrast: obstruction or structural rupture	• Abdominal: renal size and shape and renal uroliths • Contrast: obstruction or structural rupture	• Abdominal: anatomic abnormalities, calculi, tumors, or urachal diverticula • Contrast: radiolucent calculi
	MISCELLANEOUS	• Serology: leptospirosis or ehrlichiosis • Eythlene glycol concentration: + results • Ultrasound: renal uroliths and parenchymal and anatomic abnormalities • Biopsy: confirmation, cause, and severity of disease	• Biopsy: confirmation, cause and severity of disease • Blood pressure: ↑ values	• Ultrasound: anatomic abnormalities, calculi, tumors, or urachal diverticula • Prostatic fluid analysis: bacteria and neutrophils
TREATMENT	**GENERAL**	• Symptomatic • Supportive • Fluid therapy • Peritoneal dialysis • Blood transfusions • Poison antidotes (e.g., ethylene glycol) • Renal transplantation	• Symptomatic • Supportive • Fluid therapy • Peritoneal dialysis • Blood transfusions • Renal transplantation	• Symptomatic

Table 6-17 Urology (Continued)

DISEASE	Renal Failure — Acute (ARF)	Renal Failure — Chronic, (CRF)	Urinary Tract Infection (Cystitis, Urethrocystitis)
TREATMENT — MEDICATION	• Antiemetics: trimethobenzamide or chlorpromazine • Calcium gluconate • Dopamine • Diuretics: 20% mannitol, 20% dextrose, or furosemide • H$_2$-receptor antagonist: cimetidine or rantidine • Phosphate binders: aluminum hydroxide, aluminum carbonate, calcium carbonate, or calcium acetate • Potassium chloride • Sodium bicarbonate • Vasodilators: dopamine	• ACE inhibitors: enalapril or amlodipine • Androgens: stanozolol, nandrolone decanoate • Calcitriol • Erythropoietin • H$_2$-receptor antagonist: cimetidine or rantidine • Phosphate binders: aluminum hydroxide, aluminum carbonate, calcium carbonate, or calcium acetate • Potassium chloride or potassium gluconate • Sodium bicarbonate	• Antibiotics: variable
TREATMENT — PATIENT CARE	• Nutritional support • Monitor urine output, hydration, temperature, and body weight • Monitor PCV and blood values • Monitor fluid therapy for overhydration	• Treated as outpatient	• Treated as outpatient
FOLLOW-UP — PATIENT CARE	• Monitor blood values until normal	• Restrict protein, phosphorus, and sodium in the diet • n-3 Fatty acids supplementation • Fresh water at all times to increase water consumption • Subcutaneous fluids for diuresis and hydration • Nutritional support • Monitor weekly initially then monitor hydration, weight, and blood values every 1–4 months, depending on severity of CRF	• Recheck urinalysis and urine culture 5–7 days after completing antibiotics • Allow frequent access to outdoors

FOLLOW-UP

PREVENTION/ AVOIDANCE	• Anticipate ARF in susceptible animals and conduct preventative fluids and medication • Avoid use of nephrotoxic drugs • Restrict exposure to antifreeze • Maintain adequate blood pressure during anesthesia, especially in prolonged procedures and older animals	• Anticipate ARF in susceptible animals and conduct preventive fluids and medication • Avoid use of nephrotoxic drugs • Maintain adequate blood pressure during anesthesia • Selective breeding	• Avoid glucocorticoid use or urethral catheterization
COMPLICATIONS	• Seizures or coma • Cardiac arrhythmias, congestive heart failure, pulmonary edema, uremic pneumonitis, or cardiopulmonary arrest • Gastrointestinal bleed • Hypovolemia, sepsis, and death	• Hypertension • Anemia • Gastroenteritis • Urinary tract infection • Uremic stomatitis • Dehydration and constipation • Weight loss	• Pyelonephritis • Cystic calculi • Recurrence
PROGNOSIS	• Guarded to poor, but depends on severity and cause of disease	• Guarded to poor long-term because of progression of disease	• Excellent
NOTES	• Urine output: —Anuria: ≤0.1 mL/kg/hr —Oliguria: ≤0.25 mL/kg/hr —Nonoliguria: ≥2 mL/kg/hr	• Approximately 75% of the kidney must be nonfunctional before an elevation in serum BUN and creatinine is seen	• Significant bacteria count: Canine Feline Cystocentesis ≥1000 ≥1,000 Catheter ≥10,000 ≥1,000 Voided ≥100,000 ≥10,000 Expressed ≥100,000 ≥10,000

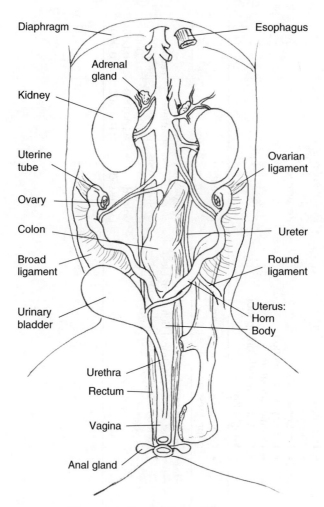

Figure 6-7 Female urogenital system.

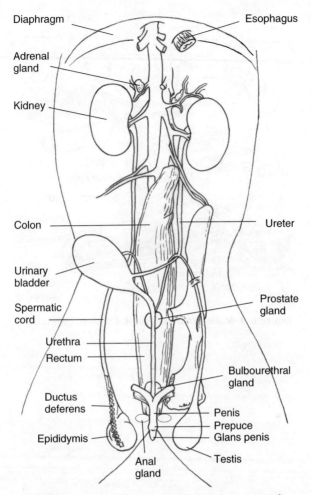

Figure 6-8 Male feline urogenital system (ventral).

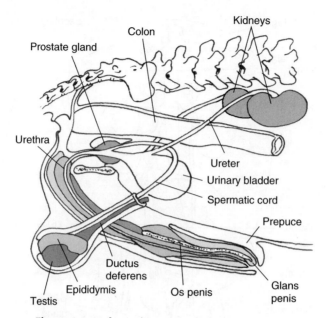

Figure 6-9 Male canine urogenital system (lateral).

Laboratory

Proficiency in laboratory skills is one of the most important needs of a veterinary hospital. Each clinic will use their laboratory to different levels, but the proper technique and understanding of each procedure should always be maintained for the most accurate results. The key to beginning the learning process of laboratory skills is to be able to recognize the normal. Having a clear understanding of what is normal allows a person to more quickly identify the abnormal.

This chapter covers two aspects to laboratory medicine. The first is proper technique to be followed in the clinic either to accomplish the laboratory task in-house or to prepare the sample to send out to a reference laboratory. The second is client education. General information is provided to allow technicians to educate clients and alleviate misunderstandings and fears.

Laboratory medicine is a critical part of each diagnosis, and this process often begins with the technician.

BLOOD CHEMISTRIES

Blood chemistries evaluate the various blood levels to reach an insight into the different bodily functions. The critical part of blood chemistries is the collection and handling of each sample. For example, allowing a blood sample to remain at room temperature may elevate some chemistries and decrease others, leading to a possible incorrect diagnosis, treatment, and outcome. Extreme care and diligence should be taken with each sample to ensure the most accurate results.

The normals for this chapter are used with permission from Phoenix Central Laboratory.

Blood Collection, Handling, Storage, and Transport Tips

Collection:

- Blood samples should be collected from a fasted patient, at least 2 hours postprandial, but preferably 4–6 hours.
- When feasible, enough blood should be collected to run the tests three times; this allows for human error, machine error, and dilution if needed.
- Always remove the needle to the syringe and the stopper of the tube to let the blood run down the inside of the tube. Sticking a needle through the rubber stopper contributes to further hemolysis, especially with a ≤25-gauge needle.

Handling:

- Gently mix any tube containing an interactive ingredient, to avoid hemolysis.
- Blood smears should be made immediately, using fresh blood after blood collection and allowed to dry at room temperature. (See Skill Box 7-6, Smear Techniques)
- Allow blood to clot in an upright position to prevent cells from sticking to rubber stopper and hemolyzing during centrifuging.
- Remove serum from contact with the cells within 30–45 minutes, to prevent altered laboratory results.
- Each tube should be clearly labeled with the patient's full name, date, and time of collection.

Storage:

- If a sample will not be evaluated in 4–6 hours, the plasma or serum should be poured off and refrigerated.
- Do not freeze whole blood, because this causes hemolysis.
- Samples to be frozen should be immediately placed in an ice bath, centrifuged, transferred into a plastic tube, and frozen.

Transport:

- Wrap ice packs or blood tubes with paper towels or newspapers to avoid direct contact and subsequent hemolysis.

Skill Box 7-1 / Blood Collection Tubes

Tube	Contents	Uses	General Information
Whole Blood (unclotted) or Plasma Samples • *Immediately invert tubes 6–10 times to prevent coagulation*			
Gray Top Tube, GTT	Potassium oxalate Sodium fluoride	• Glucose determinations	• Binds with glucose to more accurately measure blood glucose concentrations than an SST or RTT (e.g., diabetes mellitus and insulinoma)
Green Top Tube, GRNTT	Lithium heparin	• Lead determinations	• Binds with lead • Not appropriate for cell morphology
Lavender Top Tube, LTT	EDTA	• Hematology smears	• Does not alter cell morphology
Light Blue Top Tube, BTT	Buffered sodium citrate	• Coagulation determinations	• Measures clotting time (e.g., von Willebrand's disease, warfarin poisoning, activated partial thromboplastin time [APTT], and prothrombin time [PT]) • Must be a perfect venipuncture stick to avoid activation of coagulation pathways • Tube must be filled to assure proper dilution of blood with anticoagulant
Serum Samples • *Invert tube to activate clotting, stand upright for 20 minutes, and then centrifuge for 15 minutes to ensure proper separation*			
Serum Separator Tube, SST, Red/ Gray Swirl Top	Clot activator Polymer gel	• Blood chemistries	• Serum is not able to mix with clotted blood once centrifuged • The clotting activator can interfere with some lab tests (e.g., phenobarbital levels)
Red, RTT	Plain	• Blood chemistries, serology and blood banking	• Serum and clotted blood can resuspend if the tube is tilted

EDTA = Ethylenediaminetetra-acetic acid

To determine the amount of fluid in a sample, evaluate a well-hydrated patient's packed cell volume (PCV). A PCV of 50% will yield a sample with 50% cells and 50% fluid. Therefore, a 10-mL sample will yield 5 mL fluid.

Table 7-1 Blood Chemistries

Chemistry	Definition	Normal Range	Associated Conditions	Handling and Special Considerations
Alanine aminotransferase (ALT, SGPT)	*Source* • Major: hepatocytes • Minor: cardiac muscle, skeletal muscle, and pancreas *Role* • Amino acid metabolism *Notes* • Liver specific • There is a correlation between ALT levels and hepatic cell damage, but not liver function	*Canine/Feline* 5–65 U/L	(↑)Cholangitis/cholangiohepatitis, congestive heart failure, diabetes mellitus, dilated cardiomyopathy, canine/feline, ehrlichiosis, endocardiosis, exocrine pancreatic insufficiency, feline hypertrophic cardiomyopathy, hepatic disease/failure, hepatic lipidosis, hyperparathyroidism, hypertension, hyperthyroidism, hypoadrenocorticism, pancreatitis, peritonitis, pyometra, Rocky Mountain spotted fever, thrombocytopenia, toxoplasmosis	*Handling* • Hemolysis and lipemia; ↑ values *Storage* • Room temperature or refrigerator for 24 hours • 2 days at 68° F • 1 week at 32°–39° F • Do not freeze sample *Notes* • Corticosteroids and anticonvulsants; ± ↑ values (dog)
Albumin	*Source* • Hepatocytes *Role* • Maintaining osmotic pressure by retaining fluid within the vascular compartment • Binding and transport protein *Notes* • Edema and effusions = ↓ values • 35%–50% of total plasma protein • Best interpreted with globulin levels	*Canine* 2.3–4.0 g/dL *Feline* 2.6–4.0 g/dL *Danger level* 1.0	(↑)Rocky Mountain spotted fever (↓)Brucellosis, cholangitis/cholangiohepatitis, ehrlichiosis, heartworm disease, hepatic disease/failure, hepatic lipidosis, glomerular disease, hyperglobulinemia, hypertension, inflammatory bowel disease, pleural effusion, protein losing enteropathy, toxoplasmosis	*Handling* • Extreme hemolysis and lipemia; ↓ values *Storage* • Keep sample covered to prevent dehydration; ↑ values • 1 week at 68° F • 1 month at 32–39° F *Notes* • Ampicillin; ± falsely ↑ values
Albumin-to-Globulin ratio (A:G ratio)	*Source* See Albumin and Globulin *Role* See Albumin and Globulin *Notes* • First indicator of protein abnormality • Divide the albumin concentration by the globulin concentration	*Canine* 0.6–1.2 *Feline* 0.5–2.0		*Handling* See Albumin and Globulin *Storage* See Albumin and Globulin *Notes* See Albumin and Globulin

			Handling
Alkaline phosphatase (Alk phos, ALP, SAP)	*Source* • Major: liver (adult animals) and bone (young animals) • Minor: kidneys and intestines *Role* • Assist in various chemical reactions *Notes* • Dogs can often handle a 2–4-fold increase in value before significant signs of disease • Interpretation is slightly different between dogs and cats because of half-lives and amount of hepatic ALP present	*Canine* 10–84 U/L *Feline* 10–70 U/L	(↑)Cholangitis/cholangiohepatitis, congestive heart failure, diabetes mellitus, drugs (glucocorticoids, barbituates, etc.) ehrlichiosis, hepatic disease/failure, hepatic lipidosis, hyperadrenocorticism, hyperparathyroidism, hypertension, hyperthyroidism, pancreatitis, pyometra, Rocky Mountain spotted fever, thrombocytopenia, toxoplasmosis	*Handling* • Do not use EDTA or oxalate coagulants *Storage* • At room temperature >24 hours; ↑ values • 8 days at 32°–39° F *Notes* • N/A
Ammonia	*Source* • Liver and muscle *Role* • Byproduct of the breakdown of proteins, amines, amino acids, nucleic acids, and urea *Notes* • N/A	*Canine* 45–120 μg/dL *Feline* 30–100 μg/dL *Danger level* >1,000 (canine)	(↑)Cholangitis/cholangiohepatitis, hepatic disease/failure, hepatic lipidosis	*Handling* • Heparinized sample preferred • Centrifuge and pour off plasma immediately *Storage* • Store on ice and assay within 1 hour • Freeze immediately and assay within 2 days *Notes* • Vein occlusion for an extended period or strenuous exercise; ↑ values • Antibiotics, enemas, lactulose, diphenhydramine, parenteral amino acids, narcotics, diuretics, or blood transfusions may alter laboratory results

Table 7-1 Blood Chemistries (Continued)

Chemistry	Definition	Normal Range	Associated Conditions	Handling and Special Considerations
Amylase	*Source* • Major: pancreas • Minor: liver and small intestines *Role* • Breakdown of starches and glycogen in sugars *Notes* • ↑ values are not always indicative of severity of disease nor specific for pancreas	*Canine* 300–1,500 units *Feline* 500–1,500 units	(↑)Pancreatitis, peritonitis, chronic renal failure, toxoplasmosis	*Handling* • Hemolysis; ↑ values • Lipemia; ↓ values • Do not use EDTA *Storage* • 7 days at 68° F • 1 month at 32°–39° F *Notes* • Corticosteroids; ± ↓ values • Saccharogenic method; ± false ↑ values (dogs)
Anion Gap (AG)	*Source* • N/A *Role* • To differentiate causes of metabolic acidosis *Notes* • To calculate: $(Na^+ + K^+) - (Cl^- + HCO_3) = AG$	*Canine* 12–25 *Feline* 13–25		*Handling* • Refer to Na^+, K^+, Cl^-, and HCO_3 *Storage* • Refer to Na^+, K^+, Cl^-, and HCO_3 *Notes* • Drugs used in combination may blunt the gap ↑
Aspartate aminotransferase (AST, SGOT)	*Source* • Major: hepatocytes • Minor: cardiac and skeletal muscles, kidneys, pancreas and erythrocytes *Role* • Amino acid metabolism *Notes* • Not liver-specific; ↑ values may indicate liver damage, strenuous exercise, or IM injections • Tends to parallel ALT values when caused by liver disease	*Canine* 16–60 u/L *Feline* 26–43 u/L	(↑)Cholangitis/cholangiohepatitis, congestive heart failure, diabetes mellitus, endocardiosis, feline dilated cardiomyopathy, feline hypertrophic cardiomyopathy, hepatic disease/failure, hepatic lipidosis, hyperthyroidism, hypoadrenocorticism, peritonitis, toxoplasmosis	*Handling* • Hemolysis and lipemia; ↑ values *Storage* • 2 days at 68° F • 2 weeks at 32°–39° F *Notes* • N/A

Analyte	Source / Role / Notes	Reference Values	Increase/Decrease	Handling / Storage / Notes
Bicarbonate (Venous TCO_2)	**Source** • All cells **Role** • Aids in transport of CO_2 from tissues to the lungs • Bicarbonate/carbonic acid buffer system **Notes** • 95% of total CO_2 measured	*Canine/Feline* 21–31 mEq/L	(↓)Metabolic acidosis, acute renal failure	**Handling** • Chill in ice water to prevent alteration of acid–base composition **Storage** • Do not freeze, because it results in hemolysis **Notes** N/A
Bilirubin	**Source** • Hemoglobin via liver processing **Role** • N/A **Notes** • Byproduct of erythrocyte degradation • Total bilirubin is composed of conjugated and unconjugated bilirubin • Not liver specific	*Canine/Feline* 0.0–0.5 mg/dL	(↑)Cholangitis/cholangiohepatitis, hepatic disease/failure, hemobartonellosis, hemolytic anemia, hepatic lipidosis, hyperthyroidism, pancreatitis, peritonitis, toxoplasmosis	**Handling** • Lipemia; ↑ values **Storage** • Not stable when stored in the light or at 68° F • 2 weeks at 32°–39° F in the dark **Notes** • Total bilirubin may ↓ by 50%/hr with direct exposure to sunlight or artificial light
Blood Urea Nitrogen (BUN, SUN)	**Source** • Amino acids via liver processing **Role** • N/A **Notes** • Byproduct of amino acid breakdown • 75% of the kidney must be nonfunctional before ↑ values are seen	*Canine* 6–29 mg/dL *Feline* 10–35 mg/dL	(↑)Canine/feline dilated cardiomyopathy, congestive heart failure, cystic calculi, ehrlichiosis, endocardiosis, hepatic disease/failure, hypertension, hyperthyroidism, hypoadrenocorticism, mastitis, pancreatitis, pyelonephritis, renal failure, Rocky Mountain spotted fever (↓) Cholangitis/cholangiohepatitis, hepatic disease/failure, hepatic lipidosis, overhydration, dietary protein restriction	**Handling** • N/A **Storage** • 8 hours at 68° F • 10 days at 32°–39° F **Notes** • 18-hour fast is recommended, because high-protein diets can cause ↑ values

Table 7-1 Blood Chemistries (Continued)

Chemistry	Definition	Normal Range	Associated Conditions	Handling and Special Considerations
Calcium	*Source* • Bones *Role* • Maintenance of neuromuscular excitability and tone • Inorganic ion transfer across cell membranes • Blood coagulation *Notes* • Hemoglobin and bilirubin; ↑ values with chlorimetric test methods • Hypoalbuminemia; ↓ values	*Canine/Feline* 8.0–12.0 mg/dL *Danger level* ≤7.0 mg/dL or ≥16.0 mg/dL	(↑) Hyperparathyroidism, hypoadrenocorticism, neoplasia, renal failure (↓) Dystocia, eclampsia, hypoparathyroidism, pancreatitis, protein losing enteropathy, renal failure	*Handling* • Hemolysis and contact with cork stoppers; ↓ values • Lipemia; ↑ values • Citrate, oxalate, or EDTA anticoagulants; ↓ values *Storage* • 10 days at 68° F or 32-39° F *Notes* N/A
Chloride	*Source* • Extracellular fluid *Role* • Acid-base balance • Maintenance of water distribution • Osmotic pressure in blood *Notes* • Hemoglobin and bilirubin; ↑ values with chlorimetric test methods • Tends to parallel serum sodium	*Canine* 100-115 mEq/L *Feline* 117-128 mEq/L	(↑) Metabolic acidosis (↓) Canine dilated cardiomyopathy, constipation, aggressive diuretics, severe emesis, rocky mountain spotted fever	*Handling* • Hemolysis and lipemia; ↓ values *Storage* • Stable if separated from blood cells *Notes* • Potassium bromide, acetazolamide, ammonium chloride, androgens, cholestyramine, lithium, demeclocycline and amphotericin; ↑ values
Cholesterol	*Source* Major: hepatocytes Minor: adrenal cortex, ovaries, testes and intestinal epithelium *Role* • Steroid hormone production *Notes* • Helpful in screening for hypothyroidism and Cushings Disease	*Canine* 150-275 mg/dL *Feline* 75-175 mg/dL	(↑) Diabetes mellitus, hepatic disease/failure, hyperadrenocorticism, hypertension, hypoadrenocorticism, hypothyroidism, pancreatitis, Rocky Mountain spotted fever (↓) Drugs, exocrine pancreatic insufficiency, hepatic disease/failure, protein losing enteropathy (↑) Encephalitis, feline dilated cardi-	*Handling* • Hemolysis, fluoride, and oxalate; ± ↑ values, depending on testing method *Storage* • Very stable at 68° F if separated from blood cells *Notes* • Corticosteroids; ± ↑ values

Analyte	Details	Reference	Clinical Significance	Handling/Storage/Notes
Creatine Kinase (CK)	**Source** • Cardiac and skeletal muscle and brain tissue **Role** • Enzyme that cleaves creatine in muscle for energy utilization **Notes** • Peaks 12 hours after muscle injury and returns to normal in 24 hours unless damage is ongoing • Very specific, but almost too sensitive • Only large ↑ are clinically significant (≥10,000 U/L) or chronic elevations (≥2,000 U/L) indicating ongoing muscle damage	Canine/Feline 50–300 U/L	(↑) Encephalitis, feline dilated cardiomyopathy, feline hypertrophic cardiomyopathy, hypothyroidism, myasthenia gravis, polymyositis	**Handling** • Severe hemolysis, icterus, ↑ values • EDTA, citrate, fluoride, exposure to sunlight, and delayed analysis; ↓ values **Storage** • Not stable, do not freeze; analyze as soon as possible **Notes** • Exercise, recumbency, IM injections; ± ↑ values
Creatinine	**Source** • Skeletal muscle **Role** • N/A **Notes** • Byproduct of creatine degradation • 75% of the kidney must be nonfunctional before ↑ values are seen	Canine 0.6–1.6 mg/dL Feline 1.0–2.0 mg/dL	(↑) Canine/feline dilated cardiomyopathy, congestive heart failure, drugs, ehrlichiosis, endocardiosis, hypertension, hyperthyroidism, hypoadrenocorticism, severe muscle damage, pancreatitis, pyelonephritis, renal failure, Rocky Mountain spotted fever, toxoplasmosis	**Handling** • N/A **Storage** • 1 week at 86°–98.6° F **Notes** • Exercise, active muscle wasting, and meal containing meat; mild ↑ values
Fibrinogen	**Source** • Hepatocytes **Role** • Clot formation **Notes** • No fibrinogen found in serum, because it is removed from the plasma by the clotting process • Used mostly in cattle and horses	Canine 100–245 mg/dL Feline 110–370 mg/dL	(↑) Cholangitis/cholangiohepatitis, hepatic failure, severe inflammation (↓) DIC, liver failure/end stage	**Handling** • Heparin; ↓ values **Storage** • Several days at 68° F • Several weeks at 32°–39° F **Notes** N/A

Table 7-1 Blood Chemistries (Continued)

Chemistry	Definition	Normal Range	Associated Conditions	Handling and Special Considerations
Gamma glutamyltrans-peptidase (GGT)	*Source* • Major: hepatocytes • Minor: kidneys, pancreas, intestines, and muscle cells *Role* • Enzyme: function unknown *Notes* • Values typically parallel increases in ALP; can be less influenced by secondary nonhepatic conditions or enzyme-inducing drugs • Slightly more sensitive and specific for feline liver disease than canine	*Canine* 2–10 U/L *Feline* 1–8 U/L	(↑) Anterior uveitis, brucellosis, deep pyoderma, ehrlichiosis, feline immundeficiency virus, hepatic disease/failure, menigitis, pleural effusion, pyometra	*Handling* • N/A *Storage* • 2 days at 68° F • 1 week at 32°–39° F *Notes* • Corticosteroids or anticonvulsant therapy; ± ↑ values
Globulins	*Source* • α-globulins: hepatocytes • β-globulins: hepatocytes • γ-globulins: plasma cells *Role* • α- and β-globulins: transport and bind proteins • γ-globulins: antibody *Notes* • Total serum globulin concentration = total serum protein concentration – albumin concentration	*Canine* 2.7–4.4 g/dL *Feline* 2.6–5.1 g/dL	(↑) Diabetes mellitus, hepatic failure, hyperadrenocorticism, hypertension, hyperthyroidism, immune mediated disease, neoplasia, pancreatitis, polyconal gammopathies, acute renal failure (↓) Acute blood loss, heartworm disease, protein losing enteropathy/nephropathy	*Handling* • Hemolysis and lipemia; ↑ values *Storage* See Albumin and Total Protein *Notes* • Dehydration; ↑ values • Neonatal animals are 60%–80% of adult values; ↓ values

	Source / Role / Notes	Values	Conditions	Handling / Storage / Notes
Glucose	Source • Dietary intake and gluconeogenesis or glycogenolysis by the liver Role • Cellular energy Notes • Indicator of carbohydrate metabolism or endocrine function of the pancreas	Canine 65–130 mg/dL Feline 70–125 mg/dL Danger level ≤60 mg/dL	(↑) Diabetes mellitus, hypertension, hyperthyroidism, hyperadrenal, hypoparathyroidism, pyelonephritis, renal failure (↓) Dystocia, hepatic failure, hypoadrenocorticism, insulinoma, neoplasia, peritonitis, sepsis	Handling • GTT at 6–10mg/mL of blood as a glucose preservative Storage • Separate from blood cells immediately (<30 minutes) • 8 hours at 68° F • 72 hours at 32°–39° F Notes • 16–24-hour fast is recommended, except if hypoglycemia suspected • Glucose levels can drop by 10%/hr if not separated from the blood cells • Stress; ↑ values
Inorganic Phosphorus	Source • Bones Role • Energy storage, release, and transfer, carbohydrate metabolism and composition Notes • Inversely related to calcium	Canine 3.0–7.0 mg/dL Feline 3.5–6.1 mg/dL Danger level <1.5 mg/dL	(↑) Bone lesions, chronic renal failure, toxins (↓) Emesis/diarrhea, fanconi syndrome, hepatic lipidosis, hyperparathyroidism, hypoadrenocorticism	Handling • Hemolysis and lipemia; ↑ values Storage • Separate from blood cells immediately • 3–4 days at 68° F • 1 week at 32°–39° F Notes • Anabolic steroids, furosemide, mannitol, minocycline, and IV KPO_4 may alter values
Lipase	Source • Pancreas and gastric mucosa Role • Break down the long-chain fatty acids of lipids Notes • Value is not representative of severity of disease • Tends to parallel serum amylase	Canine 0-425 units Feline 0-200 units	(↑) Pancreatitis, hyperadrenocorticism, liver disease, renal disease/failure	Handling • Lipemia; ↑ values • Do not use calcium-binding anticoagulants Storage • 1 week at 68° F • 3 weeks at 32-39° F Notes • Corticosteroids; ± ↑ values

Table 7-1 Blood Chemistries (Continued)

Chemistry	Definition	Normal Range	Associated Conditions	Handling and Special Considerations
Lipids/ Triglycerides	*Source* • Diet; intestinal absorption *Role* • Fat metabolism • Stimulus of intestinal lymph flow *Notes* • Animals at an ↑ risk are obese, high dietary intake of fats and genetic predisposition (e.g., Miniature Schnauzers and Himalayan cats)	*Canine* 50–150 mg/dL *Feline* 17–50 mg/dL *Danger level* >1,000 mg/dL	(↑) Diabetes mellitus, hyperlipidemia, hypothyroidism, pancreatitis, postprandial (↓) Lymphangectasia, protein-losing enteropathy	*Handling* • Lipemia; ↑ values *Storage* • N/A *Notes* • 12-hour fast recommended
Magnesium	*Source* • Bones *Role* • Activator of enzyme systems and involved in production and decomposition of acetylcholine *Notes* • ↑ Bilirubin can cause ↑ values of magnesium	*Canine* 1.8–2.4 mg/dL *Feline* 2.0–2.5 mg/dL *Danger Level* <1.0 or >10.0 mg/dL	(↑) Hypoadrenocorticism, renal failure (↓) Metabolic conditions	*Handling* • Hemolysis and metal containers; ↑ values • Only heparin anticoagulants should be used *Storage* • Samples are very stable *Notes* • N/A
Potassium	*Source* • Intracellular fluid *Role* • Muscular function, respiration, cardiac function, nerve impulse transmission, and carbohydrate metabolism *Notes* • N/A	*Canine* 4.0–5.7 mEq/L *Feline* 4.0–5.8 mEq/L *Danger level* ≤2.5 or ≥7.5 mEq/L	(↑) Diabetes mellitus, hypoadrenocorticism, massive tissue trauma, acute renal failure, urethral obstruction (↓) Canine/feline dilated cardiomyopathy, congestive heart failure, constipation, diabetes mellitus, gastrointestinal losses, hepatic lipidosis, peritonitis, renal failure	*Handling* • Hemolysis (esp. Akitas) and refrigeration of an nonseparated sample; ↑ value *Storage* • Do not freeze nonseparated samples • Stability is not known *Notes* • Plasma is the preferred sample

Sodium	*Source* • Extracellular fluid *Role* • Water distribution, body fluid osmotic pressure maintenance, and pH balance *Notes* • "Pseudohyponatremia" seen in cases of hyperlipidemia or severe hyperproteinemia	*Canine* 140–158 mEq/L *Feline* 145–160 mEq/L	(↑)Dehydration, heat stroke (↓)Canine dilated cardiomyopathy, congestive heart failure, gastrointestinal losses, hypoadrenocorticism, chronic renal failure, Rocky Mountain spotted fever	*Handling* • Heparin; ↑ value • Hemolysis; ↓ value *Storage* • Stability is not known *Notes* • Diuretic drugs; ↓ value
Total Protein (TP)	*Source* • See Albumin and Globulins *Role* • Oncotic blood pressure, transport mechanism, and immunity *Notes* • Composed of albumin and globulins	*Canine* 5.4–7.6 g/dL *Feline* 6.0–8.1 g/dL	(↑)Dehydration, gammopathy (↓)Acute blood loss, overhydrated	*Handling* • Severe hemolysis and sample dehydration; ↑ value *Storage* • Keep sample covered to prevent dehydration • Stability is not known *Notes* • See albumin and globulins

BONE MARROW EVALUATION

Bone marrow evaluation begins with the collection of the bone marrow sample and progresses through the use of oil immersion magnification. Once each slide has been properly collected and prepared, it is often evaluated in the clinic for a preliminary diagnosis. The technician can be an integral part of this procedure by being the first to evaluate the slide and by noting any alterations, and then progressing to interpretation of the slide contents. All slides need review or confirmation by a DVM and cytopathologist.

Bone Marrow Collection, Handling, Storage, and Transport Tips

Collection:

- Bone marrow samples degenerate rapidly after collection: neutrophils are the first to take on morphologic changes resembling neoplasia
- Samples should be obtained and prepared within 30 minutes of an animal's death

---

Skill Box 7-2 / Supplies for Bone Marrow Collection

- Surgical preparation material
- 16–18-gauge, 1–1¾-inch bone marrow biopsy needle
- Scalpel blade
- Clean microscope slides
- 10–20-mL syringe with 2%–3% EDTA/isotonic fluid solution

(Injecting 0.35 mL isotonic solution into a 7-mL EDTA blood collection tube produces 0.42 mL of 2.5% EDTA/isotonic fluid solution)

Handling:

- Smears must be made within 30 seconds if an EDTA/isotonic solution is not used, to avoid clotting and cell morphology distortion.

- Allow the slides to air dry.

- Samples must be stained as soon as possible to retain accurate morphology.

- Staining typically requires 2 times the usual stain contact time to reach adequate staining.

Skill Box 7-3 / Smear Techniques

Technique	Definition/Uses	Procedure	General Information
Smear without EDTA	• Samples collected using a clean, dry syringe	1. Hold a slide at a 45–70-degree angle 2. Drip the marrow sample down the tilted slide, allowing the marrow flecks to adhere to the slide 3. With the first slide laying flat, place a second slide on top, and gently pull each slide horizontally in opposite directions	• Sample must be smeared within 30 seconds of collection
Smear with EDTA	• Samples collected using an EDTA/isotonic solution–filled syringe	1. Sample collected into an EDTA/isotonic solution syringe is expelled onto a petri dish 2. Tilt the petri dish to allow the fluid to drain to the bottom and the marrow flecks to remain adhered to the dish 3. Using a PCV tube, collect a marrow fleck/spicule and gently place it on a glass slide 4. Place a coverslip at a 45-degree angle on the slide so that the corner of the coverslip hangs off the slide 5. Pull the corner of the coverslip to make a smear of the marrow fleck • Make some slides using no pressure and some using gently digital pressure placed on the coverslip	• Sample must be smeared within a few minutes of collection

Storage:

- Slides need to be completely dry before placing in a slide holder.

Transport:

- Padding should be placed around both sides of the slide holder to prevent breakage (e.g., bubble wrap, padded envelopes)
- Do not mail slides with bottles containing formalin, because the fumes may alter the staining capabilities of the slides.

Evaluation

Once each slide has been properly collected and prepared, it is often evaluated in the clinic for a preliminary diagnosis. The technician is an integral part of this procedure by evaluating the slide and noting any alterations seen. The DVM then confirms the slide contents and makes a preliminary diagnosis. The slide is sent off to a reference laboratory for official diagnosis.

1. Collection
    a. Ease of collection
    b. Number, size, and color of flecks retrieved
2. Prepare a slide with stain.
3. Scan the slide, using 4× magnification.
    a. Verify adequate staining.
    b. Verify proper slide preparation.
    c. Cellularity
    d. Number and age of megakaryocytes
4. Examine the slide, using 10× magnification
    a. Cell size
    b. Cell type
5. Examine the slide, using 40× magnification
    a. Chromatin pattern
    b. Nucleoli
6. Examine the slide, using oil immersion magnification
    a. Myeloid:erythroid ratio

Table 7-2 Cell Type Identification (See Figures 7-1 and 7-5)

Cell Type	Appearance
Erthyrocyte Rubriblast	• 1–2 blue nucleoli • Large, round, dark purple nucleus with smooth edges • Fine granular, linear chromatin • Distinct blue tint
Prorubricyte	• Smaller than rubriblasts • Round nucleus with smooth edges • Coarse and thickened chromatin • Reddish tinge
Rubricyte	• Smaller than prorubricyte • Dark clumps of coarse chromatin that begin to disappear • Disappearing nucleoli • Redder
Metarubricyte	• Larger than a mature RBC • Very dark, pyknotic nucleus • Chromatin and nucleoli are gone
Reticulocyte	• Large • Nonnucleated • Basophilic stippling when stained • Residual, nonfunctional RNA
Granulocyte Myeloblast	• Large • Nongranular, blue–pink cytoplasm • Round to oval, red nucleus • Chromatin with stippled pattern • 1–2 pale blue nucleoli
Progranulocyte/ Promyelocyte	• ↑ Cytoplasm with small, pink granules • Dark nucleus • Chromatin is dark and lacy in pattern • ± Nucleoli

Table 7-2 Cell Type Identification (Continued)

Cell Type	Appearance

Myelocyte	• Oval nucleus
	• Chromatin is dense with a coarse pattern
	• Cytoplasm stains gray–blue
	• Granules take on stain
	   Eosinophil—red granules
	     Canine: pleomorphic
	     Feline: rod-shaped
	   Basophil—blue granules
	     Canine: round, red–purple, and few to many
	     Feline: oval, lavender, and fill cytoplasm

Metamyelocyte	• Indented or U-shaped nucleus • Cytoplasm stains light blue
Band	• U-shaped nucleus with smooth edges ± Chromatin clumps present • Cytoplasm stains light blue
Platelet Megakaryoblast	• *Not commonly distinguished in bone marrow samples because of size and number present* • 2 reddish nuclei • Small amount of basophilic cytoplasm
Promegakaryoblast	• Dividing nuclei • Deep blue cytoplasm • 2–4 Nucleoli
Megakaryocyte	• Extremely large • Abundant, deep blue to pale blue granular cytoplasm • >4 Nucleoli

Interpretation

Because of the involved information on this subject, please refer to a text dedicated to this subject matter.

CYTOLOGY

Cytology is performed in a clinical setting on a day-to-day basis. A technician well trained in cytology can quickly and easily make preliminary findings. These findings may aid in the distinction in the type of cell (i.e., adenocarcinoma), the stage of disease, and its prognosis. Although the final diagnosis must lie in the hands of the veterinarian, the technician may make crucial evaluations and interpretations of the slide material, aiding the veterinarian in the diagnosis.

Cytology Collection, Handling, Storage, and Transport Tips

Collection:

- Several slides should be made to allow different staining techniques.
- Multiple collection attempts at multiple sites from the lesion should be made to ensure a representative sample.
- Adequate pressure must be used with fine-needle aspiration (FNA) to assure retrieval of cells.
- Excessive negative syringe pressure or prolonged aspiration often leads to blood contamination and nondiagnostic slides.

Skill Box 7-4 / Collection Techniques

Technique	Uses	Procedure	General Information
Imprints	• External lesions or fresh tissue samples from a surgical biopsy or necropsy	1. Blot the lesion or area to be imprinted with a clean, dry gauze 2. Touch the lesion against a clean glass slide to make an imprint • Can repeat several times on one slide • Imprint ulcers before and after cleaning	• Collects the fewest number of cells with the greatest amount of contamination
Scrapings	• External lesions or tissues from surgical biopsy or necropsy	1. Clean lesion and blot dry 2. Hold scalpel perpendicular to lesion 3. Pull the blade toward oneself several times in a scraping motion 4. Transfer the material to the middle of a glass slide with the scalpel blade and smear	• Collects a large number of cells
Swabs	• Fistulous tracts and vaginal collections	1. Moisten a sterile swab with saline 2. Gently roll the swab against the inside wall of the tract or vagina 3. Gently roll the swab across a slide to transfer material in a thin smear	• Only alternative for tract-like lesions • ↑ Cell damage with rough or improper handling
Fine Needle Biopsy *Aspirate*	• Lesions	1. Isolate and firmly hold the tumor 2. Insert the needle into the tumor and apply strong negative pressure by pulling the plunger $^3/_4$ of the way back and release pressure 3. Redirect the needle to a different part of the tumor and again apply pressure; continue this several times in different locations 4. Quickly smear the contents, using one of the smear techniques (See Skill Box 7-6) • If the tumor is large enough, negative pressure may be maintained while the needle is being redirected	• Avoids superficial contamination, but with ↑ contamination of tissues surrounding the tumor during aspiration • ↑ Blood contamination with certain types of tumors • Allows for collection from multiple locations within the lesion
Non-aspirate	• Any mass or solid lesion that is of large enough size to isolate • Ultrasound-guided biopsy of deep tissues • Highly vascular lesions	1. Isolate and firmly hold the tumor 2. Insert the needle only into the tumor and rapidly move the needle up and down while maintaining the same track 3. Remove the needle and attach an air-filled syringe and quickly expel the contents onto a clean glass slide 4. Smear the contents, using one of the smear techniques (See Skill Box 7-6)	• Avoids superficial contamination, but with ↑ contamination of tissues surrounding the tumor during aspiration • Enough material collected for only one smear, which may reduce diagnostic yield

Skill Box 7-5 / FNB Needle and Syringe Selection

- The softer the tissue being aspirated, the smaller the gauge of needle and syringe
- Do not use needles larger than 21 gauge, because they produce core biopsies and have a greater likelihood of blood contamination
- 12-mL syringes are a safe bet for all tumors

Handling:

- The material obtained must be prepared and smeared on a slide immediately to avoid drying and clumping/clotting.
- Do not allow smear to reach the edges of the slide if possible.
- Rapidly dry the slide after smearing by waving in the air or using a blow dryer.
- Slides should be marked as to which side is the top by using the patient's information.
- 2–3 air-dried unstained slides and 2–3 air-dried stained slides should be prepared when sending to the laboratory. The stained slides are a precaution for those cells that do not hold up well for extended periods.
- Fluid samples should be sent with prepared slides if possible.

Skill Box 7-6 / Smear Techniques

The most common error in cytology is sample handling by the laboratory technician. An improperly prepared slide may contain ruptured cells or areas that are too thick to read, or the sample may dry before it is smeared. All of these errors may lead to improper evaluation, but they can be remedied by proper technique and care on the part of the laboratory technician.

Technique	Definition/Uses	Procedure
Blood Smear Technique	• Produces a thin layer of fluid material across the slide • Fluid samples	1. Expel the aspirate material onto a glass slide 2. Place the second glass slide at a 30–40-degree angle to the first slide in front of the material 3. Pull the second slide back into the material and then gently, but swiftly, push across to the end of the first slide • The end of the smear should have a feathered edge and not run off the edge of the slide
Combination Technique	• A combination using the squash preparation and the blood smear technique • Any sample	1. Expel the aspirate material onto a glass slide 2. Mentally divide the material into 3 sections and do a blood smear technique on $\frac{1}{3}$ of the slide and a squash preparation on the opposite $\frac{1}{3}$
Squash Preparation	• Produces well-smeared slides • Thicker samples (e.g., bone marrow aspirates)	1. Expel the aspirate material onto a glass slide 2. Place a second glass slide on top of the material at a right angle 3. Without applying any downward pressure, quickly and smoothly slide the top slide across the bottom slide to smear the material
Squash-modified Preparation	• Produces well-smeared slides with a ↓ tendency for cell rupture • Thicker samples (e.g., bone marrow aspirates)	1. Follow steps 1 and 2 above 2. Rotate the top slide 45 degrees and then lift up
Starfish Preparation	• Prevents destruction of fragile cells • Any sample	1. Expel the aspirate material onto a glass slide 2. Using the tip of the needle, spread the material out into the shape of a starfish

Storage:

- Slides need to be completely dry before placing in a slide holder.

Transport:

- Padding should be placed around both sides of the slide holder to prevent breakage (e.g., bubble wrap, padded envelopes).
- Do not mail slides with bottles containing formalin, because the fumes may alter the staining capabilities of the slides.
- Protect the slides from moisture, because the sample may become distorted.

Evaluation

Once each slide has been properly collected and prepared, it is often evaluated in the clinic for a preliminary diagnosis. The technician is an integral part of this procedure by evaluating the slide and noting any alterations. The DVM then confirms the slide contents and makes a preliminary diagnosis. The slide is sent to a reference laboratory for official diagnosis.

1. Prepare a slide with stain.
2. Scan the slide using 4× magnification.
   a. Verify adequate staining
   b. Check for staining features and localized areas of cellularity.
   c. Check for crystals, foreign bodies, parasites, and fungal hyphae.
3. Examine the slide, using 10× magnification.
   a. Cell size
   b. Cell type
   c. Cellularity
4. Examine the slide, using 40× magnification.
   a. Chromatin pattern
   b. Nucleoli
5. Examine the slide, using oil immersion magnification
   a. Cell inclusions
   b. Cell organisms
   c. Mitotic figures

Interpretation

Once a slide has been evaluated, the results should confirm an inflammatory and/or neoplastic process. The distinction of inflammation alone often will enable the veterinarian to determine an initial protocol and treatment plan. If the slide is found to have neoplastic cells, they are then reviewed against the criteria of malignancy. A preliminary diagnosis on cell type, associated disease, and malignancy can be made by the DVM. Often the results are sent to a cytology laboratory for confirmation and staging.

Table 7-3 Criteria of Malignancy

Any slide showing one or a combination of the following cellular changes should be carefully reviewed for potential malignancy. A cytology laboratory should be consulted for clarification if needed. Nuclear characteristics have proven to be the most reliable source of determining malignancy. However, all aspects of the cells should be evaluated. Some types of malignant cells do not routinely show any of the following characteristics; therefore all other aspects of the complete workup should be viewed simultaneously.

Cytologic Characteristics	Appearance	Tumor Cell Types
Nuclear	• Anisokaryosis • Macrokaryosis • Variation in nuclear/cytoplasmic ratio • Coarse chromatin pattern that clumps • Irregular nuclear pattern • Abnormal size, shape, and appearance of nucleoli • Irregular nuclear membrane	*Epithelial:* • Round nucleus with a smooth to slightly coarse chromatin pattern • 1 or more nucleoli *Mesenchymal:* • Variable *Round cell:* • Variable
Cytoplasmic	• Vacuolization • Variable amount of cytoplasm from cell to cell • Basophilia with Wright's stain • Abnormal cytoplasmic boundaries	*Epithelial:* • ↑ Cytoplasm with secretory products *Mesenchymal:* • Abnormal cytoplasmic boundaries and extensions *Round cell:* • Well-defined cytoplasmic boundaries
Structural	• Anisocytosis • Macrocytosis • Pleomorphism	*Epithelial:* • Large to very large cells • Round to oval to caudate cells, easily exfoliating into sheets, clusters, or clumps *Mesenchymal:* • Small to medium cells • Spindle-shaped cells hard to exfoliate • Individual cells or in disorganized clusters *Round cell:* • Small to medium cells • Round to oval cells; easy to exfoliate individual cells

Table 7-4 Specific Tumor Cells

The following chart gives a general description of common tumor types. Multiple variations can be seen because of location, duration, and malignancy. Each cell should be evaluated in lieu of the rest of the slide and the general findings of the animal. The diagnosis of a particular condition must be made by the veterinarian.

Tumor Type	Appearance
Epithelial	
Mammary Adenocarcinoma	• Basophilic cytoplasm with ± vacuoles with secretory products • Variable nuclear size and nuclear/cytoplasm ratio • Nuclei often eccentrically displaced to the periphery of the cells • Round to oval cells appearing in clusters • Variable nucleolar shape and number
Perianal Adenoma	• Hepatoid appearing in clumps • Round to oval nuclei with 1–2 nucleoli • Abundant, foamy, and gray to tan cytoplasm with ± granules
Sebaceous Gland Tumor	• Large cell • Nucleus with a slightly coarse chromatin pattern • Nuclear/cytoplasm ratio • ± Basophilic and foamy cytoplasm
Squamous Cell Carcinoma	• Basophilic cytoplasm to abundant, pale cytoplasm • Large nuclei with clumped chromatin • Variable nuclear/cytoplasm ratio
Mesenchymal	
Lipoma	• Large cells distended with fat or lacy, collapsed cells
Osteosarcoma	• Variably sized nucleus with clumped chromatin • Spindle-shaped • Abundant, foamy basophilic cytoplasm
Soft Tissue Sarcoma	• Anisocytosis or spindle shaped • Dark blue cytoplasm with ± vacuoles and pink granules • Variable number and size of nucleoli

Table 7-4 Specific Tumor Cells (Continued)

The following chart gives a general description of common tumor types. Multiple variations can be seen because of location, duration, and malignancy. Each cell should be evaluated in lieu of the rest of the slide and the general findings of the animal. The diagnosis of a particular condition must be made by the veterinarian.

Tumor Type	Appearance
Round Cell Histiocytoma	• Anisocytosis • Poikilocytosis • Variable amount of pale blue cytoplasm • ↑ Nuclear/cytoplasm ratio • Round, oval, or irregularly shaped nuclei with lacy or finely stippled chromatin pattern
Lymphoma	• Dense nuclear margins with basophilic cytoplasm • ↑ Nuclear/cytoplasm ratio • Granular chromatin • ≥1 Nucleolus
Mast cell tumors	• Anisocytosis • Round to oval nuclei; stain palely • Fine to coarse, blue-black to reddish-purple granules within cytoplasm • Variable nuclear/cytoplasm ratio depending on differentiation and grade
Melanoma	• Green-black to brown granules that are irregular in shape and size in cytoplasm • Poikilocytosis
Plasma Cell Tumor	• Oval to round cells with coarse, clumped chromatin • 1 small nucleolus • ± Basophilic cytoplasm • Non-staining Golgi apparatus eccentrically placed

Vaginal Cytology

Vaginal cytology is used in evaluating an animal's stage of estrus cycle. Because of the constant changing of cellular structures during the estrus cycle, the evaluation of vaginal cells should be done every few days and in conjunction with a thorough medical history and examination (e.g., multiple, sequential samples increase accuracy of estrus stage estimation).

Table 7-5   Classifying Vaginal Cells

Vaginal Cells	Appearance
Noncornified Squamous Epithelial Cells	
Parabasal cells	• Small round cells with a small amount of cytoplasm • Round, distinct nuclei • Uniform in size and shape
Intermediate cells	• Large round cells with a large amount of cytoplasm • Round nuclei
Superficial Intermediate cells	• ↑ Cytoplasm that is irregular, folded, and angular • Smaller nuclei, pyknotic
Cornified Squamous Epithelial Cells	
Superficial cells	• Large cells • ↑ Cytoplasm, folded and angular • Distinct edges As the cell ages: • ± Nucleus (nucleated with young cells and anuclear with older/advanced cells) and vacuoles

Table 7-6 Staging the Estrus Cycle

Estrus Stage	Definition	Cell Appearance
Anestrus	• No physical changes • Does not attract or accept males • Duration of <4.5 months	• Intermediate or parabasal cells • ± Neutrophils • ± Bacteria
Proestrus	• Swollen vulva, reddish discharge • Attracts, but will not accept males • Duration 4–13 days	Early: • Noncornified squamous epithelial cells • Neutrophils and erythrocytes • ± Bacteria Late: • Superficial intermediate cells and cornified epithelial cells • ↓ Neutrophils and ↑ erythrocytes • ± Bacteria
Estrus	• Swollen vulva and pinkish to straw-colored discharge • Accepts males • Duration 4–13 days	Early: • 90% Cornified squamous epithelial cells • ± Superficial intermediate cells • Erythrocytes • ± Bacteria Late: • ↑ Neutrophils and ↓ erythrocytes • Bacteria
Metestrus/ Diestrus	• ↓ Vulvar swelling and discharge • Does not attract or accept males • Duration of 2–3 months	Early: • Cornified squamous epithelial cells • ↑ Cytologic debris Late: • Intermediate and parabasal cells • ± Neutrophils and erythrocytes

FUNCTION TESTS

Table 7-7 Function Tests

Function tests are used to force a system in the body to perform in a specific way (i.e., suppression or stimulation) to provide predictable results. Depending on the results, the information received will help to determine whether the system is functioning correctly. Most of these procedures require a specific protocol of fasting, injections, and blood drawing times; however, individual laboratories should be consulted regarding their specific protocol. As with any laboratory test, collection and handling remain the area of biggest human error as well as the area easiest to monitor and perform correctly.

Test	Definition/Uses	Normal Range	Associated Conditions	Protocols	Handling and Special Considerations
Adrenocorticotropic Hormone (ACTH) endogenous plasma concentration Tube: LTT Amount: full tube	Distinguishes between pituitary-dependent hyperadrenocorticism (PDH) and adrenocortical tumors (AT) and primary and secondary hypoadrenocorticism	*Canine* 2.2–25 pmol/L • <2.2 = AT • 2.2–10 = nondx • >10 = PDH	• Hyperadrenocorticism and hypoadrenocorticism	• Fast for 12 hours • Collect a blood sample	*Handling/Storage* • Lipemia; may interfere with the assay • Spin sample, separate off plasma and freeze immediately • Send by overnight air on dry ice to testing laboratory *Notes* • N/A
ACTH Stimulation Test or ACTH Response Test Tube: SST or RTT Amount: 0.5 mL serum or plasma each sample	The adrenal gland will respond to exogenous ACTH stimulation by glucocorticoid release in proportion to the glands' size and development. This test measures actual cortisol hormone.	*Canine* Pretest: 0–10 µg/dL Posttest: 8–22 µg/dL *Feline* Pretest: 0.4–4.0 µg/dL Posttest: 8–12 µg/dL	• Hyperadrenocorticism and Hypoadrenocorticism—screening and monitoring therapy	• Obtain baseline sample 1. • Give dogs 0.25 mg IM and cats 0.125 mg IM cosyntropin. • Draw blood sample 1 hour post for dogs and 30 minutes and 1 hour post for cats. 2. • Give 1 unit/lb of ACTH gel IM. • Draw blood sample 2 hours post for dogs and 1 and 2 hours post for cats.	*Handling/Storage* • Delay in separation of serum/plasma from blood cells and lipemia; ↓ values • Separate and freeze serum/plasma samples immediately *Notes* • Discontinue prednisone, prednisolone, cortisone and fludrocortisone 24–48 hours before test

Table 7-7 Function Tests (Continued)

Function tests are used to force a system in the body to perform in a specific way (i.e., suppression or stimulation) to provide predictable results. Depending on the results, the information received will help to determine whether the system is functioning correctly. Most of these procedures require a specific protocol of fasting, injections, and blood drawing times; however, individual laboratories should be consulted regarding their specific protocol. As with any laboratory test, collection and handling remain the area of biggest human error as well as the area easiest to monitor and perform correctly.

Test	Definition/Uses	Normal Range	Associated Conditions	Protocols	Handling and Special Considerations
ADH response test or Vasopressin Response Test	Evaluates the effect of exogenous ADH on the renal tubular ability to concentrate urine in the face of dehydration or water deprivation	*Canine/Feline* ↑ in urine specific gravity (USG)	• Diabetes insipidus—differentiates between central and nephrogenic diabetes insipidus	• Immediately after a water deprivation test; give 0.5 U/kg vasopressin IM (max of 5 U) • Empty the urinary bladder and measure specific gravity and osmolality at 30, 60, 90, and 120 minutes	*Handling/Storage* • N/A *Notes* • Withhold all food and water until the test has been completed
Ammonia Tolerance Test (ATT) Tube: GRNTT Amount: full tube	Detect abnormal portal blood flow and liver dysfunction	*Canine* Pre-ammonia: 44–116 µg/L Post-ammonia: 85–227 µg/L *Danger level* >1000 µg/dL	• Liver disease	• Fast for 12 hours and give enemas to clear lower bowel • Obtain baseline sample 1. • Give ammonium chloride orally at 0.1 g/kg (max of 3 g) dissolved in 20–50 mL water and given by stomach tube or rectally at 0.1 g/kg as a 5% solution. • Draw heparinized blood samples at 30 to 45 minutes post. 2. • Give 0.1 g/kg (max of 3 g) as a powder in gelatin capsules.	*Handling/Storage* • Centrifuged immediately, pour plasma off and analyze within 1–3 hours or freeze at –68° F *Notes* • Not recommended for cats • Do not perform if resting ammonia levels are already increased, because it may cause hepatic encephalopathy • Oral administration may cause regurgitation

Test	Description	Reference Values	Indications	Procedure	Handling/Storage	Notes
(continued)				• Draw heparinized blood samples 45 minutes post.		• Vomiting may occur but does not invalidate test • Venous occlusion, vigorous activity before, and muscle exertion during restraint; ↑ values • 3–10-fold increase indicates ammonia intolerance
Bile acids Tube: SST Amount: 0.5 mL serum each	A dysfunctional hepatobiliary system allows increased levels of bile acids to be found systemically. A sensitive function test of the liver	*Canine/Feline* Fasted: <10 μmol/L Postprandial: <25 μmol/L	• Liver disease, portosystemic shunting, and cholestatic disorders	• Fast for 12 hours • Obtain a baseline sample • Feed ≥ 2 Tbsp of a high-fat diet to a dog and ≥ 1 Tbsp to a cat • Collect a blood sample 2 hours afterward	*Handling/Storage* • N/A	*Notes* • Ursodeoxycholic acid; altered values • Ileum disease and large-volume diarrhea; ↓ values
Canine pancreatic lipase immunoreactivity (cPLI) Tube: SST Amount: 0.5 mL serum	A direct measurement of pancreatic lipase versus the general measurement of total serum lipase activity	*Canine* 1.9–82.8 μg/L	• Pancreatitis and Pancreatic mass	• Fast for 12–18 hours • Collect a blood sample	*Handling/Storage* • Separate serum and send sample on ice with a direct carrier to Texas A&M GI Lab	*Notes* • N/A
Dexamethasone Suppression test — High-dose Tube: SST Amount: 0.5 mL serum each	The dexamethasone is expected to shut off adrenocorticotropic hormone (ACTH) production through negative feedback with pituitary-dependent hyperadrenocorticism (PDH). Differentiates PDH from adrenocortical tumors (AT) in dogs. Diagnostic screening test for hyperadrenocorticism (HAC) in cats.	*Canine* PDH: Pretest: 1.1–8.0 μg/dL Posttest: 0.1–1.4 μg/dL or ≤50% of pretest level AT: Pretest: 2.5–10.8 μg/dL Posttest: 1.4–5.2 μg/dL	• Hyperadrenocorticism	• Obtain a baseline sample • Give 0.1 mg/kg dexamethasone IV • Collect a blood sample at 4 (optional) and 8 hours post	*Handling/Storage* • N/A	*Notes* • N/A

Table 7-7   Function Tests (Continued)

Function tests are used to force a system in the body to perform in a specific way (i.e., suppression or stimulation) to provide predictable results. Depending on the results, the information received will help to determine whether the system is functioning correctly. Most of these procedures require a specific protocol of fasting, injections, and blood drawing times; however, individual laboratories should be consulted regarding their specific protocol. As with any laboratory test, collection and handling remain the area of biggest human error as well as the area easiest to monitor and perform correctly.

Test	Definition/Uses	Normal Range	Associated Conditions	Protocols	Handling and Special Considerations
Dexamethasone Suppression Test Tube: SST Low-dose Amount: 0.5 mL serum each	Used to diagnose or confirm HAC	*Canine* Pretest: 1.1–8.0 µg/dL Posttest: 0.1–0.9 µg/dL (nondiagnostic 1.0–1.4 µg/dL)	• Hyperadrenocorticism	• Obtain a baseline sample • Give 0.01 mg/kg dexamethasone IV • Collect a blood sample at 4 (optional) and 8 hours post	*Handling/Storage* • N/A *Notes* • Not recommended for cats
Folate and Cobalamin Tube: SST Amount: 1 mL serum	Folate is absorbed in the jejunum and cobalamin in the ileum. Reflect intestinal absorptive function and the status of the intestinal flora.	*Canine* Folate 3.5–11 µg/L Cobalamin 300–700 ng/L *Feline* Folate: 6.5–11.5 µg/L Cobalamin: 290–1,500 ng/L	• Intestinal bacterial overgrowth, malabsorption, exocrine pancreatic insufficiency, inflammatory bowel disease, or intestinal neoplasia	• Fast for 12 hours • Collect a blood sample	*Handling/Storage* • Folate hemolysis; ↑ value • Avoid prolonged exposure to light and heat *Notes* • N/A
Fructosamine Tube: SST or RTT Amount: 0.5 mL serum	Adjunctive test used to diagnose DM and to monitor glycemic control during insulin therapy	*Canine* 370 µmol/L *Feline* 375 µmol/L	• Diabetes mellitus	• Obtain a blood sample	*Handling/Storage* • N/A *Notes* Corticosteroids, progestins, thiazide diuretics, growth hormone, dextrose-containing fluids and morphine; ↓ value

Test	Description	Reference Values	Indications	Procedure	Handling/Storage / Notes
Prothrombin time (PTH, PT) Tube: BTT Amount: 1.8 mL whole blood	A Vitamin K–dependent coagulation protein (factor) made by the liver. Evaluates extrinsic and common coagulation pathways.	*Canine* 5–8 sec *Feline* 8–11 sec	• Liver disease and anticoagulant toxicity	• Collect a blood sample	*Handling/Storage* • Tube must be completely full • Centrifuge at 3,000 rpm for 10 minutes, remove plasma • If >24 hours to run test, spin sample and freeze plasma *Notes* • N/A
Serum Antibody Against Nicotinic AchRs Tube: SST Amount: 1 mL serum	Identifies an immune response specifically against muscle AchRs.	*Canine* <0.6 nmol/L *Feline* <0.3 nmol/L	• Myasthenia gravis	• Collect a blood sample	*Handling/Storage* • Separate serum and ship overnight on ice/chilled *Notes* • Corticosteroid therapy can lower serum antibody levels
T_3 Suppression Test Tube: RTT Amount: 0.1 mL serum	Evaluates the ability of the thyroid gland to suppress pituitary TSH secretion followed by a drop in T_4 secretion.	*Canine/Feline* • ↓ in serum T_4 after 72 hours of oral T_3	• Hyperthyroidism, occult	• Obtain a baseline sample for T_4 and T_3 • Give 25 µg/cat of T_3 orally tid, starting the next morning for 7 doses • On the morning of the 3rd day, give 25 µg orally of T_3 and redraw blood sample within 4 hours for T_3 and T_4	*Handling/Storage* • N/A *Notes* • Rise in T_3 confirms owner's compliance in giving medication
Thyroid hormone, basal serum (T_4 and T_3) Tube: SST Amount: 1 mL serum	Evaluate the resting thyroid hormone concentration, a measurement of the total T_4 or T_3.	*Canine* T_4: 1.0–4.0 µg/dL T_3: 0.5–1.8 ng/mLl *Feline* T_4: 1.8–4.5 µg/dL T_3: 0.4–1.6 ng/mL	• Hyperthyroidism and hypothyroidism	• Collect a blood sample	*Handling/Storage* • N/A *Notes* • Corticosteroids, illness and stress; altered values • T_3 is not as accurate in the early stages of disease

Table 7-7 Function Tests (Continued)

Function tests are used to force a system in the body to perform in a specific way (i.e., suppression or stimulation) to provide predictable results. Depending on the results, the information received will help to determine whether the system is functioning correctly. Most of these procedures require a specific protocol of fasting, injections, and blood drawing times; however, individual laboratories should be consulted regarding their specific protocol. As with any laboratory test, collection and handling remain the area of biggest human error as well as the area easiest to monitor and perform correctly.

Test	Definition/Uses	Normal Range	Associated Conditions	Protocols	Handling and Special Considerations
Thyroid Hormone, Free (Free T_4 and Free T_3) Tube: SST Amount: 0.5 mL serum	A measurement of thyroid hormone not bound to a protein (unbound) and available for entry into cells.	*Canine* 0.3–0.5 ng/dL *Feline* 0.8–5.2 ng/dL	• Hyperthyroidism and hypothyroidism	• Collect a blood sample	*Handling/Storage* • N/A *Notes* • Least likely to be affected by nonthyroidal diseases
Thyroid-releasing Hormone (TRH) Stimulating Test or TRH Response Test Tube: SST Amount: 0.5 mL serum each	TRH is responsible for the release of thyroid-stimulating hormone (TSH) from the anterior pituitary and the eventual synthesis of thyroid hormone.	*Canine* >2 µg/dL post-TRH or ≥0.5 µg/dL above baseline T_4 *Feline* Little to no ↑	• Hyperthyroidism (cats) and hypothyroidism (dogs)	• Obtain baseline sample • Give 0.1 mg/kg TRH IV • Collect blood sample 4 and 6 hours post for dogs and 4 hours post for cats	*Handling/Storage* • N/A *Notes* • TRH administration typically causes hypersalivation, tachypnea, and vomiting up to 4 hours post-stimulation
Thyroid-stimulating Hormone Concentration (endogenous TSH) Tube: SST Amount: 0.5 mL serum	TSH is responsible for stimulating the synthesis of thyroid hormones in the thyroid gland.	*Canine* 0.02–0.5 ng/mL	• Hypothyroidism	• Collect a blood sample	*Handling/Storage* • N/A *Notes* • N/A

Test	Description	Normal Values	Indications	Procedure	Handling/Storage · Notes
Trypsin-like immunoreactivity (TLI) Tube: SST or RTT Amount: 0.5 ml serum	Test of pancreatic digestive function. A decreased amount of serum TLI is found when there is a decrease in the amount of functioning pancreatic cells.	*Canine* 5–35 µg/L *Feline* 17–49 µg/L	• Exocrine pancreatic insufficiency and pancreatitis	• Fast for 3–12 hours • Collect blood sample	*Handling/Storage* • Allow to clot at room temperature • Serum is stored at –68° F Notes • More sensitive and specific for pancreatitis than amylase/lipase
Urine cortisol:creatinine ratio Amount: 3–4 mL urine	Although urine creatinine stays relatively constant in an animal with stable kidney function, increased urine cortisol levels are seen with hyperadrenocorticism.	*Canine* $<1.35 \times 10^{-5}$	• Hyperadrenocorticism	• Obtain urine sample • Determine cortisol and creatinine concentrations	*Handling/Storage* • N/A *Notes* • Avoid stress while obtaining urine sample • False positives are common
Urine protein:creatinine Ratio Amount: 1 mL cystocentesis sample	To determine the significance of protein in the urine; not dependent on urine concentration.	*Canine* <0.3 *Feline* <0.6	• Glomerulonephritis and renal disease	• Obtain urine sample via cystocentesis • Determine protein and creatinine concentrations	*Handling/Storage* • N/A *Notes* • N/A

Table 7-7 Function Tests (Continued)

Function tests are used to force a system in the body to perform in a specific way (i.e., suppression or stimulation) to provide predictable results. Depending on the results, the information received will help to determine whether the system is functioning correctly. Most of these procedures require a specific protocol of fasting, injections, and blood drawing times; however, individual laboratories should be consulted regarding their specific protocol. As with any laboratory test, collection and handling remain the area of biggest human error as well as the area easiest to monitor and perform correctly.

Test	Definition/Uses	Normal Range	Associated Conditions	Protocols	Handling and Special Considerations
Water-deprivation test	To dehydrate the body to the point of signaling ADH release and the subsequent concentration of urine by the kidneys.	*Canine* 1.045 *Feline* 1.075 A USG of 1.025 is considered an adequate response	• Diabetes insipidus	• Stop either test when the animal loses ≥ 5% of body weight, becomes ill, or USG is >1.025 *Gradual* • Determine unrestricted daily water intake • Measure USG and weigh animal • Reduce water intake by 5% daily (not <66 mL/kg/day) • Measure USG and weigh animal daily *Abrupt* • Empty urinary bladder and measure USG and weigh animal • Withhold food and water until the end of the test • Every 2–4 hours, empty urinary bladder, measure USG and weigh animal	*Handling/Storage* • N/A *Notes* • Contraindications: dehydration, renal disease, and azotemia • A modified water-deprivation test is the ADH response test immediately after the standard water-deprivation test. • BUN should be monitored regularly throughout both tests

HEMATOLOGY

Even though many clinics send their blood samples out to reference laboratories for evaluation or use in-house automated machines, knowledge of how to perform a manual Complete Blood Count (CBC) can be very useful in certain situations. For example, during emergency situations, when time is crucial, the technician may be asked to perform an in-house CBC—or when the automated machine is malfunctioning. The results will provide the DVM with crucial information regarding the patient's hematology status (e.g., anemia, infection, and neoplasia)

See Blood Chemistries for Blood Collection: Handling, Storage, and Transport Tips

A complete blood count consists of RBC and WBC evaluation, PCV, TP, hemoglobin (Hgb) concentration, differential, platelet estimate, RBC indices, and a reticulocyte count. These tests are all run using a whole blood sample from an anticoagulant tube, such as EDTA. (See Skill Box 7-1, Blood Collection Tubes)

Table 7-8 Complete Blood Count

Procedure	Definition/Uses	Technique	Normals	Associated Conditions
Packed Cell Volume (PCV, Hematocrit, Hct)	• Percentage of whole blood that is composed of RBCs	• Fill a capillary tube $^2/_3$–$^3/_4$ full with whole blood and plug 1 end with a clay sealant. Centrifuge and read results as a percentage • Record the color and transparency of the plasma	*Canine* 37%–55% *Feline* 24%–45% Plasma: yellow and clear	• ↑ Polycythemia, dehydration, stress, and neonates • ↓ Anemia, overhydration, and weanlings
Total Protein Concentration (TP)	• Indicates oxygen transport capacity of the blood	• Break a spun capillary tube above the buffy coat level and put the plasma onto the face of the refractometer	*Canine* 5.4–7.6 g/dL *Feline* 6.0–8.1 g/dL	• ↑ Dehydration • ↓ Overhydration

Score the capillary tube with the edge of slide just above the buffy coat to allow easy breaking. Tap the unbroken end of the tube onto the surface of the refractometer or blow air into that end to expel the plasma.

Procedure	Definition/Uses	Technique	Normals	Associated Conditions
Hemoglobin Concentration (Hgb)	• Indicates how well the blood is transporting oxygen	• Follow manufacturer's guidelines for machine's use	• $^1/_3$ of the PCV	• ↑ (Falsely) Lipemia and Heinz bodies • ↓ Hypochromic anemias
RBC Count	• Gives an accurate count of RBCs • Machine counters have shown to be more accurate than manual counting • The main use of a RBC count is to calculate indices	1. Prepare the sample (1:200 dilution) and hemacytometer (see Skill Box 7-7) 2. Find the grid at 4×, focus on the center square of the grid and then increase magnification to 10×, count the RBCs in the center square and each of the four corners using 100× 3. Average the totals from grids of both stages and add 4 zeros 4. Round to the nearest tenth place and put in scientific notation	Dog: 5.5–8.5 10^6/μL Cat: 5–10 10^6/μL	• ↑ Polycythemia and dehydration • ↓ Anemia and overhydration

Test	Purpose	Procedure	Reference Values	Significance
WBC Count (Twbc)	• Gives an accurate count of total WBCs	1. Prepare the sample (1:20 dilution) and hemacytometer 2. Count the entire grid on 10× 3. Average the totals from both grids 4. (Averaged Totals [AT] + 10% of AT) ×100 e.g., Grid #1 = 75 Grid #2 = 85 75 + 85 = 160 / 2 = 80 80 + 8 ×100 = 8,800 μL	Dog: 6,000–16,000 μL Cat: 5,000–19,000 μL	• ↑ Hemolysis, inflammation, hemorrhage, immune-mediated disease, infection, leukemia, necrosis, neoplasia, and toxemia • ↓ Bone marrow disease, radiation, drug administration, retroviruses, myeloproliferative and lymphoproliferative diseases
Differential	• Indicates the number of specific WBCs found circulating in the blood • The Twbc count should roughly equal the differential totals	1. Examine a prepared blood smear using 100× 2. Count up the different WBC (neutrophils [N], bands [B], lymphocytes [L], monocytes [M], eosinophils [E], and basophils up to 100 3. See Skill Box 7-8 Calculating a Differential	Dog: N—3,600–11,500 B—0–300 M—15–1,350 L—1,000–4,800 E—100–1,250 Cat: N—2,500–12,500 B—0–300 M—0–850 L—1,500–7,000 E—0–1,500	• Variable dependent on type of cell(s) ↑ or ↓
Nucleated RBCs (nRBC)	• Early release of immature RBCs • The corrected value should be calculated when >5 nRBCs are found and then used to calculate the differential	1. While performing the differential, keep track of any nRBCs 2. Calculate a corrected Twbc count $$\frac{\text{Observed Twbc count} \times 100}{100 + \text{nRBC}} = \text{corrected Twbc count}$$	• N/A	• Anemia, lead poisoning, or hemangiosarcoma

Table 7-8 Complete Blood Count (Continued)

Procedure	Definition/Uses	Technique	Normals	Associated Conditions
Platelet Estimate	• Indicates ability for adequate clotting	1. Examine a prepared blood smear using 100× in which the RBCs are close but not touching, typically near the periphery of the slide 2. Count 5 different fields and average 3. Multiply by 15,000 and 18,000 to obtain a range • When large areas of clumping are seen, assume adequate numbers of platelets	Dog: 200,000–500,000 µL Cat: 300,000–800,000 µL	• ↑ Myeloproliferative disorder or megakaryocytic leukemia • ↓ B_{12}, iron or folic acid deficiency, drug toxicity, acute hemorrhage, radiation, viruses, uremia or aplastic anemia

Perform the platelet count after the differential, because this allows the platelets time to settle.

Procedure	Definition/Uses	Technique	Normals	Associated Conditions
Reticulocyte Count	• Immature RBC • Used to evaluate the bone marrow's response to anemia • Perform along with a CBC when severe anemia is present PCV values: Canine: ≤30% Feline: ≤20%	1. Mix together an equal part of whole blood with new methylene blue (NMB), agitate, and let it sit for 10 minutes 2. Prepare a blood smear 3. Examine under 100× by counting 1,000 RBCs while separately keeping track of the number of reticulocytes 4. Divide the reticulocyte number by 1,000 and convert to a percentage 5. Calculate the corrected reticulocyte number $$\frac{\text{Observed retic. \% } \times \text{ PCV}}{\text{Normal mean PCV for species}} = \text{corrected retic. \%}$$	• <1%	• ↑ Regenerative anemias

RBC Indices

Test	Description	Formula	Reference	Interpretation
Mean Corpuscular Volume (MCV)	• Indicates the size or volume of RBCs • Classifies anemias as normocytic, macrocytic, or microcytic	$$MCV\ (fl) = \frac{PCV\ (\%)\ \times 10}{RBC\ count\ \times 10^{6}/\mu L}$$	Dog: 60–77 fL Cat: 39–55 fL	• ↑ Reticulocytosis, B_{12}, or folic acid deficiency • ↓ Iron deficiency
Mean Corpuscular Hemoglobin (MCH)	• The mean weight of Hgb in a RBC • Used as a lab check • ↓← MCH should see a ↑ MCV • ↑← MCH should see a ↓ MCV	$$MCH\ (PG) = \frac{Hgb\ (g/dL)\ \times 10}{RBC\ count\ \times 10^{6}/\mu L}$$	Dog: 19–24 PG Cat: 12–17 PG	• ↑↓ Hemolysis • ↓ Iron deficiency
Mean Corpuscular Hemoglobin Concentration (MCHC)	• Indicates the average hemoglobin concentration in each RBC • Classifies anemias as hypochromic or normochromic	$$MCHC\ (g/dL) = \frac{Hb\ (g/dL)\ \times 100}{PCV(\%)}$$	Dog: 32–36 g/dL Cat: 30–36 g/dL	• ↑ Hemolysis, lipemia, or Heinz bodies • ↓ Iron deficiency

Skill Box 7-7 / Hemacytometer Use

1. Prepare the WBC or RBC sample, following manufacturer's directions.
2. Shake the sample just before use to redistribute the cells.
3. Fill the stylette by squeezing the bottle and expelling any air bubbles.
4. Place the hemacytometer on the table, and place the coverslip on top.
5. While stabilizing the hemacytometer, place the stylet in the indented portion and gently squeeze just until the stage is filled

   *Caution:** overfilling of the stage will result in multilevels of RBCs and give falsely ↑ values.
6. Load up the other indented area as previously described.

Skill Box 7-8 / Calculating a Differential

1. Count up 100 WBCs and differentiate their type and record totals as %/μL

e.g.,	45 neutrophils	= 45 %/μL = .45/μL
	45 lymphocytes	= 45 %/μL = .45/μL
	7 monocytes	= 7 %/μL = .07/μL
	3 eosinophils	= 3 %/μL = .03/μL
	0 basophils	= 0
	100 WBCs	

2. Multiply each WBC type by the previously obtained Twbc count

   e.g., Twbc count = 8,650

   $$8,650 \times .45 = 3893/μL \text{ neutrophils}$$
   $$8,650 \times .45 = 3893/μL \text{ lymphocytes}$$
   $$8,650 \times .07 = 606/μL \text{ monocytes}$$
   $$8,650 \times .03 = 260/μL \text{ eosinophils}$$

   8,652/μL Twbc

3. The Twbc should roughly equal the Twbc count

   e.g., Twbc (8,652) = Twbc count (8,650)

Evaluation

Once these tests have been performed, the blood is examined and evaluated on the basis of its morphology, inclusions, and presentation.

1. Prepare a blood smear slide with stain or use the prepared slide from the differential.
2. Scan the slide, using low magnification.
   a. Platelet aggregation
   b. RBC rouleaux
   c. RBC agglutination
3. Examine the slide, using oil immersion magnification.
   a. RBC morphology
      i. Size
      ii. Shape
      iii. Color
      iv. Alterations
   b. WBC morphology
      i. Toxic changes
      ii. Nuclear degeneration
      iii. Cytoplasmic inclusions
      iv. Alterations
   c. Platelet
      i. Distribution
      ii. Alterations

RBC Morphology

The normal morphology of a canine RBC is a large, biconcave disc (7.5 μm) of uniform size with central pallor. A normal feline RBC is a slightly smaller biconcave disk (5 μm) with only slight central pallor. When observing the prepared slide for RBC morphology, the cells should be evaluated for alterations in size, shape, color, and inclusions. See Figures 7-1, 7-2, 7-3, 7-5, 7-6, 7-7, 7-8, and 7-10 in color plate section.

Table 7-9   RBC Alterations

Alteration	Definition	Appearance	Associated Conditions
Inclusions			
Basophilic Stippling	• Residual RNA	• Very small, dark-blue inclusions	• Anemia or lead poisoning
Heinz bodies	• Denatured hemoglobin caused by certain chemicals or oxidant drugs • Seen in up to 10% of normal feline RBCs	• Single, light-colored, rounded protrusions of the RBC membrane	• Lymphosarcoma, chronic renal failure, hyperthyroidism, diabetes mellitus, and oxidative toxins (e.g., onions, acetaminophen)
Howell-Jolly Bodies	• Basophilic nuclear remnants seen in young RBCs	• Dark blue to black spherical inclusions	• Splenic disorders
Morphology			
Acanthocytes (spur cell)	• Caused by cholesterol concentration changes in the cell membrane	• Irregularly spiculated	• Severe liver disease, disseminated intravascular coagulation (DIC), hemangiosarcoma, hepatic lipidosis, lymphosarcoma, portosystemic shunts, and renal disease
Anisocytosis	• Multiple possibilities (e.g., early cell release or increased cell division of RBCs)	• Variation in size	• Iron deficiency and anemia
Crenation	• pH changes associated with slow-drying blood films	• Notched or scalloped cell membrane	• Artifact • Mostly seen in cats
Echinocytes (burr cells)	• Mechanism unknown; possibly calcium or adenosine triphosphate (ATP) changes in vivo	• Evenly spaced, blunt to sharp projections of uniform shape and size	• Renal disease, lymphosarcoma, doxorubicin toxicity, electrolyte depletion, and snake bites
Keratocytes (bite or helmet cells)	• Vacuolated cells that enlarge and break open on 1 side of cell membrane	• Spiculated cells with 2 or more projections	• DIC, congestive heart failure, hemangiosarcoma, glomerulonephritis, and chronic doxorubicin toxicity
Leptocytes (target cells)	• Characterized by ↑ membrane and ↓ hemoglobin levels	• Folded or resemble a target	• Nonregenerative anemia
Nucleated RBCs (metarubricytes, normoblasts)	• Early release of RBCs still maintaining its nucleus	• Dark purple nucleus in a normal-size RBC	• Regenerative anemia, splenic dysfunction, severe stress, hyperadrenocorticism, and corticosteroid treatment

	Description	Significance
Poikilocytosis	• Variation in shape	• Liver, kidney, spleen, and other vessel problems
Schistocyte (fragments, helmet cells)	• Irregularly shaped fragments and sharp pointed projections	• Characteristic of ↑ RBC fragility • Shearing of the RBC by intravascular trauma • DIC, vascular neoplasms, severe burns, and iron deficiency
Spherocyte	• Small, dark, round RBCs with little or no central pallor	• ↓ Amount of cell membrane caused by partial phagocytosis by macrophages • autoimmune hemolytic anemia (AIHA), transfusions, parasitic infections, zinc toxicity and snake venom toxicity
Stomatocytes (mouth cells)	• Cup shaped	• Multiple possibilities (e.g., leakage of sodium and potassium from the cell membrane) • Liver disease, inherited disorders (e.g., Alaskan malamutes)
Parasites *Babesia spp.*	• Large, teardrop- or ring-shaped intercellular structures, often seen in pairs	• Rare protozoan, tick-transmitted disease of dogs • Babesiosis (acute intravascular and extravascular hemolysis with hemoglobinuria)
Cytauxzoon felis	• Small, irregular rings within RBCs, lymphocytes, or macrophages	• Rare protozoan, tick-transmitted disease of cats • Hemolytic anemia, icterus, depression, and fever
Hemobartonella canis	• Chain of small cocci or rods that stretch across the surface of a RBC • Chains may branch	• Rare rickettsial disease affecting dogs • Splenectomized or immunocompromised dogs
Hemobartonella felis	• Nonrefractile cocci, rod- or ring-like structures on the periphery of RBCs • Stain dark purple	• Common rickettsial disease of cats • Parasite is cyclic, and multiple slides may need to be evaluated for a diagnosis • Parasite rapidly disappears with antibiotic treatment (e.g., tetracyclines) • Immunocompromised cats, feline hemobartonellosis or feline infectious anemia

Blood parasites are often confused with drying artifacts and stain precipitate, but these are usually refractile.

WBC Morphology

The purpose of WBCs is to defend the body against foreign organisms, conducting their business in the tissues themselves. They are typically nonfunctional in the circulatory system. WBC morphology is significantly different between each type of cell. The frequency that they appear in the body is the order listed below. See Figures 7-4, 7-6, 7-7, 7-8, 7-9, and 7-10 in the color plate section.

Table 7-10 WBC Morphology

WBC	Definition	Appearance (stained)	Associated Conditions
Neutrophils (Polys, Segs)	• First line of defense against infection • Highly motile and phagocytic • Replaced in the body 2.5 times per day	• Convoluted and segmented nucleus • Clear to light pink cytoplasm with diffuse granules • Coarse and clumped chromatin	• ↑ Fear, exercise, stress, or inflammation • → Severe infections, infectious agents causing decreased bone marrow production, chemical toxicity, and genetic disorders
Bands	• Immature neutrophils • Hyposegmented nucleus with the constriction being <½ the width of the nucleus • Left shift is an ↑ in bands	• Nucleus is horseshoe shaped with large round ends	• ↑ Inflammation, bacterial infection, and neoplasia
Lymphocytes	• Immunity, antibody production, and interleukocyte chemical mediation	• Large, round, slightly indented, dark nucleus • Round cell with a small amount of blue cytoplasm • ± Large, pink cytoplasmic granules	• ↑ Fear, excitement, chronic infections, leukemias, and lymphosarcoma • → Corticosteroids, immunodeficiency diseases, loss of lymph, and impaired lymphopoiesis
Monocytes	• Highly phagocytic; digesting particulate and cellular debris • Antiviral and antitumor qualities • Become macrophages once in extravascular space	• Large, elongated, lobulated, or indented nucleus • Bluish-gray cytoplasm • Large cell with lacy appearance caused by vacuoles • Pink dustlike inclusions • Diffuse nuclear chromatin • Blunt, agranular, light blue cytoplasmic pseudopods	• ↑ Corticosteroids, stress, or severe infections and hemorrhages

Eosinophils	• Ingest products of antibody/antigen reactions • Replaced once daily	*Canine* • Clear cytoplasm with small to large, dull orange granules partially filling cell *Feline* • Pale cytoplasm with small, dull orange granules completely filling cell	• ↑ IgE stimulation, parasitic infections and allergies • ↓ Corticosteroids
Basophils	• Their function is still unclear, but related to immunity • Rarely seen, possibly because of rapid degranulation	*Canine* • Dark purple granules partially filling cell • Highly segmented nucleus • Gray–blue cytoplasmic vacuoles *Feline* • Violet cytoplasm with oval, non-staining granules • Highly segmented nucleus	• ↑ Hyperlipemia, chronic IgE stimulation and allergies

Table 7-11 WBC Alterations. See Figures 7-3, 7-6, 7-9, and 7-10 in the color plate section.

Alteration	Definition	Appearance	Associated Conditions
Inclusions Döhle bodies	• Retained rough endoplasmic reticulum	• Bluish–gray cytoplasmic inclusions	• Severe toxemia, inflammation, and infection
Morphology Cytoplasmic basophilia	• Persistent ribosomes	• Varying degree of solid to patchy light blue to blue-purple cytoplasm	• Severe toxemia, inflammation, and infection
Cytoplasmic vacuolation	• Disruption in bone marrow production, resulting in a loss of granule and membrane integrity	• Foamy, bubble-like, nonstaining circles	• Systemic toxicity
Reactive lymphocyte	• Immune-stimulated T- and B-cells	• ↑ Cytoplasm and basophilia and a larger, more convoluted nucleus	• Antigenic stimulation (e.g., canine ehrlichiosis)
Parasites Cytauxzoon felis	See Table 7-9, RBC Alterations		
Ehrlichia canis	• Rickettsia, tick-transmitted disease of dogs	• Small cluster in cytoplasm of monocytes and neutrophils	• Ehrlichiosis

Table 7-12   Platelet Morphology

Platelets absorb and carry plasma factors needed to form fibrin to facilitate hemostasis. These thrombocytes vary in size and shape and are non-nucleated with pale blue to lavender granules. They are often seen in clumps at the periphery or feathered edge of a prepared slide. See Figures 7-1, 7-7, 7-8, and 7-10 in the color plate section.

Alteration	Definition	Appearance	Associated Conditions
Megathrombocytes (Stress platelets, shift platelets, or giant platelets)	• Seen in cats, contributes to not being able to use an electronic counter	• Larger than an RBC	• Bone marrow disorders or myelo-proliferative disorders

Table 7-13 Coagulation Tests

Coagulation tests allow the DVM to determine whether the patient's blood clots adequately. These tests are often performed in patients with questionable hereditary backgrounds, for a diagnosis of a particular disease (i.e., von Willebrand's disease [vWD] and DIC) and in any patient having difficulty with clotting, either internally or externally. These tests can distinguish between patients with a bleeding disorder versus a patient with damaged or diseased blood vessels.

Test	Definition	Procedure	Normals
Quick Assessment Tests			
Activated Clotting Time (ACT)	• Test of intrinsic clotting mechanism • Less sensitive than APTT	1. Warm syringe and tube containing diatomaceous earth to 98° F (37° C) 2. Inject 2 mL freshly drawn whole blood into tube and invert 5 times to mix 3. Begin the clock with the injection of blood into the tube and incubate in a warm water bath for 1 minute 4. Observe at 5-second intervals for the first sign of clotting • Place the tube back in incubation between each 5-second check	*Canine* 60–120 sec *Feline* 60–75 sec • May be slightly prolonged with thrombocytopenia
Place the tube against your body (e.g., armpit or hand) for easy incubation.			
Bleeding Time **Buccal Mucosal (BMBT)**	• Making a standard wound and noting the time to the cessation of bleeding	1. Make a deep puncture at a site with no hair (e.g., buccal, gingiva, nose) 2. Begin timing when blood appears 3. Remove the blood with filter paper at 30-second intervals 4. Stop timing when there is no more blood • Do not touch the skin with the filter paper	*Canine/Feline* 1–5 minutes
Toenail (TBT)		1. Clip a toenail back past the quick to cause bleeding 2. Keeping the animal undisturbed, monitor for the bleeding to cease	*Canine/Feline* <5 minutes
Platelet Estimate	• Estimation of platelet number	1. Examine a prepared blood smear, using 100× on a place where the RBCs are close but not touching near the periphery 2. Examine at least 5 fields to assure accurate results	*Canine* 8–29/100× field *Feline* 10–29/100× field

Definitive Tests

Test	Description	Procedure	Values
Activated Partial Thromboplastin Time (APTT)	• Test of intrinsic clotting mechanism and common coagulation pathways • Measure the time in seconds for fibrin clot formation • Proper dilution is crucial to the accuracy of this test	1. Draw a fresh blood sample to fill a BTT 2. Gently invert sample 6–10 times to activate anticoagulant 3. Refrigerate if testing is < 24 hours or centrifuge sample, pipette off plasma and freeze in a plastic tube	*Canine* 8–13 sec *Feline* 13–30 sec
Fibrin split product (FSP) or fibrin degradation product (FDP)	• Measures the presence of products that result from the action of plasmin on fibrin and fibrinogen • Proper dilution is crucial to the accuracy of this test • Aids in DIC diagnosis	1. Draw a fresh blood sample to fill a FDP tube (2 ml) 2. Gently invert sample 6–10 times • Clot formation should occur shortly after blood draw	*Canine/Feline* <10 μmg/mL
Fibrinogen	• Quantitative measure of plasma fibrinogen	1. Draw a fresh blood sample to fill an LTT 2. Gently invert sample 6–10 times to activate anticoagulant	*Canine* 100–250 mg/dL *Feline* 100–350 mg/dL
Prothrombin Time (PT)	• Test of extrinsic clotting mechanism and common coagulation pathways • Measure the time in seconds for fibrin clot formation • Proper dilution is crucial to the accuracy of this test • Used for vitamin K antagonist poisons	1. Draw a fresh blood sample to fill a BTT 2. Gently invert sample 6–10 times to activate anticoagulant 3. Refrigerate if testing is < 24 hours or centrifuge sample, pipette off plasma and freeze in a plastic tube	*Canine* 5–8 sec *Feline* 8–11 sec
von Willebrand's Factor Assay (vWF)	• Measurement of vWF antigen • Proper dilution is crucial to the accuracy of this test • Do not test during pregnancy, estrus, or lactation	1. Draw a fresh blood sample, using a vacutainer needle, into a 2-mL BTT, or use a syringe containing citrate (1 part citrate to 9 parts blood) • Do not use a dry syringe and then transfer blood into a vacutainer tube 2. Centrifuge blood and gently pipette off plasma into a plastic container	Variable, dependent on bleeding time and vWF antigen percentage

IMMUNOLOGY AND SEROLOGY TESTS

Table 7-14 Immunology and Serology Tests

Immunology and serology tests are specialized laboratory tests sent out to reference laboratories, typically to follow-up on tests that have already been performed. These tests require specialized equipment and laboratory technician skills. Each laboratory has varying requirements for submission of immunology and serology samples. Refer to their specific reference guide for more information. See Blood Chemistries for Blood Collection, Handling, Storage, and Transport Tips.

Test	Technique	Associated Conditions
Coombs' Test	A species-specific Coombs' reagent is added to the blood. RBCs that are coated with antibodies will cause agglutination with the added reagent.	Autoimmune hemolytic anemia
Enzyme-Linked Immunosorbent Assay (ELISA)	A tray with antibody coated wells is filled with the sample. If any antigen is present, it will bind with the antibody in the coated wells. A second enzyme-tagged antibody is added and binds to the antibody–antigen complex. A substrate that reacts with the enzyme is then added and results in a color change if antigen is present. The color change is proportional to the amount of antigen in the sample. The antigen may be actual viral/bacterial material (e.g., FeLV) or the host's antibody vs. the pathogen (e.g., FIV)	Heartworm, canine parvovirus, FIV, FIP, FeLV, toxoplasmosis, progesterone, atopy, nonregenerative anemia, allergies, and Lyme disease
Immunodiffusion	Viral antigen and an antibody are placed into separate wells in agar. They diffuse through the agar and form a visible band of precipitation if any viral antigen is present.	Viral and fungal pathogens
Immunofluorescence Assay (IFA) **Direct**	An antibody for a specific virus is tagged with a fluorescent dye and combined with the sample. If the specific virus is present, the antibody will bind and appear fluorescent during microscopic examination.	Ehrlichiosis and Rocky Mountain spotted fever
Indirect	An antiviral antibody (immunoglobulin) that was produced in an animal (e.g., rabbit) and a fluorescent tagged antirabbit immunoglobulin are combined with a sample. The second antibody combines with the first antibody, which binds to any viral antigen present in the sample. The antibody–antibody–antigen complex will fluoresce during microscopic examination.	*Cryptosporidium*, FIV, *Giardia*, and systemic lupus erythematosus

Test	Description	Examples
Intradermal tests	Allergenic extracts are injected intradermally and observed for changes. A wheal formation indicates the presence of antibodies and an allergic reaction.	Allergies; flea allergy
Latex agglutination	Small, spherical antibody (or antigen)–coated latex particles are suspended in water. The sample is added, and any antibody–antigen complexes that form will cause agglutination. The water will be milky or contain clumps of latex particles.	Canine rheumatoid factor, Brucellosis and DIC
Polymerase Chain Reaction (PCR)	A specific nucleic acid primer reacts with a portion of the genome from the microorganism in question. The combination is amplified to produce many fragments of the DNA sequence. Electrophoresis is then used to detect the combination and to measure its size and migration pattern. • Often used to confirm results of other tests	Herpesvirus, FeLV, FIV, Coronavirus, *Bartonella, Ehrlichia,* etc.
Radioimmunoassay	An antibody for a specific virus or antigen is tagged with a radioactive element (e.g., iodine) and combined with the sample. A gamma counter is used to identify the antibody–antigen complex.	Thyroid diseases
Western blot (Immunoblot)	Antigens are separated by electrophoresis and blotted to nitrocellulose sheets. The sheets are incubated with labeled antibodies and then observed for bound antibodies by using enzymatic or radioactive methods. • Used to confirm ELISA results	FIV

MICROBIOLOGY

A small animal laboratory should only be responsible for presumptive identification of bacteria. Further tests for a definitive diagnosis should be sent to a referral laboratory, where they have access to a greater number of techniques and equipment. Skill Box 7-9 outlines basic guidelines for collection of the sample followed through to the preliminary evaluation and interpretation of bacterial growth. Books dedicated to the subject of microbiology should be consulted for further discussion of alternative tests and techniques.

Microbiology Collection, Handling, Storage, and Transport Tips

Collection:

- Collect sample aseptically.
- Collect an adequate amount of the samples to allow for complete examination.
- Samples should be attained before starting antibiotic therapy.

Skill Box 7-9 / Collection Technique

Site	Collection
Abortion	Entire fetus or multiple specimens from a range of body parts should be obtained as soon as possible after the animal has died
Abscess/Wound	Unruptured: sterile syringe with wide-bore needle Ruptured: swab near the edge of the wound and take scrapings from the inside wall of the abscess
Anaerobic bacteria	Sterile syringe with fine-gauge needle ***Caution:** Expel all air out of syringe before obtaining sample
Blood	5–10 mL of blood from at least 2 different sites and immediately place it in separate blood culture bottles. Collect multiple samples throughout the day
Ear	Swabs of both ears canals and middle ear if needed
Eye	Corneal scrapings, swab of the conjunctival sac or swab of lacrimal secretions
Fecal	1 g freshly voided or rectal examination–obtained feces ***Caution:** clean anus before collection to avoid contamination with anal skin microflora
Genital	Swab of vulvar mucosa
Leptospirosis	20 mL of midstream urine
Urine	5 mL urine via a catheter or cystocentesis

*See Cytology (Skill Box 7-4) and Urinalysis (Skill Box 7-19) sections for specimen collection techniques

Handling:

- Samples should be handled carefully to avoid human contamination.
- Separate multiple samples to avoid cross contamination.
- Maintain a clean environment in which the laboratory tests are run.
- Wood-shafted and cotton-tipped swabs should not be used with samples suspected of chlamydia.
- Sample should be clearly marked with patient's name, number, origin of the sample, time of collection and whether it was refrigerated.

Storage:

- Swabbed samples need to be placed in a transport media if they are not immediately inoculated.
- Agar plates must be stored inverted to prevent condensation buildup on the surface of the agar.

Skill Box 7-10 / Specimen Storage

Test	Specimen	Storage
Acid-Fast Stain	Tissue	Red top tube
	Slides	Slide holder
Anaerobic Bacteria	Fluid	Sterile syringe with fine-gauge needle in a rubber stopper secured with tape
Blood	Blood (5–10 mL)	Blood culture bottle (commercially prepared)
Chlamydia	Tissue or dacron swab	Chlamydia transport media
Culture and Sensitivity (bacterial)	Swab	Culturette swab or Transwab
	Fluid	Red top tube
	Tissue	Enteric transport media or red top tube
Fecal Culture	Feces	Culturette swab, enteric transport media, red top tube, or clean, dry container
Fungal culture	Hair, scrapings or swab (yeast only)	Red top tube, Culturette swab, or Transwab
	Fluid	Screw-cap tube
Gram Stain	Slides	Slide holder
	Swab	Culturette swab or Transwab
	Fluid or tissue	Red top tube
Identification only	Swab	Culturette swab or Transwab
	Fluid	Red top tube
	Tissue	Enteric transport medium or red top tube
	Plate with growth	Culture plate
KOH Preparation	Scrapings or clipped hair or nails	Red top tube
Mycoplasma	Fluid and tissue	Mycoplasma transport media or Culturette swab *Caution: mycoplasma may adhere to swabs, giving negative results
Sensitivity Only	Plate with growth	Culture plate
Urine	Fluid	Culture needs to be set up within 2 hours to avoid overgrowth of insignificant bacteria or refrigerated for no longer than 18–24 hours

Transport:

- Tape the lids and caps of inoculated tubes and plates before shipment
- Tissue submitted for fungal cultures should be frozen and marked "Caution" because of its zoonotic potential
- Empty the water that has accumulated on the lid to avoid it dropping onto the agar plate and mixing the colonies of bacteria

---

Skill Box 7-11 / Most Commonly Used Culture Media

Numerous types of culture media are available; however, most veterinary clinics use only a few. The more extensive cultures are sent to reference laboratories for growth and interpretation.

Medium	Preparation	Uses	Interpretations
Blood Agar	Trypticase soy agar Sheep's blood	• Enriched media that supports the growth of most bacteria	Observe for growth, rate of growth, morphology, and hemolytic patterns: • Gamma: no lysis or color change • Alpha: incomplete lysis of RBCs, greenish halo around the bacterial growth • Beta: lysis of RBCs, clear halo around bacterial growth
Brain–Heart Infusion Broth	Calf's brain Beef's heart Dextrose	• Enrichment media to increase the number of organisms	Subcultures are made onto agar plates after incubation of 24 hours
MacConkey agar	Crystal violet Bile acids	• Selects for gram-negative and Enterobacteriaceae	• Pink to red colonies = lactose fermenters • Colorless to light yellow colonies = nonlactose fermenters
Thioglycollate Broth	Thioglycollic acid Yeast extract Dextrose	• Supports growth of anaerobic and facultative anaerobic bacteria	Turbid or streaks if turbidity is not disturbed

- **Caution:** Thioglycollate broth should not be used as the only source of collection media.

Skill Box 7-12 / Culture Media Inoculation and Incubation

General Points for Proper Technique:

- Keep culture plates closed unless inoculating or transferring specimens.
- Do not set down the tube cap of medium to avoid contamination.
- Flame the neck of the tube before and after transferring specimens.
- When flaming the inoculation loop or wire, place the end closest to the handle in the hottest portion of the flame, the blue portion, and then move toward the loop to prevent splattering.
- When transferring the sample to the agar, use a gentle touch to avoid tearing the surface of the agar.

Plate Inoculation:

1. Mentally divide the agar plate into four quadrants.
2. Flame and cool the inoculation loop.
3. Dip the loop into the specimen to be cultured.
4. Streak the specimen in quadrant A.
5. Repeat steps 2–4 while slightly overlapping the previous quadrant and then moving around to each quadrant. Be sure to only overlap the previous quadrant's streaks 1–2 times to prevent excessive numbers of bacteria in one area. Quadrant D is expected to grow isolated colonies.
6. Remove the loop and reflame.

Slant Inoculation:

1. Flame and cool the inoculation wire.
2. Dip the wire into the specimen to be cultured.
3. Types of slant inoculations:
   a. Slant only—make a "S" shape across the slant with the tip of the inoculation wire.
   b. Stab only—stab the wire through the agar and then slowly withdraw it along the same stab path.
   c. Butt and Slant—combine the above two methods, starting with the stab method and finishing with the slant method.
4. Remove the wire and reflame.

Broth Inoculation:

1. Flame and cool the inoculation loop or wire.
2. Dip the wire into the specimen to be cultured.
3. Insert the loop or wire into the broth just below the surface and touch the side of the tube.

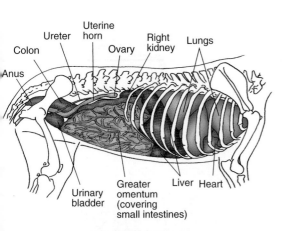

FIGURE **1-5 Left Lateral View**

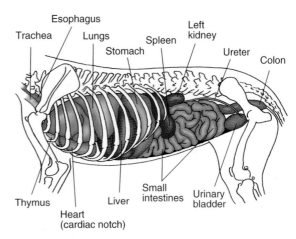

FIGURE **1-6 Right Lateral View**

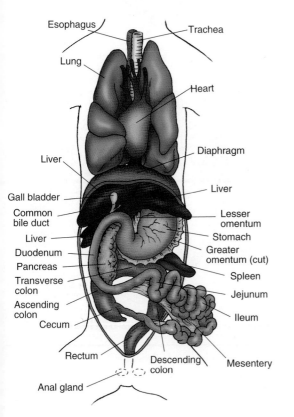

FIGURE **1-7 Ventral View**

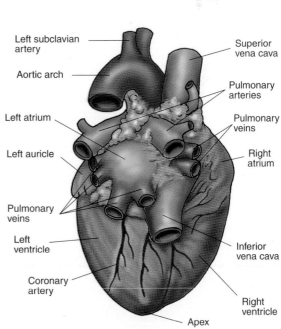

FIGURE **1-8 Dorsal View**

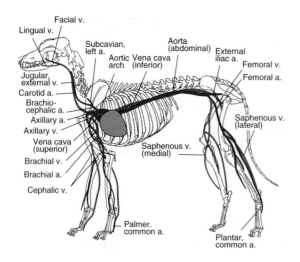

FIGURE 1-9 Lateral View

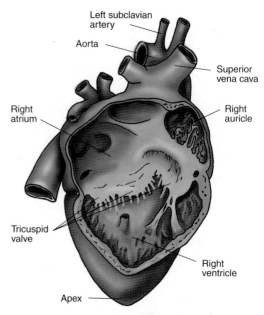

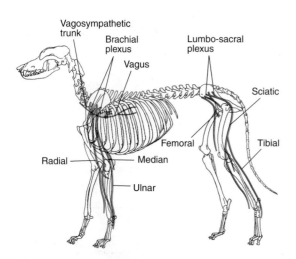

FIGURE 1-12 Lateral View

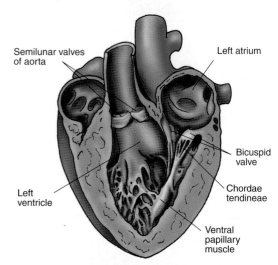

FIGURE 1-10 Inside View of Heart

Hematology

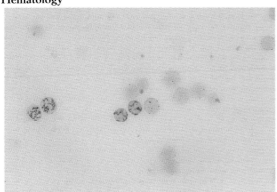

FIGURE 7-1

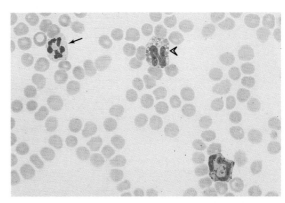

FIGURE 7-2

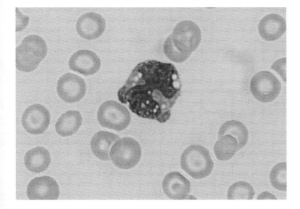

FIGURE 7-3

FIGURE 7-4

FIGURE 7-1
Feline blood smear showing reticulocytes (aggregate and punctate), platelets, and polychromatic RBCs with Heinz bodies. The Heinz bodies are also seen floating freely in the background. From Schalm's V. Hematology, page 155, figure 19.4.

FIGURE 7-2
Paired, teardrop-shaped structures of a dog infected with *Babesia canis.* From Schalm's V. Hematology, page 158, figure 27.7.

FIGURE 7-3
Small, irregular rings found in the RBCs of a cat infected with *Cytauxoon felis.* From Schalm's V. Hematology, page 160, figure 27.10.

FIGURE 7-4
Canine blood smear showing the segmented nucleus of a neutrophil (arrow), eosinophil (arrowhead) with variable sized particles and vacuoles, and a basophil with dark purple granules and a segmented nucleus. (Photo courtesy of Oklahoma State University Clinical Pathology Teaching Files.) From Schalm's V. Hematology, page 1061, figure 163.9.

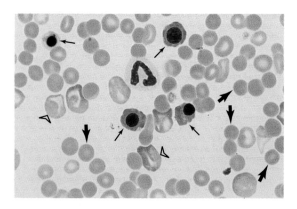

FIGURE 7-5

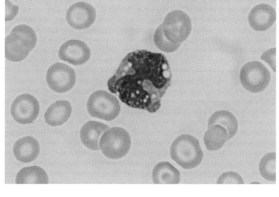

FIGURE 7-6

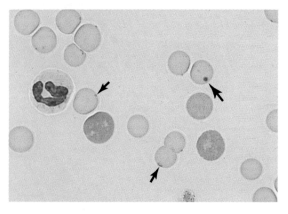

FIGURE 7-7

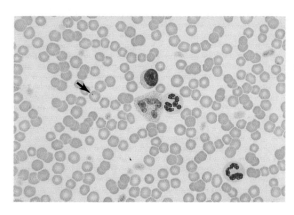

FIGURE 7-8

FIGURE 7-5
Canine blood smear showing polychromatophilic erythrocytes (arrowheads), nucleated RBCs (rubricytes and metarubriytes—thin arrows), and spherocytes (thick arrows). (Photo courtesy of Oklahoma State University Clinical Pathology Teaching Files.) From Schalm's V. Hematology, page 1058, figure 163.2.

FIGURE 7-6
Canine blood smear with a vacuolated monocyte and RBCs showing distinct central pallor. (Photo courtesy of Oklahoma State University Clinical Pathology Teaching Files.) From Schalm's V. Hematology, page 1058, figure 163.1.

FIGURE 7-7
Feline blood smear showing macrocytic gray-blue polychromatophilic and normal RBCs, neutrophil, platelets, Howell-Jolly body (large arrow), and *Hemobartonella felis* (small arrows). (Photo courtesy of Oklahoma State University Clinical Pathology Teaching Files.) From Schalm's V. Hematology, page 1066, figure 164.3.

FIGURE 7-8
Feline blood smear showing moderate anisocytosis, Howell-Jolly body (small arrow), segmented neutrophils, lymphocyte, eosinophil, and platelets. (Photo courtesy of Oklahoma State University Clinical Pathology Teaching Files.) From Schalm's V. Hematology, page 1065, figure 164.1.

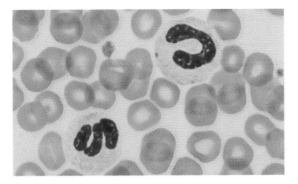

FIGURE 7-9

FIGURE 7-10

Endoparasites

FIGURE 7-11

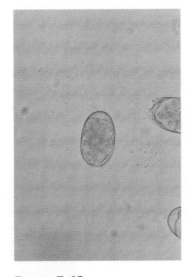

FIGURE 7-12

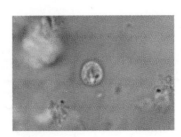

FIGURE 7-13

FIGURE 7-9
Canine blood smear showing toxic change in a segmented and band neutrophil. Toxic change showing cytoplasmic basophilia and Döhle bodies. From Schalm's V. Hematology, page 371, figure 55.5.

FIGURE 7-10
Canine blood smear showing a megathrombocyte (arrow), spherocytes, polychromatophilic erythrocytes, neutrophil, and a reactive lymphocyte. (Photo courtesy of Oklahoma State University Clinical Pathology Teaching Files.) From Schalm's V. Hematology, page 1060, figure 163.7.

FIGURE 7-11
Ancylostoma caninum. From Internal Parasites of Dogs and Cats, page 7.

FIGURE 7-12
Ancylostoma tubaeforme. From Internal Parasites of Dogs and Cats, page 7.

FIGURE 7-13
Crytosporidium. Courtesy of Gary A. Averbeck.

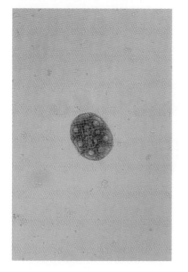

FIGURE 7-14

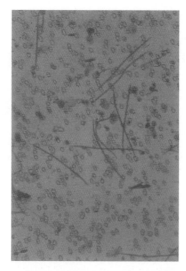

FIGURE 7-15

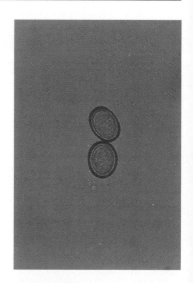

FIGURE 7-16

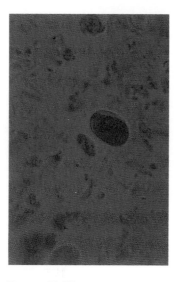

FIGURE 7-17

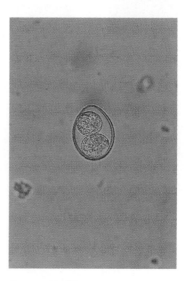

FIGURE 7-18

FIGURE 7-14
Dipylidium caninum. From Internal Parasites of Dogs and Cats, page 5.

FIGURE 7-15
Dirofilaria immitis. From Internal Parasites of Dogs and Cats, page 3.

FIGURE 7-16
Echinococcus granulosus. From Internal Parasites of Dogs and Cats, page 5.

FIGURE 7-17
Giardia spp. From Internal Parasites of Dogs and Cats, page 11.

FIGURE 7-18
Isospora spp. From Internal Parasites of Dogs and Cats, page 11.

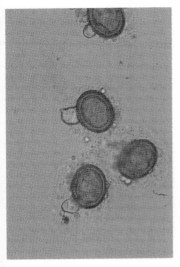

FIGURE 7-19

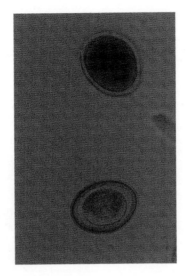

FIGURE 7-20

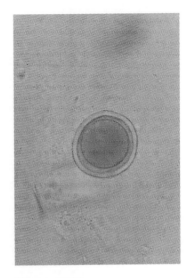

FIGURE 7-21

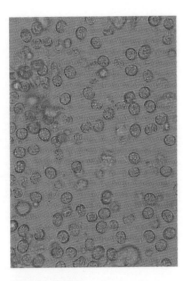

FIGURE 7-22

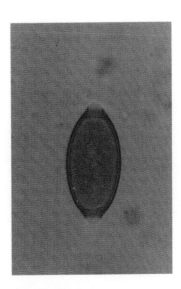

FIGURE 7-23

FIGURE 7-19
Taenia spp. From Internal Parasites of Dogs and Cats, page 6.

FIGURE 7-20
Toxocara canis (top)/Toxascaris leonina (bottom). From Internal Parasites of Dogs and Cats, page 9.

FIGURE 7-21
Toxocara cati. From Internal Parasites of Dogs and Cats, page 10.

FIGURE 7-22
Toxoplasma gondii. From Internal Parasites of Dogs and Cats, page 12.

FIGURE 7-23
Trichuris vulpis. From Internal Parasites of Dogs and Cats, page 10.

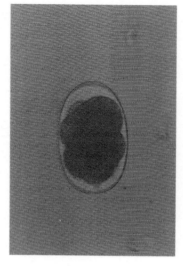

FIGURE 7-24

Ectoparasites

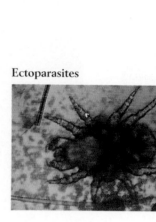

FIGURE 7-25

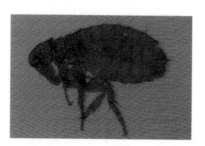

FIGURE 7-26

FIGURE 7-27

FIGURE 7-24
Uncinaria stenocephala. From Internal Parasites of Dogs and Cats, page 8.

FIGURE 7-25
Cheyletiella. From External Parasites of Dogs and Cats, page 14.

FIGURE 7-26
Ctenocephalides canis. From External Parasites of Dogs and Cats, page 3.

FIGURE 7-27
Linognathus setosus. From External Parasites of Dogs and Cats, page 10.

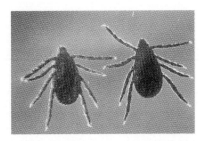

FIGURE 7-28

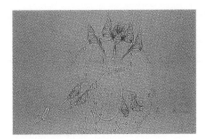

FIGURE 7-29

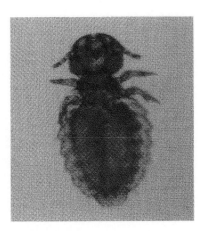

FIGURE 7-30

Urine Sediment

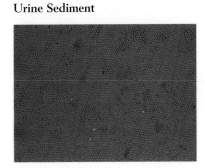

FIGURE 7-31

FIGURE 7-28
Rhipicephalus sanguineus. From External Parasites of Dogs and Cats, page 25.

FIGURE 7-29
Sarcoptes scabiei canis. From External Parasites of Dogs and Cats, page 17.

FIGURE 7-30
Trichodectes canis. From External Parasites of Dogs and Cats, page 10.

FIGURE 7-31
Bacteria. From Graff's Handbook of Routine Urinalysis, page 116, figure 3-51.

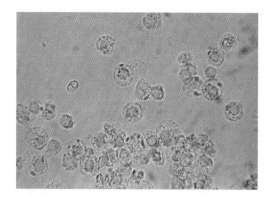

FIGURE 7-32

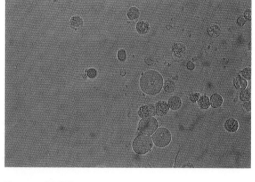

FIGURE 7-33

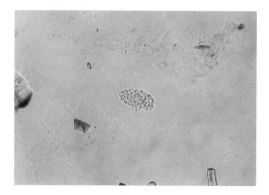

FIGURE 7-34

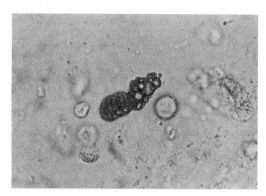

FIGURE 7-35

FIGURE 7-32
WBCs. From Graff's Handbook of Routine Urinalysis, page 77, figure 3-4.

FIGURE 7-33
Epithelial cells, WBCs, RBCs, and bacteria. From Graff's Handbook of Routine Urinalysis, page 134, figure 4-2.

FIGURE 7-34
Epithelial cast. From Graff's Handbook of Routine Urinalysis, page 113, figure 3-47.

FIGURE 7-35
Fatty cast. From Graff's Handbook of Routine Urinalysis, page 115, figure 3-50.

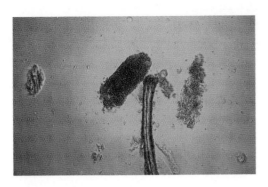

FIGURE 7-36

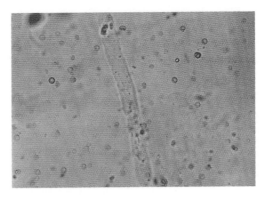

FIGURE 7-37

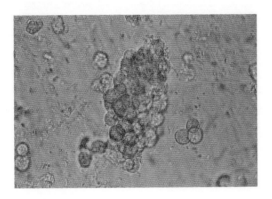

FIGURE 7-38

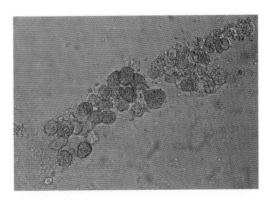

FIGURE 7-39

FIGURE 7-36
Granular cast and a hair follicle. From Graff's Handbook of Routine Urinalysis, page 127, figure 3-65.

FIGURE 7-37
Hyaline cast and RBCs. From Graff's Handbook of Routine Urinalysis, page 109, figure 3-42.

FIGURE 7-38
RBC cast and RBCs. From Graff's Handbook of Routine Urinalysis, page 110, figure 3-43.

FIGURE 7-39
WBC cast. From Graff's Handbook of Routine Urinalysis, page 194, figure 4-92.

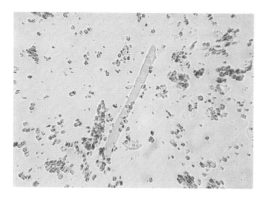

FIGURE 7-40

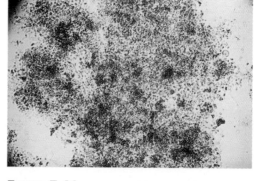

FIGURE 7-41

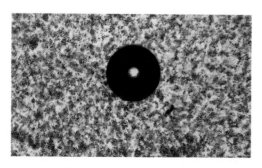

FIGURE 7-42

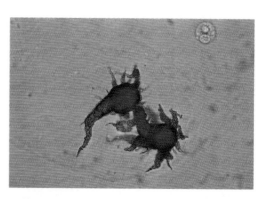

FIGURE 7-43

FIGURE 7-40
Waxy cast. From Graff's Handbook of Routine Urinalysis, page 208, figure 4-112.

FIGURE 7-41
Amorphous phosphate crystals. From Graff's Handbook of Routine Urinalysis, page 103, figure 3-36.

FIGURE 7-42
Amorphous urate crystals and an air bubble. From Graff's Handbook of Routine Urinalysis, page 128, figure 3-67.

FIGURE 7-43
Amorphous biurate crystals and mucous threads. From Graff's Handbook of Routine Urinalysis, page 180, figure 4-71.

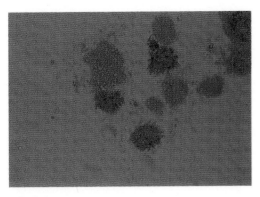

FIGURE 7-44

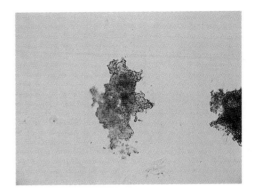

FIGURE 7-45

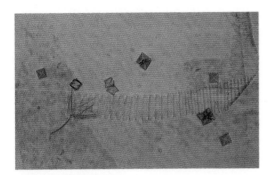

FIGURE 7-46

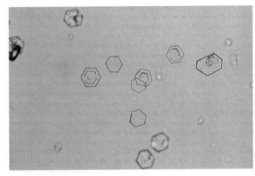

FIGURE 7-47

FIGURE 7-44
Bilirubin crystals. From Graff's Handbook of Routine Urinalysis, page 170, figure 4-55.

FIGURE 7-45
Calcium carbonate crystals. From Graff's Handbook of Routine Urinalysis, page 104, figure 3-37.

FIGURE 7-46
Calcium oxalate dihydrate crystals. From Graff's Handbook of Routine Urinalysis, page 152, figure 4-29.

FIGURE 7-47
Cystine crystals. From Graff's Handbook of Routine Urinalysis, page 93, figure 3-23.

FIGURE 7-48

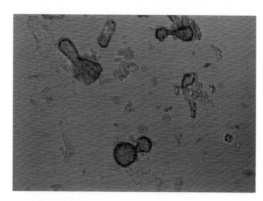

FIGURE 7-49

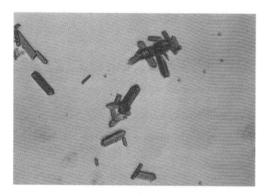

FIGURE 7-50

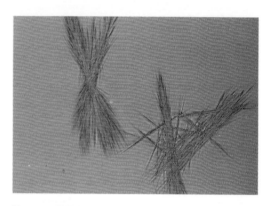

FIGURE 7-51

FIGURE 7-48
Leucine crystals. From Graff's Handbook of Routine Urinalysis, page 94, figure 3-24.

FIGURE 7-49
Sulfonamide crystals. From Graff's Handbook of Routine Urinalysis, page 163, figure 4-45.

FIGURE 7-50
Triple Phosphate crystals. From Graff's Handbook of Routine Urinalysis, page 170, figure 4-56.

FIGURE 7-51
Tyrosine crystals. From Graff's Handbook of Routine Urinalysis, page 165, figure 4-48.

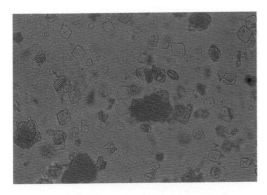

FIGURE 7-52

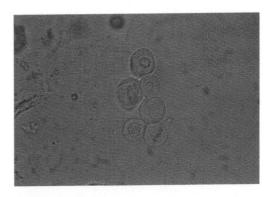

FIGURE 7-53

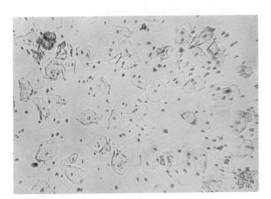

FIGURE 7-54

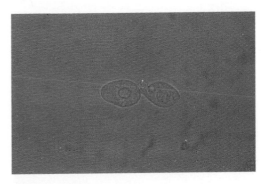

FIGURE 7-55

FIGURE 7-52
Uric acid crystals. From Graff's Handbook of Routine Urinalysis, page 144, figure 4-16.

FIGURE 7-53
Renal epithelial cells. From Graff's Handbook of Routine Urinalysis, page 139, figure 4-9.

FIGURE 7-54
Squamous epithelial cells. From Graff's Handbook of Routine Urinalysis, page 141, figure 4-12.

FIGURE 7-55
Transitional epithelial cells. From Graff's Handbook of Routine Urinalysis, page 81, figure 3-8.

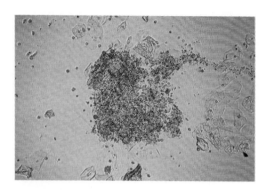

FIGURE 7-56

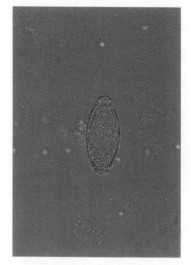

FIGURE 7-57

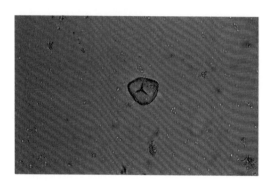

FIGURE 7-58

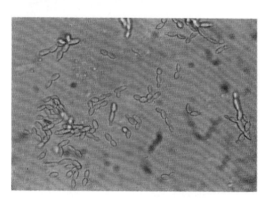

FIGURE 7-59

FIGURE 7-56
Epithelial cells and lipid droplets. From Graff's Handbook of Routine Urinalysis, page 220, figure 4-130.

FIGURE 7-57
Capillaria plica. From Internal Parasites of Dogs and Cats, page 14.

FIGURE 7-58
Starch granules. From Graff's Handbook of Routine Urinalysis, page 123, figure 3-59.

FIGURE 7-59
Yeast. From Graff's Handbook of Routine Urinalysis, page 217, figure 4-126.

4. Remove the loop or wire and reflame.

Work with two inoculation loops; one can be cooling while the other is in use.

Incubation of Cultures:

- Maintain incubator temperature at 98.6° F and humidity of 70%.
- Plates should be placed upside down to prevent the accumulation of condensation on the surface of the agar plate.
- Tube media screw caps should be left loose during incubation.
- Cultures should be incubated for 48 hours and checked after 24 hours.
- To increase the level of carbon dioxide, place the plates upside down in a glass jar with a candle on top. Light the candle and place a tightly fitting lid on top. Allow the candle to burn itself out, which will decrease the amount of oxygen and increase the amount of carbon dioxide. This does not create an anaerobic environment.

Place a bowl of water in the bottom of the incubator to maintain a high humidity.

Evaluation of Culture Growth

1. Identify the source of the sample
2. Growth

Significant	Not Significant
Only 1–2 types of bacterial growth	>3 Types of scant bacterial growth
Circular colonies with clear edges, smooth, convex, or rounded	Large, irregular, and granular colonies and spreading edges
Opaque to gray	Heavily pigmented

3. Changes to the media
    a. Hemolytic pattern
    b. Color change
    c. Odor
4. Microscopic evaluation
    a. Simple stain
    b. Gram stain
    c. Acid-fast stain
    d. Negative stain
5. Differentiation tests
    a. Catalase test
    b. Oxidase test
    c. Indole test

Skill Box 7-13 / Staining Solutions and Procedures

The first step to identification of microbiology slides is to properly prepare the slide. All staining of slides should be done on an air-dried heat-fixed slide. To heat-fix a slide, make several rapid passes of the slide over a flame source (e.g., matches, lighter, or Bunsen burner). Once the slide has been immersed in staining solution, it should be agitated to allow fresh stain to remain in contact with its surface.

Staining Technique	Uses	Preparation	Procedure	Interpretation
Differential Stains				
Diff-Quik (modified Wright's Stain)	General cytology and demonstration of bacteria	Methyl alcohol Triarylmethane dye Xanthene dye Thiazine dye mixture	1. Dip the prepared slide five times slowly in methanol fixative 2. Repeat above with eosinophilic stain and basophilic stain 3. Rinse with water 4. Air dry	• Clear differentiation of cellular morphology • Staining ranges from pale pink to dark purple
Giemsa Stain	Detection of spirochetes and rickettsiae	Methanol Giemsa powder Glycerol	1. Fix the prepared slide in absolute methanol for 3–5 minutes and air dry 2. Place the slide in diluted stain; 20–30 minutes 3. Rinse with water and air dry	• Purplish-blue stained bacteria
Gram Stain	Distinguish between gram-positive and gram-negative bacteria based on their cell wall structure	Crystal violet Gram's iodine Decolorizer Dilute carbol fuchsin	1. Flood the prepared slide with crystal violet; 30 seconds 2. Rinse with water 3. Flood the slide with Gram's iodine; 30 seconds 4. Rinse with water 5. Decolorize until the purple color is gone; 10 seconds 6. Rinse with water 7. Flood the slide with dilute carbol fuchsin; 30 seconds 8. Rinse with water 9. Air dry or blot between towels	• Purple-stained bacteria are gram-positive • Red-stained bacteria are gram-negative
Lactophenol cotton blue	Detection of fungi	Lactophenol cotton blue	Same as simple stain	• Visualization of hyphae, septae, and structure of spores

Staining Technique	Uses	Preparation	Procedure	Interpretation
Ziehl-Neelson or Acid-Fast Stain	Detection of *Mycobacterium spp* and *Nocardia*	Carbol fuchsin Acid alcohol Methylene blue	1. Flood the prepared slide with carbol fuchsin and heat over a flame until it steams and then let it sit; 5 minutes 2. Rinse with water 3. Decolorize with acid alcohol until the red color is gone; 1–2 minutes 4. Rinse with water 5. Counterstain with methylene blue; 2 minutes 6. Rinse with water and dry over low heat	• Acid-fast bacteria stain red • Nonacid-fast bacteria stain blue
Modified Ziehl/Neelson Stain with brilliant green	Same as above	Carbol fuchsin Acid alcohol Brilliant green	1. Flood the prepared slide with carbol fuchsin; 3 minutes then heat 2. Rinse with water 3. Decolorize with acid-alcohol; 3 minutes 4. Rinse with water 5. Counterstain with brilliant green; 3 minutes 6. Rinse and dry	• Acid-fast bacteria stain red • Non–acid-fast bacteria stain green
Modified Ziehl/Neelson Stain with methylene blue	Detection of *Brucella, Nocardia,* and *Chlamydia*	Carbol fuchsin Acetic acid 0.5% Methylene blue	1. Flood the prepared slide with dilute carbol fuchsin; 10 minutes 2. Rinse with water 3. Decolorize with acetic acid; 20–30 seconds 4. Rinse with water 5. Counterstain with methylene blue; 2 minutes 6. Rinse and dry	• *Brucella* and *Chlamydia* stain bright red and in clumps
Simple Stains Negative staining	Detection of capsules and difficult to stain bacteria (e.g., spirilli)	A negatively charged chromogen stain: India Ink Nigrosin	1. Prepare an air-dried slide 2. Apply 1–2 drops of stain to prepared slide 3. Apply coverslip and examine as a wet mount	• Capsules appear clear and unstained, surrounded by dark particles

Skill Box 7-13 / Staining Solutions and Procedures (Continued)

Staining Technique	Uses	Preparation	Procedure	Interpretation
Simple stain	Demonstration of bacteria and general morphology and shape arrangement	A positively charged chromogen stain: Methylene blue Safranin Carbol fuschin Crystal violet	1. Place 1 drop of stain on the coverslip and apply to prepared slide 2. Place a paper towel over the coverslip and apply gentle pressure to absorb excess stain Or 1. Place 1 drop of stain next to the coverslip on a prepared slide and allow the stain to leak under the coverslip 2. Place a paper towel over the coverslip and apply gentle pressure to absorb excess stain	• Visualization of cell shape and arrangement

Stains should be periodically filtered, using filter paper to remove any precipitate that may have formed.

Rinse slides on the reverse side to avoid disturbing the sample.

Skill Box 7-14 / Staining Problems

To avoid staining problems, use fresh clean stains and slides, do not touch the surface of the slide, and immediately stain slides after air drying.

Problem	Solution
Excessive staining	• Decrease staining time • Rinse adequately between stains and after staining • Prepare a thinner sample on the slide • Allow slide to dry before applying coverslip
Weak staining	• Increase staining time • Change stains • Stain slides sooner after air-drying • Keep the caps tightly placed on the stain containers to prevent evaporation
Uneven staining	• Use only clean and dry slides • Do not touch the sample area of the slides before or after preparation • Place slides at an angle for drying to prevent liquid from drying onto the slide • Inadequate mixing of stains • Keep the caps tightly placed on the stain containers to prevent contamination and evaporation
Slide precipitate	• Rinse adequately between stains and after staining (refer to Skill Box 7-13) • Use clean slides • Do not allow stains to dry onto slide while staining • Change or filter stains periodically and regularly • Keep the caps tightly placed on the stain containers to prevent contamination and evaporation

Replace stains monthly, more often depending on use.

Filter stains as needed to keep clear of precipitates.

Table 7-15 Bacteria Identification

Organism	General Information	Associated Conditions	Microscopic	Culture
Bordatella bronchiseptica	• Gram-negative	• Upper respiratory infection and pneumonia	• Small rods	BA = small, circular, dewdrop shape with ± beta-hemolysis; slow grower MC = weak growth
Borrelia burgdorferi	• Spirochete	• Lyme disease	Refer to reference laboratory for identification	Refer to reference laboratory for identification
Brucella canis	• Gram-negative	• Infertility, abortion, and diskospondylitis	• Small, red coccobacillus in clumps	BA = round, smooth, glistening, and translucent
Campylobacter spp.	• Gram-negative • Does not survive outside the host ≥ 3 hours	• Gastroenteritis, infertility, and abortion	• Curved rods; motile, spiral-type motion	Refer to reference laboratory for identification
Chlamydia	• Resemble gram-negative • Obligate, intracellular parasite	• Conjunctivitis and pneumonia	• Small, red, pleomorphic coccobacilli in clumps	• N/A
Clostridium	• Gram-positive • Obligate anaerobes • Resistant to most disinfectants, requires 20 minutes of boiling or 121° C in an autoclave for 20 minutes	• Gastroenteritis, otitis and tetanus	• Large, spore-forming rods with rounded ends	BA = 1–3 mm in diameter, round to slightly irregular, raised, granular, transparent with a double zone of hemolysis MC = no growth
E. coli	• Gram-negative • Facultative anaerobes • Readily killed by disinfectants, sunlight, and desiccation	• Genital tract infection, musculoskeletal infection, pneumonia, enteritis, abscesses, urinary tract infection, and sepsis	• Small, non–spore-forming rods	BA = large, smooth, gray, mucoid colonies with ± hemolysis MC = red growth, lactose fermentation, hemolytic pattern
Fusobacterium	• Gram-negative • Obligate anaerobes	• Pleuritis and abscesses	• Slender, long rods with pointed ends and long beaded filaments	BA = small, smooth, convex and whitish-yellow in color colonies with a narrow zone of alpha- or beta-hemolysis

Organism	Characteristics	Morphology	Conditions	Culture
Mycobacterium tuberculosis	• Gram-positive	• Small, straight or slightly curved acid-fast rods, singly or in clumps	• Pulmonary nodules (dogs) and gastrointestinal problems (cats)	Refer to a reference laboratory for identification
Mycoplasma spp.	• Gram-positive • Lack a cell wall; therefore do not stain adequately enough to evaluate • Readily killed by common disinfectants	• Small, coccobacillus-like, non-spore-forming, no cell wall and ± pleomorphic	• Genital tract infection, arthritis, conjunctivitis (cats) and pneumonia	Refer to a reference laboratory for identification
Nocardia spp.	• Gram-positive aerobes • Saprophyte in the soil • Partially acid-fast	• Branching, filamentous rods or coccobacilli	• Pleuritis and abscesses in multiple tissues	BA = irregularly folded, raised, smooth to rough with a dry granular texture; slow grower MC = no growth
Pasteurella spp.	• Gram-negative • Facultative anaerobes • Readily killed by most common disinfectants	• Small, non-spore-forming coccobacilli or rods	• Conjunctivitis, genital tract infection, upper respiratory infection, pneumonia, pleuritis, abscesses and urinary tract infections	BA = round, smooth, gray colonies with ± hemolysis MC = no growth
Proteus spp.	• Gram-negative • Facultative anaerobes • Readily killed by common disinfectants, sunlight and dessication	• Medium-sized non-spore-forming rods	• Cystitis, urinary tract infections, diarrhea, wounds and otitis	BA = large, smooth, gray, swarming, mucoid colonies with ± hemolysis MC = colorless growth that may spread
Pseudomonas spp.	• Gram-negative • Killed by most common disinfectants, ↑ resistance to high dilutions of quaternary ammonium compounds and phenolic compounds	• Small rods	• Conjunctivitis, otitis musculoskeletal infection, abscesses, and urinary tract infections	BA = 3–5 mm in diameter, irregular, spreading, translucent, bluish-metallic sheen, beta-hemolysis and grape-like odor MC = yellow-green pigmented growth with a grape-like odor

BA = Blood agar, MC = McConkey agar

Table 7-15 Bacteria Identification (Continued)

Organism	General Information	Associated Conditions	Microscopic	Culture
Rickettsia	• Resemble gram-negative • Obligate, intracellular parasite • Smallest organism able to reproduce on its own • Cannot live outside the host	• Rocky Mountain spotted fever, salmon poisoning disease, ehrlichia and hemobartonella	• Small, pleomorphic coccobacilli	• N/A
Salmonella	• Gram-negative • Readily killed by common disinfectants, sunlight, and dessication	• Gastroenteritis, abortion, hepatitis, and septicemia	• Small non-spore forming rods	BA = large, smooth, gray, mucoid colonies with ± hemolysis MC = colorless growth
Staphylococcus aureus/intermedius	• Gram-positive • Stable, surviving for months when dried in pus or other body fluids • ↑ resistance to common disinfectants	• Conjunctivitis, genital tract infection, mastitis, pyoderma, otitis, osteomyelitis, musculoskeletal infection, pneumonia, abscesses and urinary tract infections	• Cocci, often in grape-like clusters, non-spore forming, ± capsules	BA = 4 mm in diameter, round, smooth, glistening with a double zone of hemolysis and ± gold pigmentation MC = no growth
Streptococcus spp.	• Gram-positive • Facultative anaerobes • Remain living for weeks to months after being expelled from the body • Readily killed by common disinfectants	• Conjunctivitis, genital tract infection, otitis, pneumonia, abscesses, and urinary tract infections	• Cocci, ± singly or in chains of varying lengths and non-spore forming	BA = 1 mm in diameter, round, smooth, glistening and resemble dewdrops with beta-hemolysis (Alpha and gamma-hemolysis are typically normal flora) MC = no growth

BA = Blood agar, MC = McConkey agar

Table 7-16 Fungi Identification

Organism	Associated Conditions	Microscopic	Culture
Aspergillus	• Nasal infections • Common laboratory contaminant	Preparation: clear cellophane tape with lactophenol blue or scrapings mixed with 10% sodium hydroxide Identification: short pieces of thick, septate hyphae	Medium: Blood agar or Sabouraud dextrose agar Additive: none Incubation: 48 hours at 77°–98.6° F Identification: flat, white, and floccose, then turns green to dark green and powdery
Blastomyces dermatitidis	• Pulmonary nodules, internal ulcers and abscesses	Preparation: wet mount with 20% KOH Identification: large, oval or spherical, thick-walled with a single bud that is connected to the mother cell by a wide base	Refer to reference laboratory for confirmation by culture
Candida spp.	• Mycotic stomatitis (dogs) or enteritis (kittens)	Preparation: scrapings of lesions made as wet mounts with 20% KOH, India ink, or lactophenol cotton blue Identification: thin-walled (no capsule) oval budding yeast cells and ± pseudohyphae	Medium: Blood agar or Sabouraud dextrose agar Additive: none Incubation: 2 days at 77°–98.6° F Identification: creamy, smooth colonies with yeast-like odor
Coccidiodes immitis	• Systemic and bone infections	Preparation: unstained wet mounts Identification: thick-walled sporangia	• **Caution:** Because of its zoonotic potential, refer to a reference laboratory for culture
Cryptococcus neoformans	• Paranasal and CNS infections	Preparation: A small amount of discharge is mixed on a slide with water and India ink in a 1:2 ratio Identification: budding yeast-like cells with large capsules	Medium: Blood agar or Sabouraud dextrose agar Additive: none Incubation: 14 days at 95°–98.6° F Identification: wrinkled, whitish granular colonies to mucoid, cream to brown colonies
Histoplasma capsulatum	• Systemic, pulmonary and gastrointestinal infections • Soil borne	Preparation: Giemsa or Wright's method Identification: small oval cells surrounded by a halo seen intracellularly in monocytic cells	• **Caution:** Because of its zoonotic potential, refer to a reference laboratory for culture

Table 7-16 Fungi Identification (Continued)

Organism	Associated Conditions	Microscopic	Culture
Malassezia pachydermatis	• Chronic otitis externa (dogs) and pyoderma	Preparation: wet mounts with 10% NaOH Identification: oval or bottle-shaped, small budding cells	Medium: Blood agar or Sabouraud dextrose agar Additive: Olive or coconut oil Incubation: 14 days at 77° F in a CO_2 incubator Identification: greenish pigmentation
Microsporum canis	• Dermatophytosis	Preparation: place a few pieces of plucked hair, scales, or crust from skin scraping, 20% KOH, and black India ink on a slide, and apply a coverslip with gentle pressure • Gently heat the slide, and let it sit for 10–15 minutes Identification: chains of highly refractile arthrospores	Medium: Dermatophyte test medium (DTM, modified Sabouraud dextrose agar) Additive: Phenol red, pH indicator Incubation: 2 weeks at room temperature Identification: flat colony, white surface and silky in center, red color change to agar

PARASITOLOGY

Fecal analysis is one of the most common laboratory tests run in small animal clinics. The skills required for preparing and reading these tests are minimal and are expected of every technician. Regardless of their simplicity, the result of these tests and subsequent treatment often leads to a full recovery by the patient.

Fecal Collection, Handling, Storage and Transport Tips

Collection:

- Sample must be as fresh as possible because of rapid development of eggs once passed.
- Owner should witness animal defecating to assure freshness and observe for any straining, fresh blood, or other problems.
- Fresh samples not to be examined in 2 hours should be refrigerated for no longer than 24 hours.
- Submit the amount equal to the size of an adult male's thumb, at least 10 g.
- Sample should be clearly marked with patient's name, number, when the sample was collected, and whether it was refrigerated.

Handling:

- Samples should be handled carefully to avoid human contamination.
- Maintain a clean environment in which to run the laboratory tests.
- Maintain clear records as to the procedure performed.

Storage:

- Fecal samples can be stored in whirl pak bags, small plastic sandwich bags, plastic containers, or disposable laboratory gloves turned inside out.
- Samples can be stored indefinitely in 10% formalin (1 part feces to 9 parts formalin), with minor limitations.
- Samples should not be stored by freezing, 70% ethyl alcohol, or 100% methyl alcohol.

Transport:

- Sample should be cooled to 39.2° F in the refrigerator and then packed on ice or cold packs for 24–48 hours.

  Place important papers in a separate plastic bag in case of sample fluid leakage.

Skill Box 7-15 / Endoparasite Examination Methods

Method	Uses	Technique	General Information
Gross Examination	• Consistency • Color • Blood, mucus, or adult parasites	Visualize the feces or vomitus	• Reveals conditions (e.g., blood) not seen in other methods
Direct	• Protozoa (e.g., *Giardia*) • Parasite burden	Place a drop of saline or water with an equal amount of feces on a slide. Thoroughly mix the feces and water and smear to make a thin film over slide. Remove any large pieces of feces and add a coverslip to examine. Examine under 10× for parasite eggs and 40× for protozoal organisms. Stain can be added to the side of the coverslip for clearer identification.	• No egg distortion • Not a concentrated technique (small sample size) leading to low numbers
Standard or Simple Flotation	• Most parasites • Parasite burden	Place 1–2 g feces in a suitable container (e.g., paper cup) and add flotation solution. Mix the contents thoroughly with a tongue depressor and strain through a tea strainer or cheesecloth into a second container. Pour this mixture into a test tube and add more flotation solution until a meniscus is formed. Place a glass coverslip over the meniscus for 10–15 minutes. The coverslip is then removed, placed on a slide, and examined.	• Commercial fecal flotation kits available • Less efficiently recovers eggs than the centrifugal flotation method • Misses larvae that settle because of gravity
Centrifugal Flotation	• Most parasites • Parasite burden	Mix 1 tsp. feces in a paper cup with enough water to make a semisolid suspension. Place a tea strainer or cheesecloth over a second paper cup, and empty the contents on top of it. Push the liquid through the strainer with the tongue depressor and then discard the solid waste. Pour this mixture into a test tube and centrifuge for 3 minutes at 1,500 rpm. Decant the supernatant and add fecal solution to within $\frac{1}{2}$ inch of top. Stir the solution with a stir stick, plug with a rubber stopper and invert 4–5 times to thoroughly mix solution. Return to the centrifuge and fill the tube. Centrifuge for 5 minutes and then, without moving the tube, transfer the surface film to a slide, cover with a coverslip, and examine.	• More efficiently recovers eggs than the standard flotation method • Requires a centrifuge with a horizontal rotor and the ability to hold 15-mL tubes • Misses larvae that settle because of gravity

Method	Uses	Technique	General Information
Baermann Technique	• Nematode larvae	Fill the funnel with warmed water or physiologic saline (86° F) to cover the wire screen. Spread a piece of cheesecloth or a gauze square over the wire screen in the funnel. Place 5–15 g feces, soil, or tissue on the cheesecloth and fold any excess cloth over the sample. Make sure that the warm water covers the sample. Leave the sample undisturbed overnight (>8 hours). Place a glass slide under the cut-off pipette and allow 1 drop of the liquid to fall onto the slide. Apply a coverslip and examine. If the slide is negative, repeat several times for assurance.	• Efficient recovery of larvae
Fecal Culture	• Hookworm larvae • To distinguish between parasites that have similar-appearing eggs and cysts	Place feces in a glass jar rinsed with 0.1% sodium carbonate solution or on a piece of filter paper in a petri dish. Cover the container and place in a dark area for 7–10 days. There should be enough moisture in the container to produce condensation on the sides; if not, add a small amount of water. After 7–10 days, rinse the container with a small amount of water, collect liquid, and centrifuge. Examine the sediment with a microscope.	• Guaranteed identification

A dried tapeworm proglottid may be rehydrated by soaking in water or physiologic saline for 1–4 hours.

Skill box 7-16 / Fecal Flotation Solutions

Fecal flotation solutions are used to assist in the discovery of parasitic eggs in fecal material. The solution chosen must have a specific gravity that allows parasite eggs to float and the bulk of fecal material to sink. Because water has a specific gravity just slightly lower than many parasite eggs, sugar or salts are added to increase the solution's specific gravity and allow the eggs to float. The desired specific gravity is between 1.2 and 1.25 g/mL. Solutions with a specific gravity >1.35 g/mL will allow both debris and parasite eggs to float, making egg identification more difficult. A specific gravity <1.10 will force both debris and parasite eggs to sink, giving no diagnosis.

Solutions that are purchased premixed are preferred because of quality control. Solutions mixed in the clinical setting tend to have less quality control and give variable results. Almost all solutions will form crystals on the slide if left sitting.

Media	Preparation	Specific Gravity	General Information
Magnesium Sulfate	Magnesium sulfate: 400 g Tap water: 1,000 mL	1.20	• Readily available and inexpensive
Sodium Chloride	Sodium chloride: 400 g Tap water: 1,000 mL Stir while adding the sodium chloride to water. Heating is not necessary, but speeds the dissolution.	1.18–1.20	• Readily available and inexpensive • Corrodes expensive laboratory equipment • Severely distorts eggs
Sodium Nitrate	Sodium nitrate: 400 g Tap water: 1000 ml Stir while adding the sodium nitrate to water. Heating is not necessary, but speeds the dissolution.	1.20	• Floats the greatest percentage of eggs • Can be purchased in a ready-to-mix solution • Distorts the eggs after 15 minutes • May not be readily available and more expensive
Sugar Solution, Sheather's Solution	Granulated sugar: 454 g Tap water: 355 mL Dissolve sugar in water by heating on low heat and stirring. Add 2 mL of 37% formaldehyde or phenol crystals to prevent bacterial growth.	1.27–1.33	• Readily available and inexpensive • Does not distort eggs or crystallize • Floats an adequate percentage of eggs • Best if used with centrifugal flotation technique
Zinc Sulfate	Zinc sulfate: 371 g Tap water: 1,000 mL Stir while adding the zinc sulfate to water. Heating is not necessary, but speeds the dissolution.	1.18	• Best for intestinal protozoa (e.g., *Giardia*) • Light must be ↓ and focused immediately under the coverslip • Floats a high percentage of eggs

If a fecal sample is left for more than 1 hour, the eggs may become waterlogged, resulting in distortion or sinking to the bottom.

Skill box 7-17 / Blood Parasite Examination Methods

Method	Uses	Technique	General Information
Direct Examination	• Microfilariae	Add 1 drop of blood to a slide. Add a coverslip and examine for movement.	• Small sample volume owing to low sensitivity
Thin Blood Smear	• Trypanosomes, protozoans, and rickettsia	Place a drop of blood near one end with a glass slide laying on a flat surface, place another slide at a 30%–40% angle in front of the blood. Back the slide up until the blood runs along the edge of the second slide. Then gently and steadily push the slide forward and off the first slide, producing a smear with a feathered edge. Air-dry, ± add stain and examine.	• Small sample volume
Thick Blood Smear	• Microfilariae, protozoa, and rickettsiae	Place three drops of blood on a slide, spread the drop out with a wooden applicator stick into a 2-cm circle. Air-dry the slide. Place the slide in a slanted position in a container of distilled water. Once the smear losses its red color, remove it and allow it to air-dry. Place the slide in methyl alcohol for 10 minutes, then add Giemsa stain for 30 minutes. Rinse slide and examine.	• Larger sample volume
Buffy Coat	• Microfilariae	Fill and centrifuge an Hct tube for 3 minutes. Using a file or glass slide, score the tube just below the buffy coat and snap apart. Tap the tube until the buffy coat drops onto a glass slide. Add a drop of saline and stain, place a coverslip on, and examine.	• Does not allow differentiation of microfilariae species
Modified Knott's Technique	• Microfilariae	Mix 1 mL whole unclotted blood with 9 mL 2% formalin in a test tube. Centrifuge at 1,300–1,500 rpm for 5 minutes. Pour off the supernatant and add 2–3 drops of stain to the sediment. With a pipette, mix the sediment and stain. Place a drop on a glass slide, apply a coverslip, and examine under 10×.	• Allows differentiation of microfilariae species

Skill Box 7-18 / Ectoparasite Examination Methods

Method	Uses	Technique	General Information
Gross Examination	• Lice, mites, ticks, flies, or fleas	Visualize the ectoparasite on the animal or by using a flea comb.	• Limited number of parasites visible
Cellophane Tape	• Lice or mites	Bend the cellophane tape into a loop with the sticky side out. Press the tape against the animal's skin. Put 1 drop of water on a slide and lay tape over it and press down. Examine under a microscope.	• Limited number of parasites visible
Microscopic Examination	• Most ectoparasites	Place a drop of mineral oil on a glass slide. Roll the swab or material collected in the mineral oil to deposit any debris. Place a coverslip on the slide and examine with a microscope, using 4× magnification.	• Most thorough technique for ectoparasite diagnosis

Table 7-17 Endoparasites

Prevention of human infection from endoparasites involves proper hygiene (e.g., washing hands and properly cooking food), isolation of infected animals, and quarantine of newly acquired animals. Each fecal sample should be thought of as a zoonotic risk and treated appropriately.

Parasite	Transmission Route	Clinical Signs	Diagnostics	Common Treatments	Picture
Ancylostoma caninum **ZOONOTIC** *Common Name:* Southern hookworm *Type:* Nematode *Affected Species:* Canine *Disinfection:* Bleach *Environment:* Can live in cool, moist soil for several weeks	Eggs passed → ingestion, percutaneous, prenatal and transmammary → lungs for development → coughed up and swallowed → small intestines to mature *Prepatent period: 2 weeks*	• Anemia, weakness, inappetance, poor growth, dry cough, diarrhea, constipation, and dark tarry stools	• Fecal flotation • Egg: Oval or ellipsoid, capsule-shaped, 8-16 cells inside a thin wall • Sample must be <48 hours old because eggs larvate rapidly in the external environment	Butamisole Dichlorvos Febantel + Praziquantel Fenbendazole Ivermectin Lufenuron + Milbemycin Mebendazole Milbemycin oxime Pyrantel	See Color Plate Fig. 7-11
Ancylostoma tubaeforme **ZOONOTIC** *Common Name:* Feline hookworm *Type:* Nematode *Affected Species:* Feline *Disinfection:* Bleach *Environment:* Can live in cool, moist soil for several weeks	Eggs passed → ingestion, percutaneous, prenatal and transmammary → lungs for development → coughed up and swallowed → small intestines to mature *Prepatent period: 3-3.5 weeks*	• Interdigital dermatitis, pulmonary lesions, anemia and poor hair coat	• Fecal flotation • Egg: Oval or ellipsoid, capsule shaped, 8-16 cells inside a thin wall • Sample must be <48 hours old since eggs larvate rapidly in the external environment	Dichlorvos Fenbendazole Milbemycin oxime Mebendazole Pyrantel	See Color Plate Fig. 7-12

Table 7-17 Endoparasites (Continued)

Prevention of human infection from endoparasites involves proper hygiene (e.g., washing hands and properly cooking food), isolation of infected animals, and quarantine of newly acquired animals. Each fecal sample should be thought of as a zoonotic risk and treated appropriately.

Parasite	Transmission Route	Clinical Signs	Diagnostics	Common Treatments	Picture
Cryptosporidium **ZOONOTIC** *Common Name:* N/A *Type:* Protozoa *Affected Species:* Canine and Feline *Disinfection:* heating >131° F for 15-20 minutes, thorough drying, 5% ammonia solution and formaldehyde *Environment:* resistant for months	Oocysts passed → ingested by definitive host → develop in the ileum and cecum *Prepatent period: 2-7 days*	• Asymptomatic or diarrhea	• Fecal flotation, acid-fast staining, negative staining, ELISA and IFA tests • Oocysts: Oval to spherical, thick-walled and sporulated • **Caution:** difficult to distinguish from yeast cells on fecal flotations	Clindamycin Tylosin Azithromycin Paromomycin	See Color Plate Fig. 7-13
Dipylidium caninum **ZOONOTIC** *Common Name:* Flea Tapeworm *Type:* Cestode *Affected Species:* Canine and Feline	Proglottids passed and rupture to release thousands of eggs → ingested by intermediate host (flea and biting lice) → development → definitive host ingests the intermediate host → attaches to lining of small intestines to mature *Prepatent period: 4 weeks*	• Anal pruritus, chronic enteritis, vomiting, or nervous system disorders	• Fecal flotation or visual examination of feces, perianal area, or bedding • Egg: Double-pored, rice or cucumber seed appearance, oblong packets of 20 eggs or less	Epsiprantel Febantel + Praziquantel Praziquantel	See Color Plate Fig. 7-14

Organism	Life Cycle	Clinical Signs	Diagnosis	Treatment	Photo

Dirofilaria immitis
ZOONOTIC
 	
Common Name: Heartworm
Type: Nematode
Affected Species: Canine and Feline
	Intermediate host (mosquito) must carry the larva for 15–17 days with the temperature ≥58° F → intermediate host infects definitive host → larva passes from venous circulation to heart → resides in pulmonary arteries and right ventricle of heart → microfilaria circulate in blood and are picked up by intermediate host (mosquito)
	Prepatent period: 24 weeks
		• Murmur, lack of stamina, weight loss, chronic cough, obstruction of pulmonary vessels, and congestive heart failure	• Knott's test, buffy coat examination, direct blood smear, millipore filtration of blood, and various serologic tests for antigen of adult worm
			• Microfilaria: Straight with one tapered end and one straight end
				Adulticides:
				  Caparsolate
				  Malarsomine dihydrochloride
				Microfilariacides:
				  Diethylcarbamazine
				  Dithiazine
				  Ivermectin
				  Levamisole
				  Milbemycin oxime
					See Color Plate Fig. 7-15

Echinococcus granulosus and multiocularis **ZOONOTIC** *Common Name:* Canine and Feline Tapeworm, respectively *Type:* Cestode *Affected Species:* Canine and Feline	Proglottids passed → ingested by intermediate host (e.g., cattle, swine, sheep and rodents) → attaches to liver → definitive host ingests the intermediate host → attaches to lining of small intestines to mature *Prepatent period: 4 weeks*	• Diarrhea • Hydatid cyst disease in intermediate host	• Fecal flotation or purging the animal and collecting the clear mucus at the end • Egg: Ovoid containing a single oncosphere with 3 pairs of hooks • Caution: indistinguishable from *Taenia spp* eggs	Mebendazole Praziquantel	See Color Plate Fig. 7-16
Filaroides osleri *Common Name:* Tracheal worm and Canine lungworm *Type:* Nematode *Affected Species:* Canine	Eggs passed → ingested (passed from dam to pup through grooming or regurgitated meals)→ migrate to small intestines and then to lungs to develop→ migrate to oral cavity or passed through feces *Prepatent period: 10 weeks*	• Coughing and chronic tracheobronchitis with nodule formation in large airways	• Fecal flotation, Baerman technique, and Sputum smear • Larva: Short, with an S-shaped tail	Albendazole Ivermectin	No Photo

Table 7-17   Endoparasites (Continued)

Prevention of human infection from endoparasites involves proper hygiene (e.g., washing hands and properly cooking food), isolation of infected animals, and quarantine of newly acquired animals. Each fecal sample should be thought of as a zoonotic risk and treated appropriately.

Parasite	Transmission Route	Clinical Signs	Diagnostics	Common Treatments	Picture
Giardia **ZOONOTIC** *Common Name:* Giardia *Type:* Protozoa *Affected Species:* Canine and Feline *Disinfection:* Bleach and quaternary ammonium	Eggs passed → ingested → migrate to small intestines *Prepatent period: 5–7 days*	• Asymptomatic or diarrhea (appearing pale and greasy with a foul odor)	• Fecal flotation, direct fecal smear, and IFA • Active form: Pear-shaped with the anatomy resembling a face of crossed eyes, nose, and a mouth	Albendazole Furazolidone Metronidazole	See Color Plate Fig. 7-17

Isospora canis/felis
ZOONOTIC
 	
Common Name:
Coccidia
Type: Protozoa
Affected Species:
Canine and Feline
Disinfection:
Incineration, steam cleaning, immersion in boiling water and 10% ammonia solution
Prevention: insect and rodent control and sanitation
Environment: extremely resistant to environmental conditions
	Eggs passed, usually by mother → ingested, often by puppy or kitten → develop to a trophozoite → migration to intestines
	Prepatent period: 1–2 weeks
		• Asymptomatic or diarrhea progressing to vomiting, inappetance, and dehydration	• Fecal flotation
			• Egg:
			  Small, oval, and thin-walled
			  Sporulated: 2 sporocysts per egg
			  Unsporulated: 1 cell stage inside egg
				Furazolidone
				Sulfadiazine + trimethoprim
				Sulfadimethoxine
					See Color Plate Fig. 7-18

Nanophyetus salminocola **ZOONOTIC** *Common Name:* Salmon Poisoning Fluke *Type:* Trematode *Affected Species:* Canine	Eggs passed by definitive host (e.g., raccoon) → ingested by intermediate host (snail) → larva passed → ingested by intermediate host (salmon) → salmon ingested by definitive host (e.g., dog)→ develop in intestines *Prepatent period: 1 week*	• Lymph-adenopathy, depression, vomiting, and hemorrhagic enteritis • Caused by the rickettsial agent (*Neorickettsia helminthoica*) carried by the fluke	• Fecal flotation or fecal smear • Egg: Gold, operculum at one end and blunt point at opposite end	Fluke: Praziquantel Rickettsial organism: Chloramphenical Doxycycline Oxytetracycline Tetracycline	No Photo
Taenia pisiformis *Common Name:* Tapeworm *Type:* Cestode *Affected Species:* Canine	Proglottids passed → ingested by intermediate host (e.g., rabbit and ruminant) → attaches and develops in peritoneal cavity → definitive host ingests the intermediate host → develops in the small intestines *Prepatent period: 8 weeks*	• Enteritis and intestinal obstruction	• Fecal flotation or visual exam of feces, perianal area or bedding • Egg: Round and containing a single oncosphere with 3 pairs of hooks • Each proglottid carries many eggs	Epsiprantel Febantel + Praziquantel Febendazole Mebendazole Praziquantel	See Color Plate Fig. 7-19
Taenia taeniaeformis *Common Name:* Feline Tapeworm *Type:* Cestode *Affected Species:* Feline	Proglottids passed → ingested by intermediate host (e.g., rodent) → attaches and develops in the liver → definitive host ingests the intermediate host → develops in the small intestines *Prepatent period: 5-6 weeks*	• Diarrhea and intestinal	• Fecal flotation or visual examination of feces, perianal area, or bedding • Egg: Ovoid containing a single oncosphere with 3 pairs of hooks • Each proglottid carries many eggs	Espiprantel Febantel + Praziquantel Fenbendazole Mebendazole Praziquantel	See above

Table 7-17 Endoparasites (Continued)

Prevention of human infection from endoparasites involves proper hygiene (e.g., washing hands and properly cooking food), isolation of infected animals, and quarantine of newly acquired animals. Each fecal sample should be thought of as a zoonotic risk and treated appropriately.

Parasite	Transmission Route	Clinical Signs	Diagnostics	Common Treatments	Picture
Toxascaris leonina **ZOONOTIC** *Common Name:* Ascarid, Roundworm *Type:* Nematode *Affected Species:* Canine and Feline *Disinfection:* Bleach *Environment:* eggs can remain infective in the soil for months to years	Eggs passed → ingested by definitive hos or intermediate host (e.g., mice)→ definitive host ingests intermediate host → attaches and develops in small intestines *Prepatent period: 8–10 weeks*	• Chronic diarrhea, vomiting, constipation, and unthriftiness	• Fecal flotation or visual examination of feces • Egg: Spherical to ovoid, unembyronated, light cytoplasm, and a smooth outer shell	Dichlorvos Diethylcarbamazine Fenbendazole Milbemycin oxime Mebendazole Piperazine Pyrantel	See Color Plate Fig. 7-20
Toxocara canis **ZOONOTIC** *Common Name:* Ascarid, Roundworm *Type:* Nematode *Affected Species:* Canine *Disinfection:* Bleach *Environment:* eggs can remain infective in the soil for months to years	Eggs passed → ingested via environment or paratenic host→ hatch in small intestines and penetrate mucosa → migrate through the liver and heart until the lungs → develop in lungs → coughed up and swallowed → mature in the small intestines for 4–6 weeks *Prepatent period: 4-6 weeks*	• Distended abdomen, weakness, unthriftiness, and diarrhea	• Fecal flotation or visual examination of feces or vomitus • Egg: Spherical, unembyronated, deeply pigmented center, and a rough, pitted outer shell	Dichlorvos Diethylcarbamazine Febantel + Praziquantel Fenbendazole Mebendazole Milbemycin oxime Piperazine Pyrantel	See above

Toxocara cati **ZOONOTIC** *Common Name:* Ascarid, Roundworm *Type:* Nematode *Affected Species:* Feline *Disinfection:* Bleach *Environment:* eggs can remain infective in the soil for months to years	Eggs passed → ingested via environment or paratenic host→ hatch in small intestines and penetrate mucosa → migrate through the liver and heart until the lungs → develop in lungs → coughed up and swallowed → mature in the small intestines for 4–6 weeks *Prepatent period: 7-8 weeks*	• Stunted growth and damage caused by migrations	• Fecal flotation • Egg: Spherical, unembyronated, deeply pigmented center, and a rough, pitted outer shell	Dichlorvos Diethylcarbamazine Fenbendazole Lufenuron Mebendazole Piperazine Pyrantel	See Color Plate Fig . 7-21
Toxoplasma gondii **ZOONOTIC** *Common Name:* Toxoplasmosis *Type:* Protozoa *Affected Species:* Feline *Environment:* can live in the soil for months to >1 year	Oocysts passed → ingested via environment, intermediate host (most warm-blooded vertebrates) or transplacental → migrate to small intestines and extraintestinal dissemination elsewhere via blood and lymph *Prepatent period: 3–10 days for ingestion of cysts and 20–40 days for oocysts*	• Asymptomatic or transient diarrhea, anorexia, depression, fever, and clinical signs dependent on site and extent of injury from migration (e.g., CNS, hepatic, pulmonary)	• Fecal flotation, ELISA, or agglutination procedures • Oocysts: Oval and unsporulated	Clindamycin Pyrimethamine Sulfadiazine + trimethoprim	See Color Plate Fig . 7-22
Trichuris vulpis *Common Name:* Whipworm, Fecal jewel *Type:* Nematode *Affected Species:* Canine *Disinfection:* Diluted sodium chloride *Environment:* very resistant	Eggs passed → ingested → penetrate and develop in small intestines → migrate to cecum and develop for 60–80 days *Prepatent period: 9–12 weeks*	• Weight loss, intermittent and chronic diarrhea and typhlitis	• Fecal flotation • Egg: Thick, brown-yellow symmetrical shell with clear polar plug at each end and unembyronated	Febantel + Praziquantel Fenbendazole Ivermectin Mebendazole Milbemycin oxime	See Color Plate Fig . 7-23

Table 7-17 Endoparasites (Continued)

Prevention of human infection from endoparasites involves proper hygiene (e.g., washing hands and properly cooking food), isolation of infected animals, and quarantine of newly acquired animals. Each fecal sample should be thought of as a zoonotic risk and treated appropriately.

Parasite	Transmission Route	Clinical Signs	Diagnostics	Common Treatments	Picture
Uncinaria steno-cephala **ZOONOTIC** *Common Name:* Northern canine hookworm *Type:* Nematode *Affected Species:* Canine and Feline *Disinfection:* Bleach *Environment:* can live in cool, moist soil for several weeks	Eggs passed → ingestion, percutaneous, prenatal and transmammary → lungs for development → coughed up and swallowed → small intestines to mature *Prepatent period: 2 weeks*	• Weakness, inappetance, poor growth, and diarrhea	• Fecal flotation • Egg: Oval or ellipsoid, capsule shaped, 8–16 cells inside a thin wall • Sample must be <48 hours because eggs larvate rapidly in the external environment	Dichlorvos Fenbendazole Ivermectin Mebendazole Milbemycin oxime Pyrantel	See Color Plate Fig. 7-24

Table 7-18 Ectoparasites (Continued)

Prevention for all the human risk of ectoparasites is proper hygiene (e.g., washing hands and properly cooking food), isolation of infected animals, and quarantine of newly acquired animals. Each infected animal should be thought of as a zoonotic risk and treated appropriately.

Parasite	Transmission Route	Clinical Signs	Diagnostics	Common Treatments	Picture
Cheyletiella **ZOONOTIC** *Common Name:* Fur mite of dogs and cats and Walking Dander *Type:* Mite *Affected Species:* Canine and Feline *Human Risk:* Low	Ingest: keratin debris and tissue fluid Location: skin Transmission: direct contact and contact through inanimate objects Life Cycle: 18–21 days	• Asymptomatic, mild alopecia, dandruff, and pruritus	• Scrape margins of lesions, flea comb, visual, or cellophane tape • Adult: Body shape resembles a shield or acorn, hook-like accessory mouth parts and comb-like structures at the tip of each leg	Ivermectin Selamectin	See Color Plate Fig. 7-25
Ctenocephalides canis/felis *Common Name:* Flea *Type:* Flea *Affected Species:* Canine and Feline *Human Risk:* Low	Ingest: blood Location: head and base of tail Transmission: direct contact or through contact with inanimate objects Life Cycle: 21 days– >1 year	• Flea bite dermatitis, anemia, puritus, red lesions, hair loss, and ulcers	• Visual and flea comb • Adult: Medium brown to mahogany in color, laterally flattened body, 2–8 mm long with pronotal and genal combs • Transmit *Dipylidium* and *Hemobartonella* spp.	Dichlorvos collars Fipronil Imidacloprid Lufenuron Pyrethrins Selamectin Insect growth regulators	See Color Plate Fig. 7-26

Cuterebra
 	
Common Name: Rodent Botfly, Warbles and Wolves
Type: Fly
Affected Species: Canine and Feline
Human Risk: Low
	Ingest: N/A
	Location: face and neck region, can be found on any furred area
	Transmission: contact with rodent burrow or eggs from an adult fly
	Life Cycle: 3–4 weeks
		• Cutaneous lump with a breathing hole	• Visual
			• Larvae:
			   2nd-Stage: cream to white, toothlike spines and 5–10 mm long
			   3rd-Stage: large, coal black, heavily spined, and up to 3 cm long
				• Surgical removal of larvae
				Caution: do not crush larva when removing, because it may cause anaphylaxis
				• Wound treatment
					No Photo

Table 7-18 Ectoparasites (Continued)

Prevention for all the human risk of ectoparasites is proper hygiene (e.g., washing hands and properly cooking food), isolation of infected animals, and quarantine of newly acquired animals. Each infected animal should be thought of as a zoonotic risk and treated appropriately.

Parasite	Transmission Route	Clinical Signs	Diagnostics	Common Treatments	Picture
Demodex canis *Common Name:* Follicular Mange Mite, Red Mange, or Puppy Mange *Type:* Mites *Affected Species:* Canine *Human Risk:* none	Ingest: unknown Location: hair follicles and sebaceous glands Transmission: direct contact from dam to pup; otherwise not contagious between hosts Life cycle: 21 days	• Alopecia of muzzle, face, and forelegs, erythema, secondary bacterial pyoderma, and pruritus	• Deep skin scrapings on squeezed skin or biopsy • Adult: Cigar-shaped, 8 stubby legs at anterior end of body, and $1/4$ cm long	Amitraz 0.025% Ivermectin Milbemycin oxime Multi-vitamin/fatty acid supplement Antibiotics • Benzoyl peroxide 5% (gel or shampoo) aids in penetration in the follicles when used with Amitraz	No photo
Dermacentor variabilis/andersoni *Common Name:* American Dog Tick and Wood Tick *Type:* Tick *Affected Species:* Canine *Human Risk:* High	Ingest: blood Location: whole body Transmission: contact Life Cycle: 3 months to 2 years • Tick must be attached for 5–20 hours to transmit disease	• Asymptomatic or vasculitis • Intermediate host for Rocky Mountain spotted fever, tularemia, and other *Rickettsial spp.*	• Visual • Adults: Blue-gray with white markings on shield	Dichlorvos Fipronil Pyrethrins Selamectin	No photo
Linognathus setosus *Common Name:* Sucking louse of dogs *Type:* Lice *Affected Species:* Canine *Human Risk:* Low *Environment:* live 7 days off host	Ingest: blood Location: whole body Transmission: contact Life Cycle: 3–4 weeks	• Skin irritation, itching, dermatitis, alopecia, anemia, and roughened hair coat	• Visual • Adult: Dorsoventrally flattened, red to gray in color, head is more narrow than the widest part of the thorax, and 1st pair of claws smaller than 2nd and 3rd pairs	Ivermectin Pyrethrins	See Color Plate Fig. 7-27

Organism	Host / Transmission	Clinical Signs	Diagnosis / Identification	Treatment	Photo
Otodectes cynotis *Common Name:* Ear mite *Type:* Mite *Affected Species:* Canine and Feline *Human Risk:* N/A	Definitive host: dog and cat Ingest: epidermal debris Location: ear and base of tail Transmission: contact Life Cycle: 18–21 days	• Shaking of head, irritation, otitis media, hematomas, head tilt, circling, and convulsions	• Visual or ear swab • Adult: Oval with 8 legs, fused head and thorax, short unjointed pedicel with suckers on the end of some of the legs	• Clean the ear of all crusty debris Ivermectin Selamectin	No photo
Rhipicephalus sanguineus *Common Name:* Brown Dog Tick *Type:* Tick *Affected Species:* Canine	Ingest: blood Location: whole body Transmission: contact Life Cycle: 6 weeks to 1 year	• Anemia • Intermediate host for Babesiosis and Ehrlichiosis	• Visual • Adult: Brown with prominent lateral extensions on head, giving a hexagonal appearance	Dichlorvos Fipronil Pyrethrins Selamectin	See Color Plate Fig. 7-28
Sarcoptes scabiei canis **ZOONOTIC** *Common Name:* Mange mite or Scabies *Type:* Mite *Affected Species:* Canine *Human Risk:* low	Ingest: interstitial fluid Location: ears, lateral elbows, and ventral abdomen Transmission: contact Life Cycle: 2–3 weeks	• Severe itching, dry and thickened skin, erythema, papular rash, scaling, crusting, and excoriations	• Deep skin scraping • Adults: Oval with 8 legs, fused head and thorax, long unjointed pedicel with suckers on the end of some of the legs	Ivermectin Amitraz Benzyl benzoate Lime-sulfur Selamectin	See Color Plate Fig. 7-29
Trichodectes canis *Common Name:* Biting louse of dogs *Type:* Lice *Affected Species:* Canine *Environment:* live 7 days off host	Ingest: skin and hair Location: whole body Transmission: contact Life Cycle: 3–4 weeks	• Itching, rough hair coat, and dermatitis	• Visual • Adult: Dorsoventrally flattened, yellow, large rounded head, head is wider than any other part of the body, 2–4 mm	Pyrethrins	See Color Plate Fig. 7-30

URINALYSIS

Urinalysis is one of the most frequently performed laboratory tests in small animal clinics. Because many substances are eliminated from the body through the urologic system, it provides the DVM with a great amount of knowledge concerning many functions of the body (i.e. urinary, kidney, liver, and diabetes mellitus). This test, like fecal analysis, is a staple of every trained technician and should be performed perfectly.

Urine Collection, Handling, Storage, and Transport Tips

Collection:

- Collect before the administration of any medication, if possible.
- Morning, prepandial samples offer the most accurate specific gravity, pH and cellular components, but allow for the degeneration of casts overnight in the bladder.
- Collection containers must be clean, well-rinsed, and free of any disinfectant residues
- Collect at least 3–5 mL of urine.

Skill Box 7-19 / Collection Technique		
Method	**Procedure**	**General Information**
Voided	• Midstream sample collected in a clean container as the animal urinates • Collected from litter pan, cage floor, or examination table **Use aquarium rocks, plastic beads, or plastic packing material in a clean, well-rinsed litter pan** • **Caution:** Results can be altered by trace amounts of soaps, disinfectants, bacteria, and any debris	• Poor sample for bacterial isolation, culture, and sensitivity because of contamination from genitalia or environment
Manual Expression	• **Caution:** never use manual expression on an obstructed animal 1. Clean the vulva or prepuce, palpate the bladder in the caudal abdomen; apply gentle, steady pressure 2. Catch a midstream sample in a clean container	• Extreme pressure may cause injury or bladder rupture • Excessive pressure may send infected urine back into the ureters and kidneys • ↑ Introduction of RBCs and protein • May take several minutes of steady pressure for the sphincter to relax

Method	Procedure	General Information
Catheterization *General*	1. Clean the external urethral opening 2. Using aseptic technique, apply lubricant to the catheter tip 3. Insert the catheter into the urethra, avoiding contact with all external skin and hair 4. Gently push the catheter through the urethra until the bladder is reached 5. Aspirate urine, using a sterile syringe; the first 3–5 mL should be discarded because of possible contamination	• Urogenital tract injury with improper technique • ↑ Introduction of RBCs, protein, epithelial cells, or bacteria
Male dog	Along with the general procedure above: 1. Expose the external orifice by reflecting the prepuce away from the penis 2. Clean the penis and avoid any contact with the prepuce 3. Apply gentle pressure to advance the catheter past the level of the os penis and the point where the urethra curves around the ischial arch	
Female dog	Along with the general procedure above: 1. Place dog in standing position and flush the vagina with saline or sterilized water injected through a syringe 2. Place a speculum in the vagina to visualize the external urethral orifice Urethral orifice is 3–5 cm cranial to the ventral commissure of the vulva, just cranial to the clitoral fossa 3. Place the catheter past the clitoral fossa and advance along the ventral floor of the vagina until it enters the urethral fossa	
Male cat	Along with the general procedure above: Chemical restraint is almost always required 1. Place the cat in dorsal recumbency 2. Expose the external orifice by reflecting the prepuce away from the penis 3. Clean the penis and avoid any contact with the prepuce 4. Gently advance the catheter in a rotary motion	
Female cat	Along with the general procedure above: Chemical restraint is almost always required 1. Place the cat in sternal recumbency 2. Advance the catheter into the external orifice, applying gentle downward pressure on the catheter tip 3. Gently advance and retract the catheter until entry into the urethra	

Skill Box 7-19 / Collection Technique (Continued)

Method	Procedure	General Information
Cystocentesis	1. Animal is placed in a standing position or lateral or dorsal recumbency 2. The bladder is palpated and the needle (22- or 23-gauge 1.5" needle with a 6- or 12-mL syringe) is inserted in a caudal-dorsal direction at a 45-degree angle toward the midline Male dog: caudal to the umbilicus and to the side of the sheath Others: ventral midline caudal to the umbilicus 3. The syringe is slowly aspirated to obtain urine 4. The needle is slowly and smoothly removed • **Caution:** If blood or a dark material is aspirated, stop immediately and release all suction on the syringe, withdraw needle, reposition or advise the DVM • **Caution:** Do not palpate the bladder for several hours after cystocentesis to avoid leakage of urine into the abdomen **Bladder location: pour alcohol onto the abdomen of an animal in dorsal recumbency, and it will pool in the location of the bladder, or mentally draw an X crossing over the abdomen between the last 2 sets of mammary glands.** **These techniques must be confirmed by palpation.** **Always save ≥1 mL sterile urine for an unexpected culture**	• Sterile sample • Least amount of trauma if bladder is readily palpated • Well-tolerated with minimal restraint

Handling:

- Samples should be covered immediately to avoid pH changes and contamination.
- Thoroughly mix a sample before examination.
- Slowly warm refrigerated samples up to room temperature before examination.
- Centrifuge the sample at 500–3,000 rpm for 3–5 minutes.
- Gently pour off the supernatant to avoid disrupting the remaining pellet.
- Gently mix the pellet to avoid cellular damage.

  *__Caution:__ Applying the brake to produce an abrupt stop may resuspend the sediment and alter results.

Storage:

- Samples at room temperature should be examined within 30 minutes.
- Samples can be refrigerated for 6–12 hours in a covered container.
- Refrigerated samples tend to form crystals.
- Samples may be frozen for chemistry tests, but cellular components will be destroyed.

Transport:

- Add 1–2 drops of serum to the sample to preserve cell morphology.
- Add 1 drop of 40% formalin to each ounce of urine.

Urine Examination/ Urinalysis

All urine samples should be evaluated for the following physical properties. Each of the assessments listed below are observed through a visual examination of the sample, except the specific gravity, which is measured by using a refractometer. A refractometer accurately measures the amount of solids dissolved in a urine sample.

Table 7-19 Gross Examination

Physical Property	Observation	Definition	Associated Conditions
Color	Yellow	• Any shade of yellow is considered normal • Variations are often attributable to changes in concentration	• N/A
	Red or red/brown	• Cloudy, red urine is hematuria with intact RBCs • Clear, red urine is hemoglobinuria with free hemoglobin	• UTI, cystitis, trauma, neoplasia, or urolithiasis
	Brown	• Contains myoglobin	• Muscle cell lysis
	Yellow/brown or yellow/green	• Contains bile pigments	• Liver disease
Foam	Small amount	• Normal when sample is shaken	• N/A
	Large amount	• Contains protein	• Kidney disease, fever, or excessive exercise
	Green	• Contains bile pigments	• Liver disease
Odor	Ammonia	• Breakdown of urease	• UTI, cystitis
	Sweet, fruity odor	• Contains ketones and/or glucose	• Diabetes mellitus

Parameter	Value	Description	Associated conditions
Specific Gravity (USG)	Dog: 1.015–1.045; Cat: 1.035–1.060	• Normal • Measurement of the density of urine compared with pure water	• N/A
	Dog: ≥1.045; Cat: ≥1.060	• Hyperthenuric • If dehydrated; dog: ≥1.030 and cat: ≥1.035 • ↑ Glucose and protein falsely elevate results	• ↑ Water intake or excretion of solutes
	≤1.007	• Hypothenuric	• ↓ Water intake, pyometra, liver disease, kidney disease, diuretics, or diabetes insipidus
Transparency	Clear	• Normal	• N/A
	Cloudy or flocculent	• Contains cellular components	• UTI
Volume	Polyuria	• ↑ Urine production; pale with a ↓ USG (≤1.020)	• Nephritis, diabetes mellitus, diabetes insipidus, pyometra, liver disease, and kidney disease
	Oliguria	• ↓ Urine production	• ↓ Water intake, fever, shock, heart disease, and dehydration
	Pollakiuria	• Frequent urination	• UTI, urolithiasis, and crystalluria
	Anuria	• Complete lack of urine output • No urine output in 12 hours	• Urinary obstruction, urinary bladder rupture, and death

Preparation

Chemistry strip evaluation provides detection of elements present in an urine sample that may or may not be seen during visual examination or microscopic evaluation. Because chemistry strips provide many false-negative results, both a visual examination and a microscopic examination should always be performed.

Chemistry strip bottles should be kept at room temperature and away from intense light, moisture, and heat. Strips can be immersed in a urine sample for 2–3 seconds to allow saturation of the pads. Extended time may lead to test reagents leaking into the urine sample. A pipette or dropper also may be used to allow urine to run down the length of the strip to saturate each pad. In each technique, the strip is then run along the lip of a cup or other container to remove excess urine and to avoid chemical mixing. The results are then read in consistent artificial light to avoid the fluctuations seen with natural light.

Table 7-20 Chemistry Strip Examination

Chemical Property	Observation	Definition	Associated Conditions
Bilirubin	Bilirubinuria	• A byproduct from the breakdown of hemoglobin • Trace amounts found in dogs if USG is ≥1.030, but not common in cats • **Caution:** Exposure to light causes bilirubin degradation with subsequent false-negative results	• Hemolytic anemia, bile duct obstruction, liver disease, fever, and prolonged fasting or starvation
Blood	Hematuria	• Presence of intact RBCs • After centrifugation, urine will appear clear with a red pellet	• UTI, cystitis, renal disease, strenuous exercise, trauma, and genital tract contamination
	Hemoglobinuria	• Presence of free hemoglobin, typically caused by intravascular hemolysis • After centrifugation, urine will remain tinted red	• Hemolytic anemia, severe burns, incompatible transfusions, leptospirosis, babesiosis, systemic lupus erythematosus, and metal toxicity
	Myoglobinuria	• Presence of myoglobin typically due to muscle damage • Urine is dark brown to black	• Muscle damage
**To differentiate between hemoglobinuria and myoglobinuria, compare plasma and urine simultaneously. Plasma and urine will both appear red with the presence of hemoglobin, and only urine will appear red to brown with myoglobin.**			
Glucose	Glucosuria	• Appears if blood glucose threshold is exceeded BG values: Dog: >180 mg/dL Cat: >300 mg/dL • Not detectable in the urine of normal animals	• Diabetes mellitus, Cushing's disease, chronic liver disease, high carbohydrate meal, stress, fear, restraint, administration of IV glucose, and Fanconi's syndrome
Ketones	Ketonuria	• Formed from the breakdown of fatty acids • Not detectable in the urine of normal animals • **Caution:** Ketones will evaporate in a sample left sitting	• Diabetes mellitus, liver disease, persistent fever, high-fat diets, starvation, fasting, and long-term anorexia

Table 7-20 Chemistry Strip Examination (Continued)

Chemical Property	Observation	Definition	Associated Conditions
pH	Normal	• Concentration of H$^+$ ions, a measure of the degree of alkalinity or acidity • Dog: 5.2–6.8 • Cat: 6–7	• N/A
	Alkaline	• Increased concentration of H$^+$ ions • >7.0 • **Caution:** pH rises in a sample left sitting	• Postprandial alkaline tide, plant diets, UTI, metabolic and/or respiratory alkalosis, distal renal tubular acidosis, urine retention, and certain drugs (e.g., bicarbonate, citrate)
	Acidic	• Decreased concentration of H$^+$ ions • <7.0	• Protein diets, metabolic or respiratory acidosis, fever, starvation, excessive muscular activity, chloride depletion, and certain drugs (e.g., D,L-methionine, furosemide)
Protein	Proteinuria	• Measurement of albumin and globulins • Only found in trace amounts in normal urine • Always interpret in light of USG and contents of urine sediment	• Glomerulonephritis, glomerular amyloidosis, multiple myeloma, parturition, estrus, and UTI
Protein: Creatinine Ratio	Normal	• Quantifies level of proteinuria as significant or not • Dog: ≤0.3 • Cat: ≤0.6	• N/A
	Increased	• Increased urine protein loss • >1	• Chronic interstitial nephritis, glomerulonephritis, and amyloidosis

• **Caution:** USG may alter the degree of color change and should always be referred to when interpreting results.

Sediment Examination

A microscopic examination of the urine sediment should be a part of every routine urinalysis. It is used to confirm findings from gross examination and chemistry strip examination. Much additional information can be gained from a microscopic examination that cannot be determined in any other method. Samples collected first thing in the morning or after several hours of water deprivation provide the most diagnostic information. The increased concentration of these samples increases the likelihood of finding formed elements.

Each laboratory needs to determine their normals and urine procedures. Commonly, a standard amount of 5 mL urine is centrifuged and poured off, leaving the pellet and approximately 0.3 mL urine in the tube. The remaining urine and pellet are mixed together, and 1 drop is placed on a slide. A coverslip is placed over the drop, and the sample may be read either stained or unstained.

When examining an unstained sample, achieving proper light adjustment (e.g., lower stage slightly or partially close diaphragm) of the microscope to view refractile elements is important.

The sample is scanned with low power for casts and crystals and reported as #/lpf (low-power field). RBCs, WBCs, and epithelial cells are examined with high power and reported as #/hpf (high-power field). Bacteria and sperm are examined under high power and reported as rare through 4+.

Reporting of Bacteria and Sperm:

Rare—only a few seen after scanning numerous fields

1+ - < 1/hpf

2+ - 1–5/hpf

3+ - 6–20/hpf

4+ - >20/hpf

Table 7-21   Sediment Examination

Bacteria

Bacteria is not normally found in properly collected normal urine samples. Its presence with WBCs often indicates a bacterial infection, whereas the absence of WBCs typically indicates a contaminated sample. A sample properly collected via cystocentesis or catheterization should be sterile and any presence of bacteria is significant (e.g., diabetes mellitus, Cushing's disease, and glucocorticoid treatment). Figures 7-31 & 7-33
- **Caution:** Normal brownian movement may often be confused with bacteria in unstained sediments.

Component	Observation	Definition	Associated Conditions
Cocci	• Circular bacteria in singles, pairs or chains • Refract light and have brownian movement	• Acid pH: *Enterococci* and *Streptococcus spp.* • Alkaline pH: *Staphylococcus spp.*	• UTI, cystitis, pyelonephritis, metritis, prostatitis, or vaginitis
Bacilli	• Rod-shaped bacteria in singles, pairs, or chains • Refract light and have brownian movement	• Acid pH: *E. coli* • Alkaline pH: *Proteus spp.*	• UTI, cystitis, pyelonephritis, metritis, prostatitis, or vaginitis

Blood Cells

Blood cells are classified by number per high power field (#/hpf). Blood cells are thought to always be significant unless reviewed against other factors affecting the animal. For example, an animal with only a few RBCs and no other abnormalities may have received trauma through a catheterization procedure.

WBCs are always thought to be significant, because they typically only appear with some level of an infection, unless contamination of infected genitalia takes place. WBCs do not need to be classified into type; by the time they reach the bladder, they have degenerated to an unrecognizable state. The presence of WBCs should always result in an in-depth look for bacteria.

Component	Observation	Definition	Associated Conditions

RBCs
Figures 7-33
7-37 & 7-38
	• Smooth edges, small, and biconcave
	• Unstained: pale, yellow to orange discs without nuclei
	• Stained: varying color from light pink to dark red
	• Crenated: ruffled edges and slightly darker
	• Lysed: colorless rings of varying size
		• Normal to see a small number of RBCs
		• Normals:
		  Voided: 0–8/hpf
		  Catheter: 0–5/hpf
		  Cystocentesis: 0–3/hpf
		• Atraumatic technique will produce the above numbers, multiple attempts may ↑ the number of RBCs
			• Cystitis, neoplasia, calculi or bleeding disorder

WBCs Figures 7-32 & 7-33	• Round with granular appearance (distinct nuclei) • 1.5–2 times as big as RBCs • Presence of WBCs should cause careful consideration for the presence of bacteria and performing a culture	• Normal to see a small number of WBCs • Normals: Voided: 0–1/hpf • Neutrophils are the most common type of WBC seen	• Nephritis, pyelonephritis, cystitis, urethritis, and ureteritis

Casts

Casts are formed in the lumen of the distal and collecting tubules of the kidneys. Because of this location, they are all cylindrical with parallel sides and rounded to blunted ends. Casts are susceptible to high-speed centrifugation, rough handling, and delayed analysis (degrade when allowed to sit in alkaline urine or for long periods).

Type	Description	Clinical significance
Epithelial Figure 7-34	• Nearly transparent, clear, and highly refractile with renal epithelial cells	• Originate from the Loop of Henle, distal tubule and collecting tubule • Never observed in normal urine	• Nephrotoxicity, acute renal disease, ischemia and pyelonephritis
Fatty Figure 7-35	• Coarsely granular with fat droplets	• Signify degeneration of the renal tubules	• Diabetes mellitus and renal disease
Granular Figure 7-36	• Coarse to finely granular • Orange: bilirubin • Pink to red: hemoglobin or myoglobin	• Composed of particulate matter from renal tubular cell necrosis or degeneration • Hyaline casts containing granules • Normal to see 0-2/HPF	• Acute renal disease
Hyaline Figure 7-37	• Nearly transparent, clear and highly-refractile • Rounded ends • Stained: light pink to purple	• Composed of pure protein precipitates • Normal to see 0–2/hpf	• Fever, mild renal disease, general anesthesia, IV diuresis, and strenuous exercise
RBC/WBC Figure 7-38 & 7-39	RBC: • Contains a few to many RBCs • Deep yellow to orange WBC: • Contains a few to many WBCs • Appearance changes to granular once the cells start to degenerate	• Formed from the aggregation of RBCs and/or WBCs • Never observed in normal urine	• Intrarenal bleeding or infection, trauma, glomerulonephritis, renal tubulointerstitial inflammation and toxicity
Waxy Figure 7-40	• Highly refractile, homogenous, and translucent	• Final stage of granular cast degeneration • Most stable of all casts	• Chronic renal disease

Table 7-21   Sediment Examination (Continued)

Crystals

Crystalluria may or may not be indicative of a medical condition. Crystals may form because of sample handling (e.g., refrigeration) or through the accumulation of normal urine components. Urine pH, concentration, temperature, and solubility of the components all contributes to the type of crystal formed. Crystals can be reported as occasional, moderate, or many or by using a 1–4+ scale.

Component	Observation	Definition	Associated Conditions
Amorphous phosphate Figure 7-41	• Granular precipitate • Dull brown in color	• Typically seen in neutral or alkaline urine • Seen in normal urine • Easily confused with bacteria	• Liver disease, portosystemic shunts or breed predisposed (Dalmatians and English bulldogs)
Amorphous urate Figure 7-42	• Granular precipitate • Green-yellow in color	• Typically seen in acidic urine • Easily confused with bacteria	• Liver disease, portosystemic shunts, or breed predisposed (Dalmatians and English bulldogs)
Ammonium biurate Figure 7-43	• Round with long spicules • Resemble a thorn apple • Yellow to brown in color	• Typically seen in alkaline urine	• Liver disease, portosystemic shunts, urate urolithiasis, or breed predisposed (Dalmatians and English bulldogs)
Bilirubin Figure 7-44	• Fine elongated spicules • Red-brown or golden yellow in color	• May be seen in normal urine	• Liver disease or hemolytic anemia
Calcium carbonate Figure 7-45	• Round with lines radiating out from the center • May resemble short dumbbells	• Typically seen in alkaline urine	• N/A
Calcium oxalate dihydrate Figure 7-46	• Square with refractile lines forming an X across the surface (e.g., envelopes) • Radiopaque with hard, sharp protrusions • ± Cuboid shape	• Typically seen in neutral or acidic urine • May be seen in normal urine	• Ethylene glycol toxicity, oxalate urolithiasis
Calcium oxalate monohydrate	• Small, flat, elongated structures with pointed ends (e.g., spindles)	• Typically seen in neutral or acidic urine	• Ethylene glycol toxicity, oxalate urolithiasis
Cystine Figure 7-47	• Hexagon and flat	• Typically seen in acidic urine	• Renal tubular dysfunction

Leucine Figure 7-48	Round with concentric striations	• Typically seen in acidic urine • Not well understood	• Acute liver disease or chloroform or phosphorus toxicity
Sulfonamide Figure 7-49	• Clear to brown, eccentrically bound needles in sheaves	• Rarely seen with the newer forms of sulfonamide drugs	• Sulfonamide treatment
Triple Phosphate, Struvite, Magnesium, Ammonium and Phosphate (MAPS) Figure 7-50	• 8-sided prisms with tapered sides and ends • Resemble coffin-lids • ↑ Ammonia leads to fern leaf-like appearance	• Typically seen in neutral or alkaline urine	• Cystitis or struvite urolithiasis
Tyrosine Figure 7-51	• Very dark, very fine needles in sheaves or clusters	• Typically seen in acidic urine • Not well understood	• Acute liver disease or chloroform or phosphorus toxicity
Uric acid Figure 7-52	• Yellow-brown diamond, rosettes, or oval plates with pointed ends	• Typically seen in acidic urine	• Liver disease, portosystemic shunts, or breed predisposed (Dalmatians and English bulldogs)

Epithelial Cells

Squamous and transitional epithelial cells are seen commonly in the urine of normal animals. Squamous epithelial cells are the largest of the epithelial cells and are considered not significant. Transitional epithelial cells only prove to be significant with a large increase in number. Renal epithelial cells, however, are typically only seen with renal disease and always thought to be significant. They are the smallest of the epithelial cells and are often confused with WBCs.

Renal Figure 7-53	• Round to caudate with a large eccentric nucleus displaced near the bottom • Prominent nucleolus • Often confused with WBCs	• Epithelial cells originating from the renal tubules • Rarely found and usually indicate renal disease	• Renal disease
Squamous Figure 7-54 & 7-56	• Very large, thin, and polygonal • Tend to fold onto themselves and appear singularly or in sheets • Small, round nucleus, placed close to the center • Appears as a fried egg	• Epithelial cells originating from the urethra, bladder, vagina, and prepuce • Often seen and typically not significant	• N/A
Transitional Figure 7-55	• Round to caudate, granular with a small nucleus centrally located • Varying size	• Epithelial cells originating from the proximal urethra, bladder, ureters, and renal pelvis • Often seen and only significant in large numbers, clumps or sheets	• Cystitis, pyelonephritis, or neoplasia

Table 7-21 Sediment Examination (Continued)

Miscellaneous
Numerous artifacts can be seen in urine because of contamination. The following also can be seen with a disease condition associated with the urinary tract.

Component	Observation	Definition	Associated Conditions
Hemoglobin	• Orange globules with varying size	• Intravascular hemolysis resulting in free hemoglobin • Often confused with RBCs	• Severe hemolytic diseases or alkaline urine
Lipid droplets Figure 7-56	• Varying size, round, light green, and highly refractile • Seen in the plane of field just below the coverslip	• Commonly seen in urine associated with no disease condition • Often confused with RBCs	• Diabetes mellitus, obesity, and hypothyroidism
Mucus threads Figure 7-43	• Resemble twisting ribbons	• More commonly seen after catheterization • May be seen in normal animals	• Urethral irritation or genital contamination

Parasites
Two urinary tract parasites can be seen in the dog and cat. Fecal contamination may lead to finding an array of parasites in urine, but the following are the only ones that originate from the bladder.

Component	Observation	Definition	Associated Conditions
Capillaria plica Figure 7-57	• Clear to yellow with flattened bipolar end plugs and a roughed shell	• Bladder worm of dogs and cats • Travels through the lungs and may cause coughing	• Nonpathogenic
Dicto-phyma renale	• Barrel-shaped, bipolar, yellow-brown with a pitted shell	• Giant kidney worm of the dog • Largest nematode affecting domestic animals • Ingest the parenchyma of the right kidney, leaving only the capsule • Crayfish and fish are the intermediate host	• Kidney disease or peritonitis

Urine Artifacts

Many substances can contaminate a urine sample. They may arise from improper collection, the environment, or general anatomy. Besides the artifacts listed below, parasite eggs, fecal material, fungal spores, and fungi also may be seen. Please refer to the respective sections for identification of these items.

Table 7-22 Urine Artifacts

Urine Artifact	Definition	Appearance
Air bubbles Figure 7-47	• Result from the trapping of air during the application of the coverslip	• Varying size, round, flat, refractile with a dark border
Hair Figure 7-36	• Contaminant from environment or surrounding genitalia	• Needle-like with tapered edges
Pollen	• Contaminant from environment	• Double budding spores (e.g., Mickey Mouse®)
Sperm	• Seen in the urine of intact males or recently mated females	• Oval head with a whip-like tail
Starch granules Figure 7-58	• Contaminant from gloves	• Faceted or scallop edges with indented or dimpled center • Not refractile
Yeast Figure 7-59	• Contaminant from environment or surrounding genitalia	• Oblong, colorless budding bodies with double refractile walls • Varying size

Chapter 8

Nursing Care

FLUID ADMINISTRATION

Fluid administration is necessary when an animal is dehydrated, experiencing shock, losing blood, having a surgical procedure that may result in excessive blood loss, or has a disease that is resulting in depletion of the animal's normal fluid, electrolyte or acid–base balances. Dehydration may lead to hypovolemia and hypoperfusion.

Fluid requirements are based on an animal's hydration status, reason for fluid loss, and its physical condition. The veterinarian is responsible for prescribing the appropriate fluid therapy. Obtaining the following assessments will assist the veterinarian in the calculation of fluid requirements for the animal. Distinction between dehydration and perfusion status is an important factor in the veterinarian's choice of fluid therapy.

The following charts are to provide the technician with information to help understand the veterinarian's fluid therapy plan and to assist in the process of administration.

Table 8-1 Hydration Assessment

Assessment of Hydration	Method	Hydration Significance
Physical Examination	**Asess Dehydration Status:** • **Skin turgor**—Assess the amount of time it takes for the skin to return to the animal's body when gently pulled up and twisted at the back of the neck or along the spine. Use two to three assessment locations. • **Mucous membranes (MM)**—Assess for dryness of gums and cornea (moist, tacky, dry) • **Degree of eye sinkage** into the bony orbit **Asess Perfusion Status:** • **Capillary refill time**—Place a finger against a pink mucous membrane. Apply firm pressure for a second to the membrane and release. Count in seconds the length of time it takes for the mucous membranes to refill with blood when pressure is released (Normal = <1–3 seconds) • **Heart Rate and Pulse** (femoral and metatarsal)—Assess heart rate, pulse (amplitude and duration) Unstressed dog: HR = 80–120 beats/min Unstressed cat: HR = 170–200 beats/min • **Weight of the animal**—Well body and current weight of animal should be noted. 1 lb. body weight = 1 pint (480 mL fluid).	<5% = No obvious clinical signs, skin turgor of <2 seconds 5%–6% = Skin: Doughy with inelastic consistency Mucous membranes: dry 6%–8% = *mild dehydration:* Skin: Inelastic and leathery Twist: disappears immediately Skin turgor: >3 seconds Eyes: duller than normal and sunken Mucous membranes: tacky to dry 8%–10% = *moderate dehydration:* Skin: Inelastic and leathery Twist: disappears slowly Skin turgor: >3 seconds Eyes: duller than normal and sunken Mucous membranes: tacky to dry Heart rate: increased 10%–12% = *severe dehydration:* Skin: No elasticity Twist: remains indefinitely Skin turgor: remains indefinitely Eyes: dry, deeply sunken Mucous membranes: dry, cyanotic, and possibly cold CRT: prolonged or absent Heart rate: increased Pulse: weak 12%–15% = Patient is in shock and death is imminent
Laboratory Assessment	**Packed cell volume**—blood (Normal: Dog = 37%–55% Cat = 24%–45%) **Total protein**—serum (Normal: Dog = 5.4–7.6 g/dL Cat = 6.0–8.1 g/dL) **Specific gravity** of urine (evaluates kidney function more than hydration status) **Electrolyte assessment** (See Chapter 7: Laboratory, for normal values)	↑ Hematocrit = dehydration ↑ Total protein = dehydration Specific gravity (SG) > 1.035 for dogs SG > 1.040 for cats (only reflects dehydration if kidneys are healthy)
Medical History	Review of patient's file and conversation with the owner	Previous physical problems (i.e., heart/kidney problems) will influence fluid therapy.

Table 8-2   Calculating Fluid Requirements

Veterinarians will need to prescribe the actual amount, the type of, and the rate of the fluid to be administered.

Purpose	Basis of Calculations	Rate
Rehydration: The basic formula calculates the fixed rate of replacement fluids to correct the deficit over 4–6 hours. Then, the rate should be adjusted based on the maintenance and ongoing losses calculations given over a 12 -24 hour period.	Basic rehydration formula	% dehydrated × body weight (kg) × 1,000 mL/kg = mL of fluid replacement to be administered (Ex: Animal weighing 20 kg is dehydrated 6%. Fluid needed for basic rehydration is calculated as .06 × 20 × 1,000 = 1,200 mL).
	Maintenance calculation	Maintenance is calculated to replace fluid losses resulting from urine output, that which is contained within feces, and that lost by respiration in an animal that is not taking in fluids orally. The rate amount varies from one textbook to another but generally is between 40 and 60 mL/kg/day in a mature animal, depending on the cause of the loss and animal's condition.
	Ongoing losses	Calculation on the amount of fluid loss attributable to diarrhea or vomiting (20 mL vomit = 20 mL fluids) or excessive urination
	Calculated on expected fluid loss during surgery.	2–4 mL/kg/hr
Anesthetic Protocol		
Postoperative Protocol		9–14 mL/kg/24-hr period (adult animal)
Pediatric Protocol		60–180 mL/kg/day (Mosier, 1981)
Shock Protocol		90 mL/kg/hr if patient has adequate/normal cardiopulmonary function

Table 8-3 Routes of Fluid Administration

Fluid Administration Routes:	Appropriate Use	Possible Complications	Materials Required	Notes
Oral	• Minimal loss	• Tracheal intubation and aspiration	• Syringe • Feeding tube • Drinking bowl	• Not given in cases of vomiting, diarrhea, dysphagia, or in life-threatening situations (e.g., shock)
Subcutaneous (between scapulas or on dorsal flanks)	• Mild dehydration	• Do not use >2.5 % dextrose, as will cause sloughing and abscesses	• Large-gauge needle (18–20)	• Warmed to body temperature • Use only isotonic fluids • Use several sites; no more than 50–200 mL per site depending on the size of patient
Intravenous (cephalic, saphenous, or jugular)	• Severe dehydration • Condition of animal is severe • Perioperative precaution	• Phlebitis • Septicemia • Embolism	• IV catheter in place • Administration set • Infusion pump	• Warmed to body temperature • Requires rate calculation • Requires *closer monitoring;* especially in cardiac insufficiency cases • Flush catheter with heparinized saline every 6–12 hours; replace catheter every 72 hours (Jugular catheters can remain in place for up to 14 days)
Intraperitoneal	• When large volumes are required in mild to moderately dehydrated patients and neonates	• Peritonitis • Intra-abdominal abscess formation	• Large-gauge needle (16–18)	• Warmed to body temperature • Not common because of potential complications and slow absorption rates
Interosseous (head of femur or humerus)	• Small animals, neonates, or animals with poor venous access	• Osteomyelitis	• #15 scalpel blade • 2% Lidocaine • Heparinized saline • 16-gauge bone marrow needle • Sterile gloves • Sterile preparation materials • Clippers • Suture material • 1-inch tape • Triple antibiotic ointment	• Technique must be sterile • Flush catheter with heparinized saline every 4–6 hours if fluid therapy is discontinued • An IV catheter should be placed as soon as a site allows (24–72 hours)

Skill Box 8-1 / Calculating Drip Rates

1. Number of mL needed / the time in which the fluid can be administered (in minutes) = mL/min
2. mL/min ×drops/mL of the administration set = # drops /min
3. # drops/min divided by 6 = # drops /10 seconds - **or** –
   # drops/min divided by 60 = # drops/second if the flow rate is high

Example: Need 1,200 mL to be given over 5 hours, using a 15 drops/mL administration set;

[1,200 divided by (5 hours multiplied by 60 min/hr)] multiplied by 15 drops/mL = 60 drops/min or 1 drop/sec
[1,200/300] × 15 = 60 drops/min or 1 drop/sec

Table 8-4   Monitoring Fluid Administration

Assessment	Technique	Significance
Cardiac function	Auscultation—stethoscope	Listen for arrhythmias, abnormal rate or pulse
Central Venous Pressure (CVP) -Normal: 0–5 cm H_2O -Volume overload: >8–10 cm H_2O	• Place an indwelling IV in the cranial vena cava at the level of the right atrium via the external jugular vein (verification of proper placement = 2- to 5-mm fluctuation in CVP). • Attach a 3-way stopcock to the catheter. • Attach the open line of the stopcock to the fluid source. (Macrosize administration set) • With the patient in lateral recumbency and the zero point of the manometer positioned at the level of the sternum, take your reading. Take several readings to verify accuracy; with patient in the same position as the first reading was taken. Watch for blood clots and flush with heparinized saline if fluids are not currently being administered.	• CVP is the only method to truly assess venous return to the heart • Low pressure reflects low effective circulating volume • High pressure reflects a possible right-sided myocardial failure, restrictive pericarditis, or excessive increase in the circulating volume
Electrolyte status	Blood draw	Assesses imbalances in patient's electrolytes
Equipment	Verify all equipment is functioning properly throughout the therapy. Check fluid level in bag/bottle, patient's positioning, venous line and catheter patency.	Watch for any obstruction that may inhibit the fluid administration
Packed Cell Volume/Total Protein	Blood draw	Assesses hydration status and hemodilution effect of rapid crystalloid infusion
Respiratory Function	Auscultation—stethoscope	Listen for rales, rhonchi, or wheezing
Temperature	Rectal temperature—thermometer	Watch for hypothermia
Urine output	Urine sample	Assesses renal function and perfusion
Volume Overload Signs	Restlessness, hyperpnea, cough, moist rales, serous nasal discharge, chemosis (edema of the ocular conjunctiva), hypothermia, pitting edema, ↑ respiratory rate, ↑ lung sounds, ↑ blood pressure	Immediately notify veterinarian for reduction/reassessment of fluid therapy
Weight	Weigh animal 3 times daily	Increased weight may be a sign of developing pulmonary edema or elevated central venous pressure (e.g., volume overload)

Table 8-5 Commonly Used Isotonic Fluids

Fluid	Usage	Route	Additional Monitoring	Disadvantages
Dextran 70 (Colloid)	• Volume expansion and acute hypovolemia and shock	IV slowly	• Cardiac function	• Potential for allergic responses • No oxygen-carrying capacity
Dextrose 5% (Crystalloid)	• Supply free water and calories to the patient (1 g dextrose = 4.1 calories) as a replacement solution	IV	• Lungs for pulmonary edema	• High dosages produce pulmonary edema and dilution of electrolytes • Incompatible with penicillins
Hetastarch (Colloid) (fewer side effects than Dextran)	• Acute hypovolemia and shock • Counters hypoproteinemia by increasing osmotic/oncotic pressure of blood	IV		• Potential for allergic responses • Possible coagulopathies • Expensive
Sodium Chloride 0.9%—Normal Saline (Crystalloid)	• Replacement fluid • Increases plasma volume • Corrects hyponatremia • Bathes tissue during surgical procedures	IV, SC, IP	• Electrolyte concentrations • Pulmonary function	• Long-term infusion may cause electrolyte imbalances • Incompatible with Amphotericin B • Not recommended in patients with cardiac disease
Lactated Ringer's - (Crystalloid)	• Replacement fluid • Maintenance fluid • Shock	IV, SC		• Incompatible with cephalothin sodium and chlortetracycline
Ringer's Solution (Crystalloid)	• Replacement fluid • Corrects metabolic alkalosis	IV, SC, IP	• Electrolyte concentrations • Pulmonary pressure	
Normosol-R/ Multisol-R	• Balanced, multiple electrolyte solution	IV		• May sting when used subcutaneous

Table 8-6   Fluid Additives

Additive	Usage	Route	Additional Monitoring	Disadvantages
Sodium Bicarbonate (Alkalizing agent)	• Correction of metabolic acidosis	IV	• Blood gas measurements and acidosis status • Check for incompatibilities before mixing with other solutions	• Use with caution in patients with congestive heart failure or other edema-causing conditions • Do not use when patient is vomiting or hypokalemic
Potassium Chloride	• Correction of hypokalemia • Must be diluted before using	IV	• Rate of infusion is critical: ≥.5 mEq/kg/hr -OR- ≤3–5 mEq/kg/day) • Watch for hyperkalemia, bradycardia, or arrhythmias	
Calcium Gluconate and Calcium Chloride	• Correction of hypocalcemia (typically given diluted) • Eclampsia (typically given full strength)	IV slowly	• Watch for hypercalcemia (hypotension, cardiac arrhythmias, and cardiac arrest)	
Dextrose 50%	• Caloric supplementation	IV		

Skill Box 8-2 / Peripheral Intravenous Catheterization

Sites used: Primarily cephalic and saphenous veins. The pedal dorsal veins can be used if not using hypertonic solutions.

Materials Required:

- 3 ×3 Gauze
- Alcohol
- Adhesive tape torn into strips for attaching catheter
- Appropriately sized IV catheter flushed with heparinized saline*
- Band-Aid®
- Chlorhexidine soap
- Chlorhexidine solution
- Clippers
- Fluid bag and administration set
- Male adapter/injection cap
- Syringe with heparinized saline
- 18-gauge needle
- Vetwrap™

Technique

1. Set up all required materials.
2. Clip the area of the insertion site.
3. Scrub the area with chlorhexidine and alcohol-soaked gauze, using aseptic technique.
4. On thick-skinned animals, nick the skin with an 18-gauge needle (this will help prevent burring or fraying of the catheter tip); be careful not to perforate the vein.
5. Place a gauze square just below the insertion site to help maintain an aseptic area as well as absorb any blood.
6. Using a smooth and steady technique, insert the catheter with bevel side facing up into the vein at a 15–30-degree angle. If you have entered the vein and the patient has adequate circulation, a flashback of blood should be seen. Reduce your entry angle and advance the catheter approximately $\frac{1}{8}$–$\frac{1}{4}$ of an inch.
7. Holding the catheter with one hand and the needle with the other, advance the catheter into the vein then withdraw the needle. Blood should be seen at the hub of the catheter. If blood is seen, have the person holding off release the vein.

*Caution: Do not use heparin in catheter with patients who have coagulation disorders.

8. Screw on the male adapter/injection cap on the catheter or attach the fluid line. Aseptically place a Band-Aid® over the injection site, and secure the catheter into place with tape.

9. Flush the catheter with saline.

10. Finish wrapping the site with Vetwrap™, leaving only the cap exposed.

   A tongue depressor can be placed on the ventral side of a cat's leg before applying the Vetwrap to prohibit bending of the leg and occlusion of the vessel.

   Use EMLA on prepared skin to desensitize the animal's reaction to insertion of the catheter.

   Secure the tape by making a butterfly (leave approximately 1 inch of tape on either side of the catheter and then loop the tape back onto itself such that there is a 1-inch "wing" on either side of the catheter) and then wrapping the tape around the limb.

Troubleshooting

No flashback:

1. Assess the vein, and, if visible, try adjusting the angle of the needle and insert.
2. If too far in, try withdrawing a little.
3. If blood is not seen in the catheter, come out and start over with a fresh catheter.

Maintenance

1. Flush catheter with heparinized saline every 4–6 hours, if not administering fluids continually.
2. Check catheter site daily for phlebitis, thrombosis, swelling, and wetness, and verify patency of catheter before hookup to new fluids.
3. Change the catheter every 3–5 days.
4. Change bandaging when wet.

Skill Box 8-3 / Intraosseous Catheterization

Sites used: Greater trochanter of the proximal femur, flat medial aspect of the proximal tibia (in obese animals), and greater tubercle of the humerus.

Materials Required:
- 2% Lidocaine
- #15 or #11 scalpel blade
- 16-gauge bone marrow needle
- Alcohol-soaked gauze
- Adhesive tape torn into strips for securing catheter
- Appropriately sized IV catheter flushed with heparinized saline
- Sterile chlorhexidine-soaked gauze
- Clippers
- Fluid bag and administration set
- Gloves
- Sterile gauze—3 × 3
- Suture material
- Syringe (12 mL) with heparinized saline
- Triple antibiotic ointment

Technique

1. Set up all required materials.
2. Clip the area of the insertion site.
3. Scrub the area with chlorhexidine and alcohol-soaked gauze, using aseptic technique.
4. Inject a local anesthetic subcutaneously if the animal is responsive (0.1 mL at the catheter insertion site).
5. Place a sterile gauze square just below the insertion site to help maintain an aseptic area as well as absorb any blood.
6. Incise the insertion site with a #15 or #11 scalpel blade.
7. Using sterile technique, place one hand along the side of the femur with the thumb pointing toward the greater trochanter. Pass the catheter through the insertion site, down the medial aspect of the greater trochanter, and into the trochanteric fossa.
8. Push the catheter through the cortex by applying downward pressure and rotating a quarter turn with each rotation. A loss of resistance is felt when the catheter passes through the cortex. The catheter will bounce lightly down the bone.
9. Verify placement by rotating the femur; the catheter and femur should move as one.
10. Remove cap and stylet and attach fluid set. Secure into place by suturing tape attached to the catheter to the skin. Apply triple antibiotic ointment over the insertion site.

Prevent slippage into the muscle by extending the index finger forward toward the body wall while rotating.

Maintenance

1. Same maintenance as the peripheral catheters.
2. Change catheter sites every 72 hours.
3. Check for infection and leakage daily.

Skill Box 8-4   Jugular Catheterization

Used in patients with poor peripheral veins or circulation, measurement of CVP or serial blood glucose testing. The jugular vein should not be used on patients with coagulopathies. Generally four types of catheter are available: over-the-needle, through-the-needle, peel-away sheath, or over-the-wire (Seldinger technique).

Materials Required:

- 2% Lidocaine
- #15 scalpel blade
- 16-gauge (dogs > 35 lbs) 18-gauge (cats and dogs <35 lbs) jugular catheter
- Alcohol-soaked gauze
- Adhesive tape torn into strips for attaching catheter
- Sterile chlorhexidine-soaked gauze
- Clippers
- Flushed T-port
- Fluid bag and venoset line
- Sterile gauze—3 × 3
- Sterile surgical gloves
- Suture material (nonabsorbable)
- Syringe with heparinized saline
- Triple antibiotic ointment
- Cyanoacrylate glue
- 2–3-inch cast padding
- Elastic wrap

Technique *(The technique varies with the type of jugular catheter placed, so it is important to know what type you are using and follow the manufacturer's instructions.)*

1. Set up all required materials.
2. Hold off the jugular vein and carefully clip the area of the insertion site, avoiding clipper burn. (If the animal is in sternal recumbency, the person who is placing the catheter should hold off the vein; if the animal is in lateral recumbency, the restrainer should hold off the vein.)
3. Put on examination gloves and scrub the area with chlorhexidine and alcohol-soaked gauze, using aseptic technique.
4. Change to sterile gloves, palpate the vein again, and insert the catheter/needle ensemble smoothly and quickly into the vein about 2 mm. A "pop" should be felt. A flashback is not seen in many jugular catheters until aspirated.
5. Thread the catheter the rest of the way into the vein. If there is a needle guard, place the needle in the groove and clamp shut. Be sure the hub of the catheter is locked into the hub of the needle. Remove the stylet and attach the T-port.
6. Aspirate and then flush with 3–6 mL heparinized saline.
7. Place a butterfly tape around the catheter hub and secure the catheter. The needle guard can be used to suture the catheter in place, or a butterfly tape can be applied to provide more stability. Adhere the catheter to the skin with three simple interrupted nonabsorbable sutures (one on each side of the catheter and a third as an anchor).
8. Place triple antibiotic ointment over the catheter entry site.
9. Place a drop of glue to the catheter/needle hub if applicable to the catheter type.
10. Place a second strip of tape in a counterclockwise direction.

Skill Box 8-4   Jugular Catheterization (Continued)

11. Apply cast padding loosely around the animal's neck clockwise and then counter clockwise, keeping the T-port clear.

12. Apply the gauze wrap in the same manner.

13. Flush T-port with heparinized saline, aspirate, and then flush again.

14. Place a layer of elastic tape, testing the tightness by ensuring that 2 fingers can be inserted under the wrap.

15. Place a piece of tape to secure the T-port and write the date of placement on it. Radiographs can be taken to assess proper placement.

16. Inspect catheter daily for placement and patency.

Maintenance

1. Flush catheter with 1–2 mL heparinized saline and aspirate it back out every 4 hours, if administering fluids continuously. Aspirate blood back into the syringe to ensure catheter is patent.

2. Flush catheter with 3–6 mL heparinized saline and aspirate it back out every 4 hours, if **not** administering fluids continually.

3. Check catheter site daily for phlebitis, thrombosis, swelling, and wetness, and verify patency of catheter before hooking up to new fluids.

4. Change the infusion set every 4 days and the catheter every 14 days.

5. Change bandaging if wet.

6. Watch for signs of fever, lethargy, or changes in vital signs in the animal (which may represent sepsis), or excessive resistance when flushing (which may represent blockage or damage of the catheter).

7. Walking leads should be placed around the chest and not the neck.

NUTRITIONAL SUPPORT

Many hospitalized patients are at risk of becoming severely malnourished because they lack desire or ability to eat. In response to injury and illness, the body breaks down protein, depleting the body's protein stores. Providing protein, carbohydrate, fat, and other nutrients, slows the breakdown of lean body mass and optimizes the patient's response to therapy. Injuries and illnesses can further increase a patient's caloric requirement, making nutritional support even more crucial. There are many ways to provide this support, both enterally and parenterally. The following will give basic guidelines for choosing the correct method and ways to administer.

Encouraging Oral Intake: In many situations, coaxing a patient to eat typically involves merely stimulating their appetite. This saves the patient from having to endure enteral or parenteral nutritional support. Unless contraindicated by an illness or injury, this approach should always be tried first.

Environment:

- If possible, move the patient to a quiet area, away from barking dogs and loud noises.
- Spray the environment with feline facial pheromones (for cats).
- Try various shapes and types of bowls; plastic may have a strange smell to cats.

Patient:

- Make sure the patient is capable of oral intake.
- Hand-feed or pet the animal during feeding.
- Make sure the nasal passages are clear of exudate to allow sufficient olfactory senses.

Diet:

- Warm the food; stir the food well before feeding to avoid hot spots.
- Add water to either dry food (to moisten) or to canned food (to make a slurry).
- Use top dressings: baby food or canned food.
- Use foods that have a strong odor or flavor.
- Offer a variety of foods with differing flavors and textures, both canned and dry.
- Appetite stimulants for the short term: anabolic steroids, Cyproheptadine, Diazepam, Inteferon

Table 8-7   Enteral Nutrition

Method	Advantages	Disadvantages	Indications	Contraindications
Syringe	• Noninvasive	• Patient tolerance	• Patients requiring coaxing to eat	• Patients with difficulty swallowing
Orogastric tube	• Ease of procedure • Rapidly deliver high quantities	• Patient tolerance • Increased restraint and stress on patient • Aspiration • Repeated intubation; trauma	• Patient in beginning stages of anorexia	• Patients with disorders of the oral cavity, pharynx, larynx, or esophagus
Nasoesophageal/ Nasogastric Tube	• Easy placement • Patient tolerance • Placement without general anesthesia • Tube can be left in for several weeks • Easily removed • Patient can eat and drink around the tube • Tube removal can be performed anytime after placement	• Size restriction of tube • Need for a liquid or highly blended food because of tube clogging	• Any patient experiencing malnutrition	• Patients undergoing oral, pharyngeal, esophageal, gastric, or biliary tract surgery
Pharyngostomy Tube	• Large-bore tube	• A tube placed too close to the laryngeal apparatus may cause irritation and obstruction, resulting in dysphagia or dyspnea • May cause coughing, laryngospasm, and/or aspiration	• Anorexic patient • A patient unable to or unwilling to ingest food orally • Patient with cleft palate, jaw fractures, or oral masses	• Patients with esophageal disorders; esophagitis, esophageal stricture, recent esophageal surgery, postesophageal foreign body removal, or esophageal neoplasia
Esophagostomy Tube	• Easy placement • Patient tolerance • Slurried food can be used • Patient can eat and drink around the tube • Easy tube care for owner • Tube removal can be performed anytime after placement • Large-bore tubes	• General anesthesia	• Anorexic patients with a functional gastrointestinal tract (GIT) • Patients with disorders of the oral cavity or pharynx	• Patients with an esophageal dysfunction; esophageal stricture, esophagitis, megaesophagus • Patients with esophageal foreign body removal or esophageal surgery

Type				
Gastrotomy Tube	• Patient tolerance • Patient can eat and drink with tube in place • Large-bore tube • Easy tube care for owner • Tube can be maintained for weeks to months	• General anesthesia • Specialized equipment • Feeding cannot take place until 24 hours after tube placement • Tube must remain in for 10–14 days before removal	• Anorexic patients with functional GIT distal to stomach • Patients undergoing surgery of oral cavity, larynx, pharynx, or esophagus	• Patients with primary gastric disease: gastritis, gastric ulceration, or gastric neoplasia • Patients with disorders causing vomiting
Surgical placement with Gastropexy	• No special equipment • Ease of finding the stomach in an anorexic patient • Ensures immediate seal between stomach wall and body wall • Confirmation of tube placement during procedure • Tube can be safely removed at any time	*Same as Gastrotomy Tubes*	*Same as Gastrotomy Tubes*	*Same as Gastrotomy Tubes*
Surgical placement without Gastropexy	• Easy placement • No special equipment needed	• Stomach is not fixed to body wall • Tube must remain in for 10–14 days • Confirmation of tube placement must be done by endoscopy or radiography	*Same as Gastrotomy Tubes*	*Same as Gastrotomy Tubes*

Table 8-7 Enteral Nutrition (Continued)

Method	Advantages	Disadvantages	Indications	Contraindications
Endoscopic Placement without Gastropexy	• Direct visualization of the tube during placement	• Inability to perform gastropexy to ensure seal between stomach wall and body wall • Tube must remain in for 10–14 days	*Same as Gastrotomy Tubes*	*Same as Gastrotomy Tubes*
Laparotomy Placement	• Ability to perform gastropexy to ensure seal between stomach wall and body wall	• Performing a laparotomy	*Same as Gastrotomy Tubes* • *Patients already undergoing surgery for a biopsy or mass removal*	*Same as Gastrotomy Tubes*
Jejunostomy	• Immediate feeding of a highly digestible, low-bulk diet allowed	• General anesthesia • Performing a celiotomy	• Patients undergoing oral, pharyngeal, esophageal, gastric, pancreatic, duodenal, or biliary tract surgery where the GI tract is functional past the lesion or disease • Patients whose neurologic status prevents postoperative feeding • Patients with gastric, intestinal, or pancreatic disease	• Patients with lower GI disorders or diseases

Table 8-8   Enteral Nutritional Procedures

The methods and procedures listed below (with the exception of the syringe and orogastric tube methods) should only be performed by a licensed DVM. The procedures below are meant only as a general description of how the procedure is performed, not complete instructions.

Method	Set up	Sedation	Procedure	Complications	Removal
Syringe	• 12-mL curved tipped syringe • High-calorie diet that has a texture allowing easy passage through the syringe	• None	Cut the end of the curved tip syringe about $\frac{1}{4}$–$\frac{1}{3}$ inch to allow easier passage of food. Insert the syringe into the cheek pouch of the patient's mouth positioned toward the back of the mouth. Slowly begin filling the mouth according to the speed of swallowing and allowing breaks to breathe.	• Aspiration • Vomiting	• None
Orogastric Tube	• 3.5–5 Fr feeding tube • High-calorie diet that has a texture allowing easy passage through the tube • Lubricant • Mouth speculum	• None	Measure the feeding tube from the tip of the nose to the 9th or 10th intercostal space and mark with tape. Lubricate the end of the tube and position the patient's head in a slightly flexed position. Begin inserting the tube into the patient's mouth, allowing them to swallow the tube. Continue to insert tube until the premeasured tape mark. Check for correct placement by attempting to aspirate air into the syringe. If no air is withdrawn or the patient is coughing, remove tube and try again.	• Patient biting tube in pieces • Endotracheal placement: kittens do not have a gag reflex, allowing easy endotracheal intubation and aspiration • Vomiting • Stressful to some patients	• Immediately following each procedure • Pull the tube straight out, sealing the end of the tube to prevent leakage and aspiration

Table 8-8 Enteral Nutritional Procedures (Continued)

The methods and procedures listed below (with the exception of the syringe and orogastric tube methods) should only be performed by a licensed DVM. The procedures below are meant only as a general description of how the procedure is performed, not complete instructions.

Method	Set up	Sedation	Procedure	Complications	Removal
Nasoesophageal/ Nasogastric Tube	• Topical anesthetic (Proparacaine hydrochloride 5%) • 3.5–5 Fr feeding tube • Tape to mark the proper length of the tube • 5% viscous lidocaine • 3-5 mL syringe • Sterile saline • Stethoscope • Needle drivers • Suture material • Elizabethan collar	• Topical anesthetic or light sedation • Cats may require light general anesthesia	Place 2 (0.5–1 mL) applications of local anesthetic in the nasal cavity by tilting the head up to encourage coating of the nasal mucosa. Select proper tube size and measure from the nares to the 7th or 8th intercostal space for nasoesophageal placement or the last rib for nasogastric placement and mark with tape. Lubricate the end of the tube with 5% viscous lidocaine and hold the head in a normal functional position. Be sure to avoid hyperflexion or hypoflexion of the neck. Place the tube in the ventrolateral aspect of the external nares and pass it in a caudoventral medial direction into the nasal cavity. The tube will drop into the oropharynx and stimulate a swallowing reflex. Pass the tube to the desired location. Confirm proper placement by either injecting 3–5 mL of sterile saline into the tube and eliciting a cough, placing 6–12 mL of air into the tube and auscultate for borborygmus at the xyphoid, or by taking an x-ray. Once proper placement is established, secure the tube. Place the tube directly over the dorsal aspect of the nose and forehead and secure it with sutures. Finally, place an Elizabethan collar on.	• Tube should not pass through the lower esophageal sphincter because this may cause sphincter incompetence, esophagitis, or esophageal reflux	• Tubes can be left in place for several weeks • Cut sutures and gently pull

Pharyngostomy Tube	• Surgical site preparation materials • Mouth speculum • 20–24 Fr polyvinyl chloride feeding tube • Tape to mark proper length of tube • Scalpel blade • Large, curved forceps • Suture material • 3-cc syringe	• General anesthesia	Administer general anesthesia. Place the patient in lateral recumbency. Aseptically prepare the area just caudal to the angle of the mandible. Place a mouth speculum. Measure the tube from the point of exit to the 7th or 8th intercostal space. Using your index finger or a pair of curved forceps, locate the pharynx near the base of the tongue and flex finger toward the neck making a visible bulge on the outside skin. Making a 1–2-cm skin incision, dissect down to your finger or forceps. Insert tube and pull it into the oral cavity, then reinsert it and correctly place it into the mid-esophagus. Suture the tube at its exit point for security.	• Vomiting the tube • Improper placement may cause coughing, gagging, partial airway obstruction, or reflux esophagitis	• Immediate or after several weeks or months • To remove, cut the skin sutures and pull • Exit site does not need further care; the holes will seal in 1–2 days and heal in 7–10 days
Esophagostomy Tube	• Surgical site preparation materials • Mouth speculum • 16–24 Fr polyvinyl chloride feeding tube • Tape to mark proper length of tube • Eld™ feeding tube placement device • #15 scalpel blade • Suture material • Sterile, water-soluble lubricant • 3-cc syringe	• General anesthesia	Administer general anesthesia. Place the patient in right lateral recumbency. Aseptically prepare the lateral midcervical area from the angle of the mandible to the thoracic inlet. Place a mouth speculum and slightly extend the neck. Measure the tube from the point of exit (midcervical region) to the 7th or 8th intercostal space. Using the Eld™ feeding tube placement device, make an incision through the cervical musculature and place the tube into the esophagus according to manufacturer's guidelines. Suture the tube to the cervical skin. The exit site can be bandaged or left open.	• Patient inadvertently removing tube • Patient chewing off the end of the tube • Vomiting the tube	• Immediate or after several weeks or months • To remove, cut the skin sutures and gently pull the tube out • Exit site does not need further care; the holes will seal in 1–2 days and heal in 7–10 days

Table 8-8 Enteral Nutritional Procedures (Continued)

The methods and procedures listed below (with the exception of the syringe and orogastric tube methods) should only be performed by a licensed DVM. The procedures below are meant only as a general description of how the procedure is performed, not complete instructions.

Method	Set up	Sedation	Procedure	Complications	Removal
Gastrotomy Tube					
Surgical Placement with Gastropexy	• Surgical site preparation materials • Large-bore stiff plastic stomach tube • Mouth Speculum • General surgical pack • #11 scalpel blade • Suture material • 18–20 Fr Foley catheter • Large curved forceps • 6-cc syringe	• General anesthesia	Administer general anesthesia. Aseptically prepare the skin of the left flank. Place a stomach tube into the stomach and palpate the left flank until the stomach tube can be felt and grasped. The tube should be felt 1–2 cm past the last rib and 3–4 cm ventral to the transverse processes of lumbar vertebrae 2, 3, and 4. While holding the tube, make a 2-cm incision over the end of the tube. Dissect down to the outside of the stomach and then with a scalpel blade insert tube. Inflate bulb on Foley catheter, withdraw stomach tube, and tighten purse string. Suture stomach wall to the body wall and place some subcutaneous sutures. Suture tube to abdominal skin.	• Leakage of gastric contents into the abdominal cavity resulting in peritonitis • Vomiting • Peristomal infection	• Immediately
Surgical placement without Gastropexy	• Surgical site preparation material • Large-bore stiff stomach tube • Mouth speculum • General surgical pack • 18-g needle • 18-g sovereign catheter • 20 Fr Pezzer urinary catheter • Suture material • Sterile water-based lubricant • Sterile saline • 6-cc syringe	• General anesthesia	Administer general anesthesia. Place a stomach tube or feeding tube placement device from the oral cavity to the stomach. Palpate the tube bulging against the left body wall. Direct it 1–2 cm caudal to last rib. Pass an 18-g needle through the abdominal wall and into the lumen of the stomach tube. Thread the needle with suture and direct through to oral cavity. Remove the stomach tube. Thread the end of the suture through the 18-g sovereign catheter and tie it to the proximal end of the Pezzer urinary catheter. Pull the suture and the attached catheter back into the stomach cavity, enlarge the exit hole and pull sovereign catheter out until the mushroom tip of the Pezzer catheter is snugly against the body wall. This will ensure a seal between the stomach wall and body wall. Secure the catheter to the skin with sutures.	• Early removal of tube, causing leakage of gastric contents into the abdominal cavity resulting in peritonitis • Vomiting • Peristomal infection	• 10–14 days after placement

Endoscopic placement without Gastropexy	*Same as Surgical Placement without Gastroplexy*	• General anesthesia	Placed the same as Surgical Placement without Gastroplexy except the suture is retrieved endoscopically instead of via a stomach tube.	• Early removal of tube causing leakage of gastric contents into the abdominal cavity resulting in peritonitis • Vomiting • Peristomal infection	• 10–14 days after placement
Laparotomy Placement	• Surgical site preparation materials • 18–20 Fr Foley or Pezzer catheter • General surgical pack • #11 scalpel blade • Suture material • Sterile saline • 6-cc syringe	• General anesthesia	Administer general anesthesia. With a midline laparotomy approach, incise into the stomach. Place the Pezzer catheter directly into the stomach and place through the stomach and body wall as above. Fix the stomach wall to the body wall with sutures. Suture the abdomen closed.	• Leakage of gastric contents into the abdominal cavity resulting in peritonitis • Vomiting • Peristomal infection	• Immediate
Jejunostomy Tube	• Surgical site preparation materials • 5 Fr feeding tube • General surgical pack • #11 scalpel blade • Suture material • Bandaging material	• General anesthesia	Administer general anesthesia. Make a 2–3-mm stab incision through the abdominal wall. Through the celiotomy, select a section of jejunum that can be easily moved within the stab incision in the body wall. Incise into the jejunum and place the distal end of the feeding tube through the incision and pass 25–30 cm of the tube aborally into the jejunum. Suture the exit site of the jejunum and fix to the body wall. Secure the exit portion of the tube to the outside skin. Incorporate the tube into an abdominal bandage.	• Early removal of tube • Tube-induced jejunal perforation • Peritoneal leakage • Subcutaneous leakage	• 10–14 days after placement

Table 8-9   Enteral Nutrition Administration

Method	Tube Care	Feeding
Syringe	• Rinse syringe with water after administration	• Fill syringe with desired food and place the tip of the syringe in the cheek pouch directed toward the back of the mouth. Gently depress plunger of syringe and deposit food. Speed will depend on the rate of swallowing and patient tolerance.
Orogastric Tube	• Rinse tube with water after administration	• Once tube is in place (see Table 8-11), attach food-filled syringe to the end of the tube. Begin depressing plunger to administer required amount.
Nasoesophageal/ Nasogastric Tube	• Place a column of water in the tube and cap it at the end of each feeding. This will prevent the intake of air, reflux of esophageal contents, and occlusion of the tube by the diet	• Give 25%–50% volume on day 1, 50%–75% volume on day 2, 75% volume on day 3, and total volume on day 4, depending on patient tolerance • Divide the total daily volume by 3–4 feedings • Warm the food to body temperature in a microwave. Make sure it is not too hot or it will burn the stomach lining • Remove the cap on the tube and draw back on syringe to observe for any food or fluid. If more than 0.5 mL/lb withdrawn, do not feed • Infuse 5–10 mL water to assure the tube is patent • Infuse the allotted food slowly over a few minutes • Infuse 5–10 mL water to clear tube and recap
Pharyngostomy Tube	• Place a column of water in the tube and cap it at the end of each feeding. This will prevent the intake of air, reflux of contents, and occlusion of the tube by the diet • The site of tube exit should be periodically cleaned with an antiseptic solution	*Same as Nasoesophageal/Nasogastric Tube*
Esophagostomy Tube	*Same as Pharyngostomy Tube*	*Same as Nasoesophageal/Nasogastric Tube*
Gastrotomy Tube	*Same as Pharyngostomy Tube*	*Same as Nasoesophageal/Nasogastric Tube*
Jejunostomy Tube	*Same as Pharyngostomy Tube*	• May feed immediately after surgery • Dilute for 1:1 on day 1, 1:0.5 on day 2, and full strength on day 3 • Give 25%–50% volume on day 1 and gradually increase over the next 3–4 days • Infuse continuously with an infusion pump, but check regularly for back pressure • Do not hang bag for more than 24 hours; it may cause bacteria to grow

Table 8-10 Parenteral Nutrition

	Advantages	Disadvantages	Indications	Contraindications
Total (TPN)	• Provides 100% nutritional support	• Expensive • Difficulty of inserting and maintaining a central venous catheter • Increased risk of infection • Central venous thrombus • Metabolic disturbances • Mechanical complications • Associated with increased permeability of the GIT	• Nonfunctional GIT • Postoperatively for some surgeries • Prolonged ileus • Severe malassimilation • Patients with vomiting or regurgitation	• Patients of marginal nutritional status • Well-nourished animals undergoing elective surgery or diagnostic procedures
Peripheral (PPN)	• Administered via a cephalic or saphenous vein • Easier, fewer complications, and less expensive than TPN	• Expensive • Venous thrombosis • Inflammation of the limb • Mechanical failure • Associated with increased permeability of the GI tract	• Patients of marginal nutritional status • Patients who cannot receive a jugular catheter • Patients needing supplemental feeding to enteral feeding • Patients benefiting from nutritional support before surgery for gastrotomy or jejunostomy tube • Nondebilitated animals needing IV support for >7 days • Patients with vomiting or regurgitation	• Debilitated patients needing full nutritional support • Well-nourished animals undergoing elective surgery or diagnostic procedures

Table 8-11   Parenteral Nutrition Administration

	Patient Care	Administration
TPN	• Patient fluid, electrolyte, and acid–base abnormalities should be corrected before administration • Check body weight and temperature twice daily • Evaluate serum electrolytes, glucose, total protein, serum lipids, packed cell volume (PCV), and blood urea nitrogen (BUN) daily • Change neck bandage every 48 hours and clean entrance site of catheter with iodine solution • Change administration set every 48 hours • Catheter should be placed in a new vein if there is any questions to its patency, sterility, or tissue irritation around site • Patient should have a dedicated TPN catheter	• Administered over a 24-hour period • Solutions should be refrigerated and hung at room temperature for no more than 48 hours • Homemade TPN solutions should be mixed in an all-in-one container with separate sterile transfer lines for each solution • Inline filters should be used in the administration set • Infusion pumps should always be used to avoid bolus administration • Calculation is critical and should be verified • Drugs should not be included in the TPN solution to avoid incompatibility • A bag of TPN should not be shared between patients
PPN	• Dehydrated patients should be rehydrated • Crystalloid fluids should continue to correct ongoing fluid loss • Discontinue PPN after patient consumes >50% of its energy requirement orally • Patient should have a dedicated PPN catheter • Line should only be disconnected to change the bag every 24 hours • Catheter bandaging should be sterilely changed every 24 hours when bag and line are changed • Catheter site should be checked daily for swelling, redness, or irritation • Catheter should be placed in a new vein if there is any question of its patency, sterility, or tissue irritation around site • If no interest in self-feeding in 3–5 days, TPN or enteral feeding should be started • Monitor weight gain or loss	• Administered over a 24-hour period • Solutions should be refrigerated and hung at room temperature for no more than 24 hours • A bag of PPN should not be shared between patients • Inline filters should be used in the administration set • Infusion pumps should always be used to avoid bolus administration • Calculation is critical and should be verified

Table 8-12 Nutritional Support Diets And Calculations

Method	Formulas	Calculations
Enteral		
Syringe Orogastric Tube	• If diet is hyperosmolar (>350 mOsm/kg water) it will need to be diluted with water to make it hypoosmolar • Commercial diets not requiring blenderizing (e.g., CliniCare, Ensure, Jevity, Osmolite HN, Promote, Vital HN, Vivonex HN)	• Calculate the maintenance energy requirement (see Skill Box 8-5) • Divide the total daily volume by 3–4 feedings

Nasoesophageal/ Nasogastric Tube Pharyngostomy Tube Esophagostomy Tube Gastrotomy Tube	• Commercial diets typically requiring blenderizing (e.g., CNM-CV Feline, Iams NRF, Eukanuba Feline Max, Hill's A/D, Hill's P/D)
	• Homemade diets:
	  Dog/Cat: 1 jar cooked baby food, 1 cooked egg, 15 mL corn oil, 15 mL corn syrup, 100 mL water
	  Cat: #1) 3 oz egg yolk, 3 oz strained baby food, 3 oz water, 1 tsp cooking oil, 1 T corn syrup- #2) 3 cans (5.5 oz) CNM-CV Feline, 8 oz water, 2 oz Wesson oil, and 16 mEq Tumil K
	• Blend at high speed for 60 sec and strain twice through a strainer
		• Calculate maintenance energy requirement (see Skill Box 8-5)
		• Give 25%–50% volume on day 1, 50%–75% volume on day 2, 75% volume on day 3, and total volume on day 4, depending on patient tolerance
		• Divide the total daily volume by 3–4 feedings

Jejunostomy Tube	• Commercial liquid diets (e.g., Ensure) • Liquid formulas are required to prevent tube clogging • Dilution with water is not needed if a hypoosmolar formula is used	• Calculate the maintenance energy requirement (see Skill Box 8-5) • Dilute for 1:1 on day 1, 1:0.5 on day 2, and full strength on day 3 • Give 25%–50% volume on day 1 and gradually increase over the next 3–4 days
Parenteral		
TPN/PPN	• Commercial solutions purchased from human hospitals and health care suppliers • Homemade solutions consisting of amino acid solutions (e.g., 8.5% Travesol Injection with Electrolytes), lipid emulsions (e.g., Intralipid 20%), dextrose (e.g., 50% Dextrose), and vitamin supplements (e.g., vitamins B, A, D, E, K) • Refer to a parenteral reference for proper calculations	• Calculate the maintenance energy requirement (see Skill Box 8-5) • Give 50% the first day and 100% the second day

Skill Box 8-5 / Nutrition Calculating Worksheet for Nutritional Support

Step 1: Calculate Resting Energy Requirement (RER)

Animals weighing <2 kg and >45 kg:

$$70 \ (\underline{\hspace{1cm}} \ kg)^{0.75} = \underline{\hspace{1cm}} \ Kcal/day$$
$$(RER)$$

Animals weighing between 2 and 45 kg:

$$70 + 30 \ (\underline{\hspace{1cm}} \ kg) = \underline{\hspace{1cm}} \ Kcal/day$$
$$(RER)$$

Step 2: Calculate Maintenance Energy Requirement (MER) using the Illness Energy Requirement (IER) factor

Takes into account the severity of the illness; ranges from 1.0 for minor conditions, to a maximum of 1.4 (cat) to 1.6 (dog) for conditions such as sepsis or severe thermal burns.

$$\underline{\hspace{1cm}} \times \underline{\hspace{1cm}} = \underline{\hspace{1cm}} \ Kcal/day$$
$$(IER) \quad (RER) \quad (MER)$$

Step 3: Calculate Volume of Formula Required

$$\underline{\hspace{1cm}} \ Kcal/day \ / \underline{\hspace{1cm}} \ Kcal/ml \ of \ formula = \underline{\hspace{1cm}} \ mL \ formula/day$$
$$(MER)$$

Step 4: Calculate Amount of Each Feeding

$$\underline{\hspace{1cm}} \ mL \ formula/day \ / \ 3\text{--}4 \ feedings \ per \ day = \underline{\hspace{1cm}} \ mL \ formula/feeding$$

PAIN MANAGEMENT

Animals respond to painful stimuli both behaviorally and physiologically. Research shows that a patient's normal functions return sooner and they recover and heal quicker with pain control. In the past, the hardest part of pain control was trying to decide when the patient was truly in pain. It is now thought that preemptive treatment is the best method. Do not wait for the patient to prove they are in pain; assume, after surgical procedure, and during illness and injuries, that a patient is experiencing pain. To ensure a patient's comfort, continual observation and appropriate treatment are needed, especially in the first 12–24 hours.

After a discussion of the basic pain mechanics, we list a few myths surrounding the use of pain control in animals. Much research has shown these myths to be unsubstantiated. This section explains a few of these myths and provides clear and safe ways of dealing with these concerns.

The pain pathway begins with the stimulation of receptors and peripheral nerves through the conversion of a chemical, mechanical, or thermal insult into a nerve impulse. The signal is then conducted through the spinal cord to the brain, where it is perceived as pain. The degree of pain is related to the number of receptors in the injured tissue. The skin, periosteum, joint capsule, muscle, tendon, and arterial wall contain the highest density of pain receptors.

The peripheral nervous system is the source of the intense sharp pain felt with an injury. This is directly related to the number and location of pain receptors. The central nervous system produces burning, throbbing pain because of the low density of pain receptors found there. The internal organs require a major insult on the organ to produce intense pain. Typically it is hard to locate diffuse pain in contrast to the easily located intense pain associated with the peripheral nervous system.

Pain Management Myths:

1. *Analgesics mask the physiologic indicators of patient deterioration.*
   Evidence exists in both human and veterinary medicine showing that this is not the case. In fact, if the patient were treated adequately for pain, any changes in physiologic indicators would indeed be attributable to patient deterioration rather than a pain stress response.

2. *Potential for toxicity or adverse reactions associated with drug administration.*
   With our current level of understanding, there is no longer an overpowering reason to avoid the use of analgesics. Many drug options exist for both dogs and cats, with proven guidelines to allow safe administration.

3. *Pain is hard to recognize.*
   It is best to think of pain in terms similar to human pain. Treat for this level of pain regardless of whether you think the animal is truly showing signs of pain. Assume that invasive procedures, trauma, and illness result in a need for analgesics. Merely being aware and observing for behavioral signs of pain will make recognition easier.

Table 8-13 Potential Complications and Suggested Solutions

Concern	Solution
Physiologic	
Cardiovascular compromise	• Increase cardiovascular monitoring
Respiratory compromise—sedation may inhibit movement, leading to respiratory complications	• Increase respiratory monitoring • Provide proper nursing care (e.g., rotating patient)
Overdose/Toxicity	• Be aware of all options of pain control available and make wise choices • Be aware of the effects and toxicity of each drug • Double-check the dosage calculation
Complicated evaluation and monitoring because of the masking of physiologic signs and sedation altering cardiovascular parameters	• Obtain baseline parameters of behavior, heart rate, and respiratory rate before and immediately after the procedure • Maintain pain relief; animals with continual changes in pain experience continual changes in cardiovascular parameters
Activity	
Increased activity—animals that feel no pain will be more inclined to move around, causing further damage	• Use sedation or confinement
Slower recovery—pain drugs may cause sedation and therefore a slower recovery to normal function	• Accept a slower recovery in an animal's return to normal activities (e.g., walking, eating)

Nondrug Approach to Decrease Pain and Anxiety: Along with the use of analgesics and sedatives, proper nursing care will also help alleviate pain. The following should be observed in every patient that might possibly be experiencing pain or anxiety.

Environment:

- Provide familiar toys and blankets
- Quiet—away from loud animals and human noise
- Decrease anxiety; anxiety increases the perception of pain

Contact:

- Visits from owners
- Interactions with staff
- Talking, petting, stroking

Nursing Care:

- Schedule the least interruptions possible; combine monitoring, medication administration, and cage moving
- Offer multiple opportunities for dogs to urinate or defecate

Table 8-14   Drugs Commonly Used to Reduce or Alleviate Pain

This is a partial list of the many drugs currently used to alleviate pain. Each patient should be evaluated, and the proper drug (or often combination of drugs) should be decided on by the veterinarian.

Drug	Indications	Contraindications	Dose/Duration	Comments
Opioids				
Morphine Sulfate	• Moderate to severe pain	• Shock • Severe head injury • Any disease that compromises respiratory function • Intraocular ophthalmic surgery • Severe renal or hepatic disease	• *Dog:* 0.25—5.0 mg/kg IM, SC • *Cat:* 0.1 mg/kg IM, SC *Duration:* 1–4 hours IV, 2–6 hours IM, SC	• High doses may cause excitement in cats; give lower doses combined with a tranquilizer
Oxymorphone HCl	• Moderate to severe pain	• Use with caution in patients with hypothyroidism, Addison's, severe renal disease, head injury, intracranial pressure, respiratory disease, or acute respiratory dysfunction	• *Dog:* 0.05–0.2 mg/kg IV, IM • *Cat:* 0.02–0.1 mg/kg IV, IM *Duration:* 2–6 hours	• May cause auditory sensitization, increased body temperature, and bradycardia • Use atropine or glycopyrrolate for the bradycardia • Placement of cotton balls in the patient's ears and a quiet environment may alleviate signs of sound sensitivity
Meperidine HCl	• Mild to moderate pain • Preoperative sedation	• Postoperative pain control • Same as oxymorphone HCl	• *Dog/Cat:* 2–10 mg/kg IM, SC *Duration:* 20–30 minutes	• IM administration is painful • Rapid IV administration may cause severe hypotension

Drug	Indications	Contraindications/Cautions	Dosage	Notes

Fentanyl Citrate	• Moderate to severe pain	• Use with caution in patients with fevers, geriatric, very ill, debilitated, or preexisting respiratory problems	• *Dog/Cat:* 0.001–0.01 mg/kg
			• *Duration:* 30–45 minutes
			• Transdermal patch:
			  <11 lb = 12.5 μg (½ patch)
			  11–22 lb = 25 μg
			  22–44 lb = 50 μg
			  44–66 lb = 75 μg
			  >66 lb = 100 μg
			• *Duration:* at least 72–104 hours
				• May cause auditory sensitization, increased body temperature, and bradycardia
				• Use atropine or glycopyrrolate for the bradycardia
				• May cause bradycardia, hypotension, and respiratory depression if used with barbiturates
				• Cotton in the ears and a quiet environment may alleviate signs of sound sensitivity

Butorphanol tartrate	• Mild to moderate pain
	• Dog: visceral pain
	• Cat: skin pain
		• Somatic pain
		• Same as oxymorphone HCl
			• *Dog:* 0.3–0.5 mg/kg SC, IM, IV
			• *Cat:* 0.8 mg/kg
			• *Duration:*
			  Dog: 20–60 minutes
			  Cat: 2 hours
				• Has an anesthetic ceiling effect in which an increased amount will not decrease the pain further

NSAID
Aspirin (acetylsalicylic acid)
	• Mild to moderate pain
	• Peripheral inflammation
	• Muscle or joint pain
		• Deep or visceral pain
		• Bleeding disorders
		• Asthma
		• Renal insufficiency
		• GI sensitivity
			• *Analgesia:*
			  Dogs: 10–25 mg/kg PO 2–3 times daily
			  Cats: 10 mg/kg PO every other day
			• *Arthritis, Anti-inflammatory:*
			  Dog: 10–25 mg/kg PO q8h
			  Cat: 81 mg PO three times weekly
				• Buffered aspirin should be used to protect stomach lining
				• Enteric-coated aspirin does not get broken down and absorbed in the GIT
				• Caution should be used in cats; inability to rapidly metabolize and excrete salicylates

Flunixin meglumine	• Moderate to severe pain • Relief of persistent, severe inflammation and pain associated with degenerative joint disease	• Cats • Preexisting GI ulcers, renal, hepatic or hematologic diseases	• *Dogs:* 1.0 mg/kg SQ • *Duration:* repeat once in 8–12 hours	• May cause severe GI bleed

Ketoprofen	• Moderate to severe pain
	• Treatment of inflammation
		• Late pregnancy; premature closure of patent ductus	• *Surgical pain:*
			  Dog: 2 mg/kg IV, SC, IM initially, then 1 mg/kg daily
			  Cat: 2 mg/kg SC initially, then 1 mg/kg daily
			• *Chronic pain:* 2 mg/kg PO initially, then 1 mg/kg daily
				• May mask signs and symptoms of infection

Table 8-14 Drugs Commonly Used to Reduce or Alleviate Pain (Continued)

This is a partial list of the many drugs currently used to alleviate pain. Each patient should be evaluated, and the proper drug (or often combination of drugs) should be decided on by the veterinarian.

Drug	Indications	Contraindications	Dose/Duration	Comments
Carprofen	• Moderate to severe pain • Treatment of inflammation	• Bleeding disorders • Chronic disease; inflammatory bowel disease, hepatic or renal disease • GI sensitivity	• Surgical pain: Dog/Cat: 4 mg/kg IV initially once; 2.2 mg/kg PO, IV, SC, or IM; repeat in 12 hours if needed • Chronic pain: Dog/Cat: 2.2 mg/kg PO q12h	• Monitor blood values when using long-term • Give with food
Etodolac	• Moderate to severe pain • Treatment of inflammation associated with osteoarthritis	• GI, hepatic, cardiovascular, or hematologic abnormalities • GI sensitivity	• Dog: 10–15 mg/kg PO daily	• Very difficult to accurately dose dogs <5 kg • Caution should be taken in animals that are dehydrated, on diuretics, or that have renal, hepatic, or cardiovascular dysfunction
Meclofenamic Acid	• Treatment of chronic inflammatory disease of the musculoskeletal system • Hip dysplasia or chronic osteoarthritis	• GI, renal, or hepatic disease • Late pregnancy	• Dog: 1.1 mg/kg PO daily	• Vomiting, decreased hemoglobin, leukocytosis, tarry stools, and small intestinal ulcers have all been reported after therapy at usual effective doses
Local Anesthetics Lidocaine	• Mild to moderate pain	• Bradycardia • Congestive heart failure • Liver disease • Shock • Hypovolemia • Severe respiratory depression or marked hypoxia • Malignant hyperthermia	• Dog/Cat: 1–2 mL infiltration • *Duration:* 2 hours	• Cats are very sensitive to the CNS effects—use with caution
Ketamine HCl	*See Chapter 2 — Anesthesia*	*See Chapter 2 — Anesthesia*	• Dog/Cat: 1-4 mg/kg IV • *Duration:* 30 minutes	*See Chapter 2 — Anesthesia*

Table 8-15 Behaviors Suggesting Pain And Anxiety

Each behavior that an animal portrays may have a variety of meanings. Often a behavior may be indicative of both pain and a normal behavior. When evaluating whether a patient is in pain, look for multiple behaviors to assure a correct assessment of pain. Remember, it is always best to err on the side of pain and administer a pain medication, most likely a patient is always experiencing some level of pain after a surgical procedure, or during an illness or injury.

Behavior	Pain	Poor General Health	Apprehension/Anxiety	Normal Behavior
Posture				
Hunched up guarding abdomen	X			
Tensing abdomen and back muscles	X			
Splinting of abdomen	X			
Reluctance to lie down	X		X	
Leaning against cage wall	X		X	
Sitting or lying in an abnormal position	X		X	
Resting in abnormal position	X		X	
Praying position (forequarters on ground, hindquarters in air)	X			
Weak tail wag	X		X	
Low carriage of tail	X		X	
Head hangs down	X		X	X
Gait				
Limping	X			
Non-weight bearing (partial or complete)	X			
Stiff	X			
Unwilling to walk	X		X	
Unable to walk	X			

Table 8-15 Behaviors Suggesting Pain And Anxiety (Continued)

Each behavior that an animal portrays may have a variety of meanings. Often a behavior may be indicative of both pain and a normal behavior. When evaluating whether a patient is in pain, look for multiple behaviors to assure a correct assessment of pain. Remember, it is always best to err on the side of pain and administer a pain medication, most likely a patient is always experiencing some level of pain after a surgical procedure, or during an illness or injury.

Behavior	Pain	Poor General Health	Apprehension/Anxiety	Normal Behavior
Movement				
Restless, agitated	X		X	X
Trembling, shaking	X		X	X
Thrashing	X		X	
No movement when sleeping	X			X
Lying quietly and not moving for hours and doesn't dream	X			
Stuporous	X			
Recumbent and unaware of surroundings	X	X		
Slow to rise	X	X	X	
Reluctant to move head (eye movement only)	X	X	X	
Stretching all 4 legs when abdomen is touched	X			X
Pacing	X		X	
Repetitively lying down, getting up, lying down	X		X	X
Attitude				
Bite or attempts to bite caregivers	X		X	X
Looking, licking, chewing at painful area	X		X	
Hyperesthesia/hyperalgesia	X			
Allodynia	X		X	X

Sitting in back of cage		X		X	X
Hiding under blanket (cat)		X		X	X
Cleaning/licking wound		X			X
Aggressiveness		X		X	X
Inability to sleep regardless of obvious exhaustion		X		X	
Vocalization					
Screaming		X		X	X
Whining		X	X	X	X
Crying		X	X	X	X
None		X		X	X
Barking/growling (dog)		X		X	X
Growling/hissing (cat)		X		X	X
General Appearance					
Not grooming		X	X	X	X
Dull eyes		X	X		
Ears pulled back		X		X	
Penile prolapse		X	X		
Stare into space		X	X	X	X
Grimacing		X	X	X	X
Sleepy		X	X		X
Photophobic					
Ruffled greasy fur		X	X		

Table 8-15   Behaviors Suggesting Pain And Anxiety (Continued)

Each behavior that an animal portrays may have a variety of meanings. Often a behavior may be indicative of both pain and a normal behavior. When evaluating whether a patient is in pain, look for multiple behaviors to assure a correct assessment of pain. Remember, it is always best to err on the side of pain and administer a pain medication, most likely a patient is always experiencing some level of pain after a surgical procedure, or during an illness or injury.

Behavior	Pain	Poor General Health	Apprehension/Anxiety	Normal Behavior
Physiologic				
Tachypnea/panting	X	X	X	X
Tachycardia	X	X	X	X
Dilated pupils	X		X	
Hypertension	X		X	
Increased body temperature	X	X	X	
Increased salivation	X	X	X	
Appetite/elimination				
Inappetance	X		X	
Decreased appetite	X		X	
Picky appetite	X		X	X
Makes no attempt to move to eliminate	X			

Table 8-16   Pain Levels Associated with Surgical Procedures, Injuries, and Illnesses

Surgical procedures, illnesses, and injuries are known to cause pain in humans and are thought to do so in animals also. This chart can be used to preemptively treat animals for expected pain. It will also help to choose the correct drug or combination of drugs to administer when there is an understanding of the level of pain each procedure may produce.

	Mild to Moderate	Moderate	Moderate to Severe	Severe to Excruciating
Surgical Procedure	• Chest drains • Urinary catheterization • Dental cleaning • Ear examination and cleaning • OVH (young animals) • Castration (young animals) • Mass removal	• Cystotomy (inflamed) • Anal sacculectomy • Dental extractions • Laparotomy (short procedure with minimal manipulation and no inflammation) • Enucleation • OVH (older, obese, or pregnant animals) • Castration (older or obese animals) • Mass removal • Inguinal hernia repair	• Onychectomy • Limb amputation • Thoracotomy • Exploratory laparotomy • Total ear ablation • Laminectomy	• Postsurgical pain when extensive tissue injury or inflammation
Injury	• Abscess lancing • Removing cutaneous foreign bodies • Laceration repair-minor	• Laceration repair (severe) • Soft tissue injury • Extracapsular cruciate repair • Diaphragmatic hernia repair (acute, simple with no organ injury)	• Fracture repair • Frostbite • Mesenteric, gastric, testicular, or other torsions • Corneal abrasion or ulceration • Trauma (orthopedic, extensive soft tissue injury, head injury) • Rewarming after accidental hypothermia • Traumatic diaphragmatic hernia repair (organ and extensive tissue injury) • Intra-articular surgical procedure (large dogs or extensive manipulation)	• Multiple fracture repair with extensive soft tissue injury • Neuropathic pain (nerve entrapment, cervical intervertebral disk herniation, inflammation)
Illness	• Cystitis • Otitis	• Pancreatitis (early or resolving) • Urethral obstruction	• Osteoarthritis, acute polyarthritis • Peritonitis	• Meningitis • Bone cancer (especially after biopsy) • Pathologic fractures • Necrotizing cholecystitis • Necrotizing pancreatitis • Extensive inflammation (peritonitis, fasciitis, cellulitis)

WOUND TREATMENT AND BANDAGING

Inevitably pets end up with wounds, either self-inflicted or caused by another source. These wounds may be intentional, such as a surgical incision, or an accident. A technician plays a valuable role in the setup, preparation, cleaning, and the actual bandaging of these wounds. An understanding of the wound healing process, supplies to use, and the expected final outcome is necessary for proper treatment and care. These items are included in this chapter to facilitate excellent nursing care by the technician.

Table 8-17 Wound Healing Process (These stages are not stationary, but rather overlap one another.)

Inflammatory →	Repair →	Wound Contraction →	Maturation
1. Vasoconstriction in first 5–10 minutes that allows the small vessels to clot. 2. Vasodilation permits the leakage of plasma and proteins necessary for clotting. 3. White blood cells leak out (~6 hours after initial trauma) to engulf and remove bacteria, foreign debris, and necrotic tissue.	4. Fibroblasts and new capillaries fill the wound producing granulation tissue (~3–5 days), which protects the wound from infection and provides a surface for the attachment of epithelial cells to connect the two sides of the wounds. 5. New epithelial cells reproduce at wound edge covering the granulation bed resulting in a scab.	6. Fibroblasts pull the wound edges together (~5–9 days)	7. Remodeling of fibrous tissue to strengthen the scar and reduce the scab (begins ~4 weeks after the initial trauma).

Table 8-18   Classification of Wounds

Classification	Characteristics
Tissue Integrity	
1. Open	1. Lacerations or skin loss
2. Closed	2. Crushing injuries and contusions
Etiologic Force	
1. Abrasion	1. Loss of epidermis and portions of dermis. Usually attributable to shearing between two compressive surfaces.
2. Avulsion	2. Tearing of tissue from its attachment because of forces similar to those causing abrasion but of greater magnitude.
3. Incision	3. Created by a sharp object. Wound edges are smooth, and minimal tissue trauma is present in surrounding tissue.
4. Laceration	4. Irregular wound caused by tearing of tissue with variable damage to superficial and underlying tissue.
5. Puncture	5. Skin penetration by a missile or sharp object. Superficial damage may be minimal. Damage to deeper structures may be considerable. Contamination by hair and bacteria with subsequent infection is common.
Degree of Contamination and Duration	
1. Class I	1. Zero to 6 hours duration with minimal contamination.
2. Class II	2. Six to 12 hours duration with significant contamination.
3. Class III	3. Twelve hours or longer with gross contamination.
Degree of Contamination	
1. Clean wound	1. Surgically created under aseptic conditions. No invasion of respiratory, alimentary, or genitourinary tracts, or of the oropharyngeal cavities.
2. Clean contaminated wound	2. Minimal contamination, and contamination can be effectively removed. Includes operative wounds involving the respiratory, alimentary, and genitourinary tracts.
3. Contaminated wound	3. Open traumatic wound with heavy contamination and possibly foreign debris. Includes operative wounds with major breaks in aseptic technique, and incisions in areas of acute nonpurulent inflammation adjacent to inflamed or contaminated skin.
4. Dirty/infected wound	4. Old traumatic wounds and wounds with clinical infection or perforated viscera.

From Small Animal Wound Management, 2nd edition, Chapter II, page 14 by Steven F. Swaim and Ralph A. Henderson Jr. Baltimore: Lippincott Williams & Wilkins.

Table 8-19 Factors Affecting the Healing Process

Factor	Effect on Healing
Blood Supply	• Low blood supply means less ability to naturally cleanse and heal the wound and therefore an increase in the infection rate. Dehydration, trauma to the area, tight bandages, or location of the wound may have an effect on this factor.
Dead Space	• Separation of tissue can result in fluid accumulation, resulting in a loss of blood supply to the wound, thereby increasing the infection rate. • Sutures and drains reduce the dead space
Diseased, Geriatric, Overweight, or Malnourished Animals	• Condition of kidneys, liver, and total protein level contribute to efficient healing. Diseased, debilitated, or stressed organs hinder the healing process.
Foreign Material	• Foreign material (debris or suture material) results in prolonged inflammatory phase of healing and increases the risk of infection.
Healing Method: (Dependent on the age and condition of the wound)	
First Intention Wound Healing (Wound is sutured closed) • Used when wounds are 6–8 hours old, with minimal tissue damage and minimal contamination	• May necessitate debridement of wound edges
Second Intention Wound Healing (Wound is left to heal open) • Used when wounds are 5 or more days old, have significant tissue damage and loss, or are excessively contaminated	• Allows gradual debridement and optimal drainage • New skin may not contain hair follicles

Third Intention Wound Healing—
Delayed Primary Closure
(Wound is sutured closed after the granulation tissue has formed)
• Used when wounds are 3–5 days old and are heavily contaminated or infected

• Allows controlled debridement and optimal drainage

Hemostasis

• If bleeding is not stabilized effectively, a seroma or hematoma may form. Extra fluid in a wound slows down the healing process because the body must reabsorb/breakdown old blood/fluid during the inflammatory phase.
• Can predispose to sepsis of wound

Infection

• Overgrowth of bacteria prolongs the inflammatory phase.

Medications: (Corticosteriods; Anti-Inflammatory, Chemotherapeutic or Radiation)

• Medications may inhibit connective tissue building and epithelial cell turnover rate (especially chemotherapy)

Necrotic Tissue

• Dead tissue prolongs the inflammatory phase and predisposes the animal to sepsis

Table 8-20   Wound Care

If the owner calls before arriving at the clinic, advise them to cover the wound with a clean, dry cloth, gauze, or bandage.

Setup:
- Chlorhexidine solution
- Clippers
- Cold tray instruments (hemostats, needle holder, scissors, thumb forceps)
- Gloves
- Suture material
- Sterile water-soluble lubricant
- Wound cleaning fluids

Step I: Preparing the Wound for Treatment
1. Clean out any debris. This may involve gently picking out debris piece by piece.
2. Protect the wound with a water-soluble lubricant (K-Y Jelly™) or close with clamps.
3. Clip the hair from around the wound.

Scissors dipped in mineral oil can be used so that the hair will stick to the scissors.

4. Prepare the area, being careful not to get soap in the wound.
5. Remove the lubricant.

Step II: Cleaning
1. Lavage the wound with warm sterile normal saline or other wound cleaning solution (see Table 8-21): do not use soaps, because they can damage the tissue.
   To lavage:
   a. Assemble an intravenous administration set with a 3-way stopcock attached to the syringe and needle . . . OR . . .
   b. Use a plastic squeeze bottle or trigger-style bottle . . . OR . . .
   c. A 30–35-cc syringe w/18–19-gauge needle, using moderate pressure to thoroughly clean the wound, *except when using hydrogen peroxide because of potential tissue damage.* All debris should be removed and at times must be handpicked out.

Step III: Debridement (Performed by the veterinarian.)

Step IV: Closure (Performed by the veterinarian.)
Type of closure is dependent on: time lapse, degree of contamination, tissue damage, thoroughness of debridement, blood supply, animal's health, closure without skin tension or dead space, and location of wound.
1. Primary wound closure (suture or graft)
2. Delayed primary closure (1–3 days post trauma)
3. Contraction and epithelialization (dirty or contaminated wounds)
4. Secondary closure (3–5 days post trauma)

Table 8-21 Wound Management Medications

Medication	Uses				Type of Wound									Disadvantages/Concerns
	Lavage	Antimicrobial	Sporicidal	Other	Grossly Contaminated	1st-Degree & 2nd-Degree Burns	Lacerations	Dermal Ulcers	Abrasions	Thermal and Electrical Burns	Frostbite	Distal Dying Flaps	Repair Stage	
SOLUTION Tap Water	X				X		X							• May cause cellular damage
Hydrogen Peroxide	X		X		X									• Minimal bactericidal activity
Isotonic Saline and Lactated Ringer's	X				X	X	X	X	X					• No antimicrobial activity
Chlorhexidine	X	X			X	X	X	X	X	X				• Synovial inflammation with joint lavage • Precipitates in lactated Ringer's or saline solutions
Povidone Iodine	X	X			X									• Toxic to wound-healing cells • Systemic absorption resulting in metabolic acidosis, hypothyroidism, or hyperthyroidism • Inactivated by blood cells and other wound organic matter and tissue

Table 8-21 Wound Management Medications (Continued)

Medication	Lavage	Antimicrobial	Sporicidal	Other	Grossly Contaminated	1st-Degree & 2nd-Degree Burns	Lacerations	Dermal Ulcers	Abrasions	Thermal and Electrical Burns	Frostbite	Distal Dying Flaps	Repair Stage	Disadvantages/Concerns
TOPICAL OINTMENT														
Nitrofurazone		X			X									• Water soluble; so will leech out of contact bandaging • Blood and serum cause slight reduction of antibacterial activity (in vitro)
D-glucose polysaccharide-maetodexin				hydrophilic agent	X									• No direct antimicrobial activity
Trypsin—Balsam of Peru—Castor Oil				enzymatic debridement and healing stimulant	X									• Possible brief stinging, local inflammation, pyogenic reaction • No antimicrobial activity
Bacitracin Neomyxin														• Not for use in large wounds because of its possible toxicities

Agent	Notes	Comments
Gentamicin Sulfate		• Inhibition of neutrophil oxidative burst • Inactivated by purulent exudates (pus)
Silver Sulfaciazine		• In large wounds: possible bone marrow suppression, depression of lymphocyte proliferation, and inhibition of neutral oxidative
Aloe Vera Cream	antithromboxane	• Requires neuroleptanalgesia for application • Expensive for large area burns
Live Yeast Cell Derivative		• No antimicrobial and possibly mild stinging
WOUND DRESSING Topical Hydrogel	Healing stimulant	• No direct antimicrobial activity

(Modified from Small Animal Wound Management, Second Edition, Steven F. Swaim and Ralph A. Henderson, Jr.)

Table 8-22 Wound Bandaging

Bandaging increases the acidity of the wound environment, resulting in an increase in oxygen dissociation from hemoglobin, thereby increasing oxygen to the wound, which promotes healing.

Bandage Layer	Purpose	Material Type	Change
1. Primary (contact layer)	Protect the wound and in some cases for debridement	See below	Daily
• Adherent:	To promote debridement of wounds in the inflammatory or debridement stages:		Daily
	a. Dry/dry: absorbs exudate and allows debris to adhere to bandage	a. Gauze pads, cling gauze, disposable baby diapers	
	b. Wet/dry: loosens dried exudate/debris by rehydration of wound	b. Same as dry/dry, but soaked in saline just before application	
• Nonadherent	Minimal disruption of granulation tissue to wounds in the repair stage	Telfa pads; polyurethane foam sponges	Daily
-Occlusive	Used when no exudate is present; in the repair stage	Hydrocolloid dressing; hydrogel dressing	2–3 days
-Semiocclusive	Prevents tissue dehydration, but allows fluid absorption	Telfa pads; coated gauzes	1–2 days
2. Secondary layer	To protect the wound from further impacts/trauma and provide absorptive area for heavy secretions/exudates	Roll cotton—heavy padding Cast padding—moderate padding Stretch bandage—light padding	1–4 days
3. Tertiary layer	To provide consolidation of the secondary layer	Stretch gauze	1–4 days
4. Protective layer	To protect the bandaging from contamination	Elastic wrap (Coban™, VetWrap™) followed by adhesive tape.	1–4 days

AFTER CARE

Client Education:

1. Bandage should be kept dry. A plastic bag can be used when the pet is going outside, but should be removed within a 30-minute period to permit maximum breathing space around the bandage and reduce build-up of moisture.
2. Wet bandages should be changed immediately.
3. An Elizabethan collar should be worn until the stitches are removed.
4. Daily monitoring of toes for warmth, color, swelling and foul odor is essential.
5. Follow instructions of the veterinarian for bandage changes and removal.

Skill Box 8-6 / Basic Bandage

Usage: Bandaging of basic wounds

1. Place two adhesive tape strips on either side of the wound from where you expect the bandage to start to the distal portion of the limb.

   A tongue depressor assists in keeping the two adhesive strips from sticking to one another.

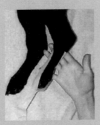

2. Apply primary bandage layer over the wound—wet or dry, depending on the veterinarian's decision.

3. Apply secondary bandage layer starting two-thirds up from the expected bottom of the bandage such that the layers overlap one another by 50% and are taut, but not constricting. Place extra padding over the depression areas and be careful not to permit wrinkles. Toes can be covered to inhibit edema or they can be left exposed to check on temperature of limb, permit drainage of fluids, and permit assessment of the healing environment. Care must be taken to ensure that the bandages are not too tight, because this could cut off circulation.

   Always end the bandage at the bottom of the area to alleviate pressure.

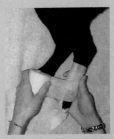 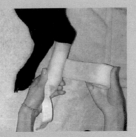

4. Place 1 layer of tertiary bandage layer on next, twist adhesive strips back over this layer, and finish with final layer of tertiary bandage.

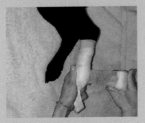

Skill Box 8-6 / Basic Bandage (Continued)

5. Place protective layer of elastic wrap.
6. Place adhesive tape around top of bandage, partially adhering to fur and around the bottom of bandage for reinforcement of the toe area.

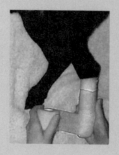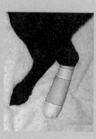

Skill Box 8-7   Robert Jones Bandage

Usage: Temporary immobilization of fractures before surgery by providing rigid stabilization (Remove after 1 day)

1. Place two adhesive tape strips on either side of the wound from where you expect the bandage to extend to the distal portion of the limb.
2. There is no primary layer unless sutures or wounds are present; then a nonadherent dressing can be placed.
3. While maintaining normal flexion of the limb, wrap thick roll cotton around the limb to constitute the secondary layer.

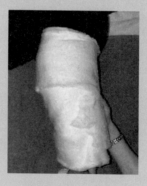

4. Compress with a conforming gauze (3–4-inch) secondary layer. Keep tension on the conforming gauze throughout application.

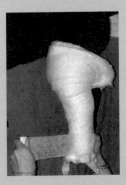

5. Twist adhesive strips back over the secondary layer.
6. Place protective layer of elastic wrap as the tertiary layer.
7. Place adhesive tape around the top of the bandage, partially adhering to fur and around the bottom of the bandage for reinforcement.

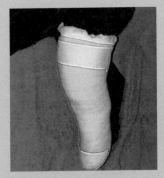

A well-applied Robert Jones bandage should make a dull thud sound when tapped by a finger. Not typically used on a femur or humerus fracture.

Skill Box 8-8 / Modified Robert Jones Bandage

Usage: To reduce postoperative swelling of the limbs

1. Place two adhesive tape strips on either side of the wound from where you expect the bandage to extend to the distal portion of the limb.
2. There is no primary layer unless sutures or wounds are present; then a nonadherent dressing can be placed.
3. While maintaining normal flexion of the limb, wrap "cast padding" around the limb to constitute the secondary layer, which is compressed with a conforming gauze tertiary layer.
4. Twist adhesive strips back over the tertiary layer.
5. Place protective layer of elastic wrap.
6. Place adhesive tape around top of bandage, partially adhering to fur and around the bottom of bandage for reinforcement.

Skill Box 8-9 / Chest/Abdominal Bandage

Usage: To control abdominal bleeding; effective for 1–2 hours and should be removed before 4 hours

1. Apply primary bandage layer over the wound if necessary.

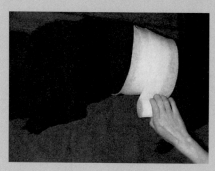

2. Apply secondary bandage layer, starting mid-thorax such that the layers overlap one another by 50% and are taut but not constricting. The bandage should extend to the pelvis. On male dogs, be sure to leave the animal's prepuce exposed. Care must be taken to ensure that the bandages are not too tight, because this could cut off circulation.

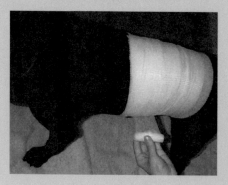

3. Place protective layer of elastic wrap.

4. Place adhesive tape around the cranial aspect of the bandage, partially adhering to fur, to prevent slippage.

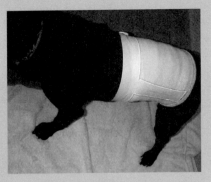

Skill Box 8-10 / Distal Limb Splint

Usage: Temporary immobilization or definitive stabilization for certain fractures

1. Place two adhesive tape strips on either side of the wound from where you expect the bandage to extend to the distal portion of the limb.

2. There is no primary layer unless sutures are present; then a nonadherent dressing can be placed.

3. While maintaining normal flexion of the limb wrap "cast padding" around the limb to constitute the secondary layer, which is compressed with a conforming gauze tertiary layer. Layers should cover and pad the area the splint will be resting on. Assure that *all edges are well padded* to avoid pressure sores.

4. Place the *appropriate sized splint* on the caudal aspect of the limb after the tertiary layer. There should be no gaps between cast padding and splint.

5. Adhesive strips are reflected onto the splint.

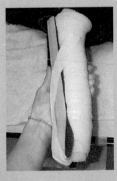
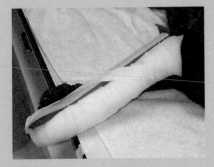

Skill Box 8-10 / Distal Limb Splint (Continued)

6. Place a layer of gauze over the splint.
7. Place protective layer of elastic wrap.
8. Place adhesive tape around top of bandage, partially adhering to fur and around the bottom of bandage for toe reinforcement.

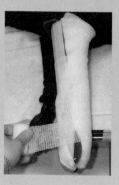 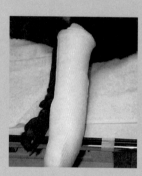

Skill Box 8-11 / Casts

Usage: for stabilization of simple fractures and immobilization of limbs (usually on for 4–5 weeks)

1. Have a bowl of warm–hot water ready for the cast material and examination gloves ready for the application process of the cast material.
2. Place two adhesive tape strips on either side of the wound from where you expect the bandage to start to the distal portion of the limb. Tape strips are reflected over the cast.
3. Apply a stockinette as a primary layer (Must be smooth, no wrinkles).
4. Apply secondary bandage layer, starting two thirds up from the expected bottom of the bandage such that the layers overlap one another by 50% and are taut, but not constricting. Pad the PROMINENCES on the leg, not the depressions. Toes can be covered to inhibit edema OR they can be left exposed to check on temperature of limb, permit drainage of fluids, and permit assessment of the healing environment. Care must be taken to ensure that the bandages are not too tight, because this could cut off circulation.
5. The cast material is used as the tertiary layer. Cast materials vary, and manufacturer's guidelines should be followed.
6. Twist adhesive strips and stockinette edges back over the top layer of the cast material.
7. Protective tape is applied over the ends of the cast. A walking stick can also be applied.

Skill Box 8-12 / Ehmer Sling

Usage: Immobilization of the hind limb after reduction of a craniodorsal coxofemoral luxation and prevention of weight bearing after pelvis surgery (typically changed every 5–7 days)

1. Place minimal padding on the metatarsal area (use secondary layer material).

2. Using 2-inch adhesive tape, wrap the tape around the medial aspect of the metatarsal and attach the tape end to the tape roll. Continue medially around the flank and back around the metatarsus. Keep the limb with stifle and hock in maximum flexion for 1–2 passes.

3. On next pass, go around the flank and twist behind the hock.

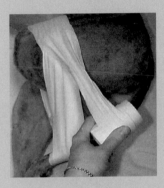

4. Pass over the front of the metatarsal area.

5. Repeat steps 3 and 4 for 3–4 passes.

6. Note: Correct application results in the internal rotation and adduction of the coxofemoral joint.

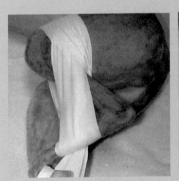
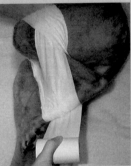
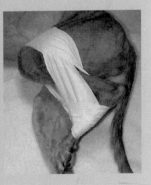

Skill Box 8-13 / 90–90 Flexion

Usage: After distal femoral fracture surgery in young patients and for prevention of weight bearing after hindlimb surgeries

1. Stifle and hock are in a 90-degree flexion. No attempt to adduct or internally rotate the coxofemoral joint is made.

2. Place minimal padding on the metatarsal area.

3. Same as Ehmer sling, step 2.

4. The tape is passed horizontally around the tibia to hold the layers in place.

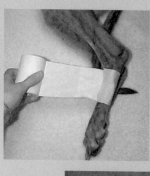 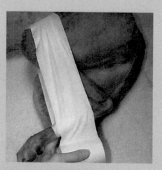

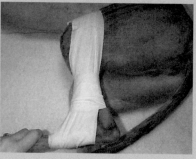

Skill Box 8-14 / Velpeau Sling

Usage: Holds flexed forelimb against the chest; non–weight-bearing sling for the forelimb; reduction of scapulohumeral joint luxation; immobilization of a scapular fracture

1. Cover the chest wall and shoulder with a lightly padded secondary layer and gauze tertiary layer.

2. Bandage the forelimb in same manner, keeping the foot exposed and pad the depressions of the limb.

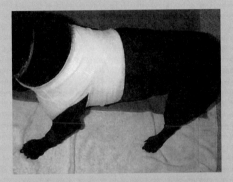

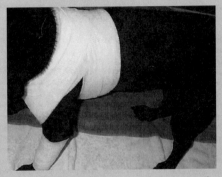

3. Gently flex the forelimb against the chest wall and attach adhesive tape (2–4-inch width) around the chest and flexed forelimb, creating a sling.

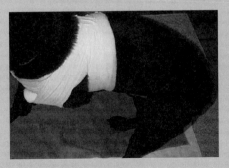

Skill Box 8-15 / Hobbles

Usage: **To prevent excessive abduction of the hindlimbs; specifically indicated after reduction of ventral coxofemoral luxation; to relieve excessive tension in the inguinal region; to prevent excessive activity after pelvic fracture repair, or nonsurgical, conservative management of pelvic fractures**

1. Stand the animal with the hindlimbs equal distance to the width of the pelvis.

2. Pass the adhesive tape (which needs to be wide enough to cover half of the metatarsal area) around the two limbs. Press the tape together in the area between the two limbs.

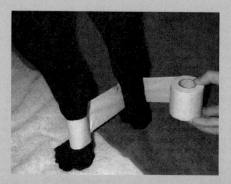

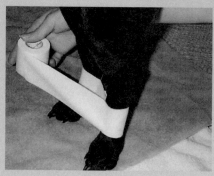
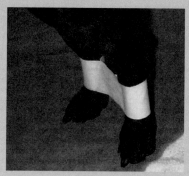

Pharmacology

Although all drugs are prescribed by the veterinarian, the technician is often the person administering the drugs. An awareness of the purpose of the drug used and its interaction with other drugs is essential for monitoring the patient and answering clients' questions regarding these drugs. All dosages should be double-checked before administration as should all other medications the patient is currently using and their interactions. New products are constantly being brought to market, and every technician should be reviewing information for new products that are purchased for use in their clinic. Every clinic must have a current veterinary drug book on site. This chapter is meant only to give pertinent technician information. A veterinary drug book should always be consulted if there are any questions regarding a medication's side effects or interactions.

Chart 9-1   Cross Reference for Drugs

Key:

CAN	Cancer
CAR	Cardiovascular
D	Dermatologic
GI	Gastrointestinal
M	Metabolic
MS	Musculoskeletal
N	Neurologic
OP	Ophthalmic
OT	Otic
R	Respiratory
REP	Reproductive
RU	Renal/Urinary
T	Toxicologic

Drug	Category
Acepromazine	GI: antiemetic, N: phenothiazine
Acetazolamide	OP: carbonic anhydrase inhibitor
Acetylcysteine	R: mucolytics
Acetylsalicylic acid	MS: NSAID
Actinomycin-D	CAN: antibiotic
Activated charcoal	GI: protectant
Albendazole	Antinematodal
Albuterol	R: bronchodilator
Allopurinol	RU: enzyme inhibitor
Aluminum hydroxide	GI: anti-ulcer
Aluminum carbonate	GI: anti-ulcer
Amikacin	Anti-infective
Aminopentamide	GI: antidiarrheal, antiemetic
Aminophylline	GI: bronchodilator

Drug	Category
Amitriptyline	RU: Tricyclic antidepressant
Amlodipine besylate	CAR: anti-arrhythmic
Ammonium chloride	RU: acidifier
Amrinone	CAR: contractility enhancer
Antacids	GI: anti-ulcer
Anticoagulant	CAR: antiarrhythmic
Apomorphine	GI: emetic
Atenolol	CAR: hypotensive
Atropine	GI: antidiarrheal, antiemetic, OP: mydriatic/cycloplegic
Azathioprine	CAN: antimetabolite
Benzoyl peroxide	D: antiseborrheics
Bethanechol chloride	RU: cholinergic
Bismuth subsalicylate	GI: antidiarrheal

Drug	Category
Butorphanol tartrate	R: antitussives
Calcitroil	MS: parathyroid
Calcium carbonate	GI: anti-ulcer
Calcium chloride	CAR: calcium supplement
Calcium gluconate	CAR: calcium supplement
Captopril	CAR: vasodilator
Carbachol	OP: miotic
Carboplatin	CAN: alkylating agent
Carprofen	MS: NSAID
Catecholamines	CAR: contractility enhancers
Cephalosporins	Anti-infective
Chlorambucil	CAN: alkylating agent
Chloramphenical	Anti-infective OT: anti-infective

Drug	Classification
Chlorinated hydrocarbons	Ectoparasitic
Chlorpheniramine maleate	D: antipruritic
Chlorpromazine	GI: antiemetic
Cholinergic	R: antihistamine
Cimetidine	GI: anti-ulcer
Ciprofloxacin	Anti-infective
Cisapride	GI: antiemetic
Cisplatin	CAN: alkylating agent
Clindamycin	Anti-infective
Clotrimazole	Antifungal
Coal tar	D: antiseborrheics
Codeine phosphate	R: antitussives
Corticosteroids	MS: anti-inflammatory
Cyclophosphamide	CAN: alkylating agent
Cyclosporine	OP: immunosuppressant
Cyproheptadine	N: appetite stimulant; R: bronchospasm manager
Danazol	CAN: synthetic hormone
Desmopressin acetate	M: pancreatic
Desoxycorticosterone acetate (DOCA; DOCP)	M: adrenal cortex
Dextromethorphan	R: antitussives
Diazepam	N: anesthetic, anticonvulsant; appetite stimulant; toxicologic
Dichlorphenamide	OP: carbonic anhydrase inhibitor
Diethylstilbestrol	REP: estrogen
Digoxin	CAR: contractility enhancer
Dihydrostreptomycin	Anti-infective: Antibiotic-aminoglycoside
Diltiazem	CAR: antiarrhythmic
Dimercaprol	T: chelating
Dimethylsulfoxide	OT: anti-infective
Diphenhydramine	R: antihistamines
Diphenoxylate	GI: antidiarrheal
Dobutamine hydrochloride	CAR: contractility enhancer
Docusate sodium succinate	GI: stool softener
Dopamine	CAR: contractility enhancer
Doxapram	R: stimulant
Doxorubicin	CAN: antibiotic
d-Penicillamine	T: chelating
Ectoparasitics	Anti-parasitic
Edrophonium chloride	N: cholinergic
Enalapril	CAR: vasodilator
Enrofloxacin	Anti-infective
Ephedrine	N: adrenergic
Epinephrine	CAR: contractility enhancer; R: bronchodilator; OP: adrenergic agonist
Epsiprantel	Anticestodal
Erythromycin	Anti-infective
Erythropoietin	CAR: anti-anemia
Etodalac	MS: NSAID
Famotidine	GI: anti-ulcer
Febendazole	Antinematodal
Ferrous sulfate	CAR: anti-anemia
Fipronil	Ectoparasitic
Fludrocortisone	M: adrenal cortex
Flumethasone	MS: anti-infective
Flunixin meglumine	MS: NSAID
Fluorescein	OP: stain
Fluoroquinolones	Anti-infectives

Chart 9-1 Cross Reference for Drugs (Continued)

Key:		
CAN	Cancer	
CAR	Cardiovascular	
D	Dermatologic	

GI	Gastrointestinal	
M	Metabolic	
MS	Musculoskeletal	
N	Neurologic	

OP	Ophthalmic	
OT	Otic	
R	Respiratory	

REP	Reproductive	
RU	Renal/Urinary	
T	Toxicologic	

Drug	Category	Drug	Category	Drug	Category
Fluoroquinolones	Anti-infectives	Imidacloprid	Ectoparasitic	Lufenuron	Ectoparasitic
Fluorouracil	CAN: anti-metabolite	Imidazole	Anti-fungal	Magnesium hydroxide	GI: anti-ulcer and laxative
Fomepizole	T: synthetic alcohol dehydrogenase inhibitor	Insulin	M: pancreatic	Mannitol	CAR: diuretics
		Interferon	CAN: immunomodulating	Marbofloxacin	Anti-infective
Furosemide	CAR: diuretics	Isoproterenol	CAR: contractility enhancer	Mebendazole	Antinematodal
Gentamicin sulfate	OT: anti-infective	Ivermectin	Antinematodal	Meclizine	R: antihistamines
Glucosamine + Chondroitin	MS: supplement	Kaolin-pectin	GI: protectant	Medroxyprogesterone	REP: progestin
Gonadorelin	REP: gonadotropin	Ketoconazole	Antifungal	Megestrol acetate	REP: progestin
Griseofulvin	Antifungal	L-asparaginase	CAN: enzyme	Melarsomine	Antinematodal
Heparin	CAR: anticoagulant	Lactulose	GI: laxative	Methimazole	M: thyroid
Hydralazine	CAR: vasodilators	Levothyroxine sodium	M: thyroid	dl-Methionine	RU: acidifier
Hydrocodone	R: antitissuves	Lidocaine	N: anesthetic–numbing agent CAR: antiarrhythmic	Methocarbamol	N: muscle relaxant
Hyrdocortisone	MS: anti-inflammatory			Methotrexate	CAN: anti-metabolite
				Methoxamine	N: adrenergic
Hydrogen peroxide	GI: emetic	Lincomycin	Anti-infective	Methylprednisolone	MS: anti-inflammatory
Hydroxyzine	D: antihistamine	Loperamide	GI: antidiarrheal		

Drug	Category
4-Methylpyrazole	T: synthetic alcohol dehydrogenase inhibitor
Methyltestosterone	REP: androgen
Methylxanthines	R: bronchodilators
Metoclopramide	GI: antiemetic
Metoprolol	CAR: anti-arrhythmic
Metronidazole	Anti-infective/anti-protozoal
Mibolerone	REP: androgen
Milbemycin oxime	Antinematodal
Misopristol	GI: anti-ulcer
Mitotane	M: adrenal cortex
Mitoxantrone	CAN: antibiotic
Moxidectin	Antinematodal
Naloxone	R: stimulant
Nandrolone deconate	RU: anabolic steroid
Neomycin	Anti-infective
Neostigmine methylsulfate	N: cholinergic
Nitroglycerin ointment	CAR: vasodilators
Norfloxacin	Anti-infective
Nystatin	Antifungal
Omeprazole	GI: anti-ulcer
Orbifloxacin	Anti-infective
Organophosphate	Ectoparasitic
Oxytocin	REP: hormone
Pancreatic enzyme replacement	GI: enzyme
Paramethasone	MS: anti-inflammatory
Penicillin	Anti-infective
Pentobarbital	N: anticonvulsant, anesthestic, euthanasia solution
Phenobarbital	N: anticonvulsant
Phenoxybenzamine	RU: alpha-adrenergic
Phenylbutazone	MS: NSAID
Phenylpropanolomine	RU: beta-adrenergic
Physostigmine	N: cholinergic
Piperazine	Antinematodal
Piroxicam	MS: NSAID
Polysulfated glycosaminoglycans	MS: protectant
Potassium bromide	N: anticonvulsant
Praziquantel	Anticestodal
Prazosin	CAR: vasodilator
Prednisolone	MS: anti-inflammatory
Procainamide	CAR: antiarrhythmic
Prochlorperazine	GI: antiemetic
Promethazine	GI: antiemetic
Propantheline	GI: antidiarrheal
Propranolol	CAR: hypotensive
Proparacaine	OP: anesthetic
Prostaglandins	REP: muscle stimulant
Psyllium	GI: laxative
Pyrantel	Antinematodal
Pyrethrins	Ectoparasitic
Quinidine	CAR: anti-arrhythmic
Ranitidine	GI: anti-ulcer
Salicylic acid	D: antiseborrheic
Selamectin	Ectoparasitic
Selegiline (l-deprenyl)	M: adrenal cortex
Sodium influx inhibitors	CAR: anti-arrhythmic
Stanozolol	RU: anabolic steroid
Sucralfate	GI: anti-ulcer

Chart 9-1 Cross Reference for Drugs (Continued)

Key:

CAN	Cancer
CAR	Cardiovascular
D	Dermatologic
GI	Gastrointestinal
M	Metabolic
MS	Musculoskeletal
N	Neurologic
OP	Ophthalmic
OT	Otic
R	Respiratory
REP	Reproductive
RU	Renal/Urinary
T	Toxicologic

Drug	Category
Sulfonamides	Anti-infective
Sulfur	D: antiseborrheic
Syrup of ipecac	GI: emetic
Terbutaline	R: bronchodilator
Testosterone: (cypionate, enanthate, propionate)	REP: androgen

Drug	Category
Tetracyclines	Anti-infective
Theophylline	R: bronchodilator
Thiabendazole	OT: anti-infective
Tobramycin	Anti-infective
Triamcinolone	MS: anti-inflammatory
Trimethobenzamide	R: antihistamine
Tylosin	GI: antidiarrheal

Drug	Category
Vasopressin	M: pancreatic
Vincristine	CAN: vinca alkaloid
Verapamil hydrochloride	CAR: anti-arrhythmic
Warfarin	CAR: anticoagulant
Xylazine	GI: emetic / N: anesthetic
Yohimbine	N: stimulant

Skill Box 9-1 / Basic Calculations

Type of Calculation	Equation	Example
Dosage Calculation using pure drug form	Dose = (animal's weight × dosage rate for the drug)/ concentration of the drug	A 5 kg cat requires 2.7 mg/kg dosage of Cestex (12.5 mg/tablet): D = (5 kg × 2.7 mg/kg)/(12.5 mg/tablet) D = (13.5 mg)/(12.5 mg/tablet) D = 1.08 mg tablet Give the cat 1 tablet Cestex (12.5 mg)
Solutions (denoted by their strength as percentages or ratio) • 5% denotes 5 parts of solute in 100 parts solution • 1:5 ratio denotes 1 part of solute in 5 parts of solution	Amount of pure drug needed = (amount of solution needed) × (strength required)	*Liquids:* Make 125 mL of 4% bleach solution: D = 125 mL × (4 mL/100 mL) D = 500 mL/100 mL D = 5 mL of bleach Add 5 mL of bleach to 120 mL of water* *Solids:* Make 200 mL of 5% dextrose solution using the powdered form of dextrose and lactated ringers: D = 200 mL × (5 grams/100 mL) D = 10 grams Add 10 grams powdered dextrose to 200 mL lactated ringers*
Dilution of Stock Solution (changing a concentration of solution)	$\dfrac{\text{Desired concentration (C1)}}{\text{Available concentration (C2)}} = \dfrac{\text{Volume to use (V1)}}{\text{Volume to make (V2)}}$ Or noted as: $(C1 \times V2) = (C2 \times V1)$	Prepare 600 mL of 5% dextrose solution using 50% stock solution and sterile water. You need to find the volume of the stock to use: (5% = 5 mL/100 mL) V1 = (C1 × V2)/C2 V1 = (5 mL × 600 mL)/50 mL V1 = 3000 mL/50 mL V1 = 60 mL Add 60 mL of the 50% stock solution to 540 mL sterile water*

When dealing with liquids, always extract an equal volume from the container that you are going to put the solution in (i.e., Remove 100 mL saline before adding 100 mL of dextrose solution.)

ANTI-FUNGAL DRUGS

Table 9-1   Anti-Fungal Drugs

Drug Class	Anti-Fungals			
DRUG (TRADE NAME)	• Clotrimazole (Lotrimin, Mycelex) • Imidazole (Enilconazole)	• Griseofulvin (Fulvicin, Gris-actin, and Grifulvin)	• Ketoconazole (Nizoral)	• Nystatin (Panalog and Mycostatin)
ACTION	• Inhibits membrane synthesis	• Inhibits mitosis of fungi	• Inhibits ergosterol synthesis in the fungal cell membrane	• Fungistatic and fungicidal
INDICATIONS	• Candida stomatis, localized dermatophytosis, and canine nasal aspergillosis	• Mycotic infections (trichophytosis and dermatophytosis)	• Systemic mycotic infections (*Malassezia canis*, candidiasis and dermatophytosis) and superficial skin infections	• Candidiasis and *Malassezia canis*
DISPENSIBLE FORMS	• Topical	• Tablet	• Tablet and topical	• Topical
PRECAUTIONS		• Cats and pregnant animals have ↑ toxicity due to metabolizing difficulties	• May ↓ testosterone and fertility in stud dogs	
CONTRAINDICATIONS			• Animals taking antisecretory drugs, antacids, anticonvulsants, cyclosporine, and cisapride • Pregnant animals	
PATIENT CARE/ CLIENT EDUCATION	• Monitor for local irritation, salivation, sneezing, and weight loss	• Monitor for toxicity (anorexia, vomiting, diarrhea and lethargy) • Provide a high-fat diet to facilitate absorption	• Monitor for vomiting, diarrhea, decreased appetite, and liver dysfunction (jaundice) • Administer with food	
NOTES		• Phenobarbital ↓ absorption • Reaches high concentrations in skin, hair, and nails • Drug effects are seen ≥6 weeks after initiation • Vaccinations are not recommended during treatment		• Usually combined with other drugs

ANTI-INFECTIVE DRUGS

Antibiotics should typically be given with food, unless specifically stated in drug insert. The signs of an allergic reaction are shock, skin rash, facial or site swelling, swollen lymph nodes, or fever.

Table 9-2   Anti-Infective Drugs

Drug Class	Aminoglycosides	Cephalosporins	Chloramphenicol
DRUG (TRADE NAME)	• Amikacin (Amiglyde-V, Amikin) • Gentamicin (Gentocin, Garasol, Garacin) • Neomycin (Biosol, Mycifradin) • Dihydrostreptomycin (Ethamycin) • Tobramycin (Nebcin)	• *1st Generation:* cefadroxil, cephalexin, cephradine, cephalothin, cefazolin, cephapirin (Kefsol, Ancef, Zolicef, Cefa-drops, Cefa-tabs, Cefazolin) • *2nd Generation:* cefamandole, cefaclor, cefoxitin (Mandol, Ceclor, Mefoxin) • *3rd Generation:* cefixime, cefotaxime, ceftoperaxone, ceftazidime, moxalactam (Suprax, Claforan, Fortaz) • *4th Generation:* cefepime	• Chloramphenicol (Amphicol, Chloramphenicol Ophthalmic Ointment, Vedichol Tablets; Amphicol Capsules; Bemocal)
ACTION	• Bactericidal	• Bactericidal	• Bacteriostatic

INDICATIONS	• Broad spectrum (mainly G-); but not against anaerobic bacteria
	• Genitourinary tract infections
	• Leptospirosis (Ethamycin)
		• *1st Generation:* G+
		  • *2nd/3rd Generation:* G-/G+
		  • *4th Generation:* G-/G+
		• Cystitis, respiratory, skeletal and genitourinary, skin and soft tissue infections
			• G- & G+ bacteria, *Rickettsia spp.*
			• Respiratory illnesses
			• Need central nervous system (CNS) penetration

DISPENSIBLE FORMS	• Injectable	• Tablet, injectable, and oral suspensions	• Tablet, capsule, ointment
PRECAUTIONS	• Do not mix with penicillin in the same syringe as it renders them ineffective	• Animals (especially cats) may vomit on an empty stomach	• May cause bone marrow suppression (idiosyncratic) • Cats tend to show more sensitivity to the adverse effects of this drug

Table 9-2 Anti-Infective Drugs (Continued)

Drug Class	Aminoglycosides	Cephalosporins	Chloramphenicol
CONTRA-INDICATIONS	• Ruptured eardrums (topically) • Kidney disease (parenterally) • Pregnant or young animals • Animals taking furosemide	• Animals taking bacteriostatic drugs • Allergies to penicillin	• Animals taking bactericidal drugs • Pregnant animals • Impaired liver function (drug is a potent liver enzyme inducer) or myocardial dysfunction
PATIENT CARE/ CLIENT EDUCATION	• Monitor for respiratory paralysis, cardiovascular depression, vestibular toxicity, deafness, and nephrotoxicity • Use with Fluid Therapy to support kidneys	• Monitor for allergic reactions	• Monitor for allergic reactions
NOTES	• Administer parenterally or topically because of poor absorption in the GIT • Accumulates in the inner ear and kidneys • Metabolized through the kidneys • Neostigmine is the reversal agent	• Execreted by kidneys	• Do not use for >3 weeks • Metabolized in the liver and excreted through the kidneys

Table 9-3   Anti-infective: Fluoroquinolones—Metronidazole

Drug Class	Fluoroquinolones	Lincosamides	Metronidazole
DRUG (TRADE NAME)	• Ciprofloxacin (Cipro) • Enrofloxacin (Baytril) • Marbofloxacin (Zeniquin) • Norfloxacin (Noroxin) • Orbifloxacin (Orbax)	• Clindamycin (Antirobe) • Lincomycin (Lincocin) • Erythromycin (Erythro-100)	• Metronidazole (Flagyl)
ACTION	• Bactericidal	• Bacteriostatic	• Bacteriostatic • Non-specific anti-inflammatory for in-testines
INDICATIONS	• G-/G+ bacteria • Genitourinary tract, respiratory, and ex-ternal auditory infections • Need for soft tissue penetration	• G+ and anaerobic bacteria • Chronic skin, bone, oral and bladder in-fections • *Neospora caninum* and *Babesia canis*	• G- anaerobic bacteria and *Giardia* • Diarrhea
DISPENSIBLE FORMS	• Tablet and injectable	• Tablet, capsule, solution	• Tablet, powder, and injectable
PRECAUTIONS	• Concurrent use with NSAIDS may cause seizures		• Toxicity can occur even at recom-mended doses
CONTRA-INDICATIONS	• Growing animals, because it causes ar-ticular/physeal damage • Pregnant animals	• Animals taking kaolin (lincomycin) • Candidiasis infection • Liver insufficiency or cholestasis	• Pregnant animals
PATIENT CARE/ CLIENT EDUCATION	• Administer 1–2 hours before feeding • Monitor for vomiting, diarrhea, polydip-sia, dehydration, and CNS dysfunction • Keep animals well hydrated	• Monitor for vomiting and diarrhea	• Monitor for anorexia, hepatotoxicity, neutropenia, vomiting, diarrhea, and CNS signs
NOTES	• ↓ Dosages with kidney disease • Metabolized by the liver and excreted by kidneys	• Metabolized by the liver and excreted in bile or urine	• Clinical signs of toxicity can manifest 7–12 days after initiating therapy • Do not crush the pills, because they have a bitter taste

Table 9-4 Anti-infective: Penicillin—Tetracyclines

Drug Class	Penicillin	Sulfonamides	Tetracyclines
DRUG (TRADE NAME)	• Amoxicillin (Amoxi-tabs, Biomox, and Robamox-V) • Ampicillin (Polyflex, Amcill, Omnipen) • Potentiated Amoxicillin (Clavamox with clavulinic acid)	-Short Acting: • Sulfadiazine (Tribissen, Di-Trim) • Sulfamerazine • Sulfamethazine • Sulfamethoxazole -Intermediate Acting: • Sulfisoxazole • Sulfadimethoxine (Albon)	• Chlortetracycline (Auroemycin) • Doxycycline (Vibramycin) • Minocycline (Minocin) • Oxytetracline (Terramycin, Liquamycin) • Tetracycline (Panmycin Aquadrops, Tetracycline Soluble Powder-324, Oxy-Tet 100 Injectable)
ACTION	• Bactericidal	• Bacteriostatic	• Bacteriostatic
INDICATIONS	• G+ bacteria • Respiratory, skin, and soft tissue infections	• G-/G+ bacteria and protozoa • Respiratory, urinary tract, meningeal, enteric and soft tissue (sulfadimethoxine) and coccidial (sulfadimethoxine) infections	• G-/G+ bacteria, *Rickettsia spp.* and *Bordetella spp.*
DISPENSIBLE FORMS	• Tablet and injectable	• Tablet and solution	• Tablet, powder, solution, and injectable
PRECAUTIONS	• Do not mix with aminoglycosides • Resistance to amoxicillin with *Bordetella spp.* and some *E. coli* strains	• Ineffective in the presence of pus • Bone marrow suppression with extended use • Use with caution with kidney and thyroid disease • Not recommended for use in cats for more than 14 days	• Dairy products, antidiarrheal agents and antacids will interfere with absorption
CONTRA-INDICATIONS	• Animals taking bacteriostatic drugs	• Liver disease, blood diseases or sulfonamide sensitivity	• Kidney disease (oxytetracycline and minocycline) • Animals taking bactericidal drugs
PATIENT CARE/CLIENT EDUCATION	• Administer 1–2 hours before feeding • Monitor for allergic reactions (shock, skin rash, facial swelling, swollen lymph nodes, and fever)	• Maintain adequate hydration • Monitor for pruritis, photosensitivity, alopecia, allergic reactions, and keratoconjunctivitis sicca (KCS) (dogs) • Monitor for anemia (Tribissen)	• Monitor for vomiting, diarrhea, hypotension, and anorexia
NOTES	• Metabolized by the kidneys in a mostly unchanged form	• Metabolized in the liver and excreted in the urine	• Causes yellow discoloration of teeth and bones in young animals during enamel development • Metabolized by the kidneys

ANTI-PARASITIC DRUGS

Table 9-5   Anti-Parasitic Drugs

Drug Class	Antinematodals			
DRUG (TRADE NAME)	*Benzimidazoles* • Albendazole (Valbazen) • Febendazole (Panacur) • Mebendazole (Telmin)	• Ivermectin (Ivomec and Heartgard)	• Milbemycin oxime (Interceptor, Sentinel)	• Melarsomine (Immiticide)
ACTION	• Interferes with parasite's energy metabolism	• Interferes with parasite's CNS	• Interferes with parasite's CNS	• Interferes with parasite's metabolism
INDICATIONS	• Ascarids, Hookworms, Whipworms and *T. pisiformis* tapeworms	• Heartworm microfilariacide (dogs) • Most parasites except Demodex, cestodes, and liver flukes • Ear mites	• Hookworms, whipworms, and ascarids • Heartworm preventative	• Heartworm adulticide
DISPENSIBLE FORMS	• Tablet, paste, and powder	• Tablet and injectable	• Tablet	• Injectable
PRECAUTIONS	• ± Liver toxicity (mebendazole)	• Collies and most herding breeds are very sensitive and may develop toxic signs	• Shock-like symptoms in dogs with a high level of microfilaria (rare)	• ± Vessel blockage by dead worms • Wear gloves and wash hands after administering
CONTRA-INDICATIONS		• Puppies <6 weeks		
PATIENT CARE/ CLIENT EDUCATION	• Monitor for vomiting and diarrhea	• Monitor for mydriasis, ataxia, vomiting, diarrhea, hypersalivation, tremors, and depression		• Monitor for swelling or tenderness at the injection site, coughing, emesis, depression, lethargy, fever, and anorexia
NOTES		• Passes through the blood-brain barrier • Pretesting for heartworm infection should be done before administering	• Retroactive action on larval forms recently acquired	• Dimercaprol may be used as an antidote

Table 9-6   Anti-Parasitic Drugs: Antinematodals

Drug Class	Antinematodals		
DRUG (TRADE NAME)	• Moxidectin (Pro Heart 6)	• Piperazines (Pipa-Tabs, Sergeant's Worm Away, Purina liquid wormer)	*Tetrahydropyrimidines* • Pyrantel (Strongid-T and Nemex)
ACTION	• Interferes with parasite's CNS	• Paralyzes the worms	• Interferes with parasite's CNS
INDICATIONS	• Heartworm preventative	• Ascarids	• Ascarids, hookworms
DISPENSIBLE FORMS	• Injectable	• Tablet and solution	• Tablet and solution
PRECAUTIONS	• Heartworm testing is recommended before initiation of treatment		• Use with caution in animals with liver dysfunction, dehydration, malnutrition, or anemia
CONTRA-INDICATIONS		• Chronic liver disease or kidney disease	• Organophosphates and piperazines
PATIENT CARE/ CLIENT EDUCATION	• Monitor for depression, ataxia, and swelling at the site of injection	• Monitor for tremors, ataxia, seizures, emesis, and weakness	• Monitor for ↑ respiration, sweating, and incoordination
NOTES		• Live worms are passed, and appropriate environmental control should be followed	

Table 9-7 Anti-Parasitic Drugs: Anticestodals

Drug Class	Anticestodals	
DRUG (TRADE NAME)	• Epsiprantel (Cestex)	• Praziquantel (Droncit)
ACTION	• Reduces worm's resistance to host's digestive system	• Reduces worm's resistance to host's digestive system
INDICATIONS	• Tapeworms except *Echinococcus spp.*	• Tapeworms and *Paragonimus* infections in dogs
DISPENSIBLE FORMS	• Tablet	• Tablet and injectable
PRECAUTIONS		
CONTRAINDICATIONS	• Animals <7 weeks	• Puppies < 4 weeks old and kittens < 6 weeks old
PATIENT CARE/ CLIENT EDUCATION	• Monitor for vomiting, diarrhea, anorexia and lethargy	• Monitor for vomiting, diarrhea, anorexia, and lethargy
NOTES	• Effective with a single dose	• Effective with a single dose • Eggs are passed in feces; so appropriate environmental cleanup should be implemented

Table 9-8 Anti-Parasitic Drugs: Ectoparasitics

Drug Class	Ectoparasitics			
DRUG (TRADE NAME)	• Fipronil (Frontline, Frontline–Top Spot)	• Imidacloprid (Advantage)	• Lufenuron (Program)	• Organophosphates (Proban) • Chlorinated hydrocarbons (Duratrol, Paramite Dip) • Carbamates (Sevin)
ACTION	• Disrupt parasite's neuro-transmission	• Adulticide	• Protein inhibitor in flea egg that prevents the eggs from hatching or the larvae from developing	• Disrupts parasite's neuro-transmission
INDICATIONS	• Fleas and ticks	• Fleas	• Fleas	• Fleas, lice, and ticks
DISPENSIBLE FORMS	• Liquid	• Liquid	• Tablet and injectable (cats)	• Liquids and powders
PRECAUTIONS	• Avoid contact with eyes and mouth • Wear gloves when administering or wash hands thoroughly	• Avoid contact with eyes and mouth • Wear gloves when administering or wash hands thoroughly		• Do not combine the use of multiple organophosphates • Cats show ↑ sensitivity • Wear gloves when administering
CONTRA-INDICATIONS	• Animals < 10 weeks old	• Animals < 7 weeks old	• Puppies < 6 weeks old	• Animals < 12 weeks old • Pregnant or nursing animals
PATIENT CARE/CLIENT EDUCATION	• Monitor for skin irritation at application site			• Monitor for bradycardia, respiratory depression, salivation, muscle tremors, convulsions, paralysis, constricted pupils, vomiting, and diarrhea
NOTES	• Effective for 4 weeks for ticks and 3 months for fleas	• Effective for 4 weeks	• Takes 30–60 days to reach full effectiveness because of life cycle disruption	• Atropine can ↓ toxic effects

Table 9-9   Anti-Parasitic Drugs: Ectoparasitics continued

Drug Class	Ectoparasitics	
DRUG (TRADE NAME)	• Pyrethrins and synthetic pyrethroids (Ovitrol, Sectrol, Kiltix)	• Selamectin (Revolution)
ACTION	• Stimulates parasite's CNS	• Adulticide and inhibits eggs from hatching
INDICATIONS	• Fleas, ticks, ear mites, and flies	• Fleas, ear mites, heartworm prevention, sarcoptic mange (dog) and nematode treatment (cat)
DISPENSIBLE FORMS	• Liquid	• Liquid
PRECAUTIONS		
CONTRAINDICATIONS	• Animals <6 weeks	• Animals < 6 weeks old
PATIENT CARE/ CLIENT EDUCATION	• Hypersalivation is common	• Monitor for alopecia at the site of administration, vomiting, diarrhea, anorexia, lethargy, salivation, tachypnea, and muscle tremors
NOTES	• Some are degraded by ultraviolet light, and some lose effectiveness when in contact with synthetic fibers	

CANCER/CHEMOTHERAPY DRUGS

Table 9-10   Cancer/Chemotherapy Drugs

Drug Class		Alkylating Agents	
DRUG (TRADE NAME)	• Carboplatin (Platinol)	• Cisplatin (Cisplatin, Para-platin)	• Cyclophosphamide (Cyto-toxan, Neosar)	• Chlorambucil (Leukeran)
ACTION	• Interrupts DNA replica-tion	• Interrupts DNA replication	• Interrupts DNA replication and inhibits DNA synthesis and base pairing	• Inhibits DNA and RNA synthesis and base pair-ing
INDICATIONS	• Adenocarcinomas, squa-mous cell carcinoma and osteosarcomas	• Canine osteosarcoma, nasal adenocarcinoma, squamous cell carcinoma, transitional cell carcinoma, thyroid car-cinoma, mesothelioma, and testicular and ovarian neo-plasia	• Lymphosarcoma, heman-giosarcoma, mammary gland carcinoma, mastocy-toma, and mammary ade-nocarcinoma	• Lymphocytic leukemia, lymphoma, poly-cythemia vera, multiple myeloma, ovarian ade-nocarcinoma, and macroglobulinemia
DISPENSIBLE FORMS	• Injectable	• Injectable	• Tablet and injectable	• Tablet
PRECAUTIONS	• Requires saline diuresis 4 hours before and 2 hours after treatment • Use with caution in pa-tients with active infec-tions, hearing impair-ment, or preexisting renal/hepatic disease	• **Wear gloves and protective clothing** when preparing solution (skin contact may cause local reaction)	• **Wear gloves** when splitting or crushing tablets • Use with caution with pa-tients with hepatic/renal dysfunction, leukopenia, thrombocytopenia, im-munosuppression, or previ-ous radiotherapy	• Use with caution in pa-tients with bone marrow depression

CONTRA-INDICATIONS	• Severe bone marrow suppression or sensitivity to platinum containing compounds	• Use in cats, renal impairment, myelosuppression, and sensitivity to platinum-containing compounds		
PATIENT CARE/ CLIENT EDUCATION	• Monitor for GI upset, bone marrow suppression, ototoxicity, alopecia, neuropathy, nephrotoxicity, and emesis (rarely) • Use with caution in patients with active infections, hearing impairment and preexisting renal/hepatic disease	• Monitor for vomiting, anemia, bone marrow suppression with bimodal nadir, nephrotoxicity, and rarely neuropathy (ototoxicity)	• CBC should be assessed weekly for first 2 months and then monthly • Monitor for vomiting, gastrointestinal toxicity, bone marrow depression, hemorrhagic cystitis, and alopecia	• Monitor CBC on a regular basis • Monitor for leukopenia, thrombocytopenia and anemia, cerebellar toxicity, bone marrow suppression, alopecia, and gastrointestinal toxicity
NOTES	• Less nephrotoxic than carboplatin (does not require diuresis) • Do not refrigerate	• Response may take 1–4 weeks • Only use 4–5 months	• Alopecia is more profound in Poodles and Kerry Blues	

Table 9-11 Cancer/Chemotherapy Drugs: Anthracycline Antibiotics

Drug Class	Anthracycline Antibiotic		
DRUG (TRADE NAME)	• Actinomycin D; dactinomycin (Cosmegen)	• Doxorubicin hydrochloride (Adriamycin)	• Mitoxantrone (Novantrone)
ACTION	• Inhibits DNA, RNA, and protein synthesis	• Disrupts DNA and RNA synthesis	• Disrupts DNA and RNA synthesis
INDICATIONS	• Bone and soft tissue sarcomas, lymphoma	• Lymphoma, osteosarcomas, solid neoplasia, and sarcomas (hemangiosarcoma, thyroid carcinoma, mammary adenocarcinoma, and mesothelioma)	• Leukemia, lymphoma, mammary adenocarcinoma, thyroid carcinoma, and squamous cell carcinoma
DISPENSIBLE FORMS	• Injectable (IV)	• Injectable (IV—given slowly over 10-minute period in a free-flowing line)	• Injectable (IV)
PRECAUTIONS	• Use with caution in animals that have had radiation therapy within the past 3–6 months or bone marrow suppression, infection, obesity, or renal/hepatic impairment. If skin is contaminated, rinse with running water for 10 minutes, then rinse with buffered phosphate solution. If solution gets into the eyes, wash with water immediately; then irrigate with water or isotonic saline for 10 min. **Wear gloves and eye shield.**	• **Wear gloves and eye shield.** If skin is contaminated, wash with soap and rinse thoroughly • **Pregnant women should not be handling this drug** • Monitor for **immediate hypersensitivity reaction** (facial swelling, urticaria, vomiting, arrhythmias, and/or hypotension)	• Do not mix with heparin
CONTRA-INDICATIONS	• Viral infection		• Myelosuppression, cardiac dysfunction, infection, or prior cytotoxic treatment
PATIENT CARE/ CLIENT EDUCATION	• Monitor for GI upset, anorexia, anemia, alopecia, bone marrow suppression, and gastrointestinal toxicity	• CBC should be analyzed 10 days after initiation and before each treatment • Monitor for head shaking, pruritis, erythema, vomiting, diarrhea, weight loss, leukopenia, alopecia, bone marrow suppression, and gastrointestinal toxicity	• Monitor for depression, vomiting, diarrhea, anorexia, thrombocytopenia, leukopenia, anemia, and sepsis
NOTES			• Related to doxorubicin

Table 9-12 Cancer/Chemotherapy Drugs: Antimetabolites

Drug Class	Antimetabolite		
DRUG (TRADE NAME)	• Azathioprine (Imuran)	• Fluorouracil (Adrucil)	• Methotrexate
ACTION	• Suppresses primary and secondary antibody responses and is an anti-inflammatory	• Interferes with DNA synthesis	• Inhibits DNA, RNA, and protein synthesis
INDICATIONS	• Autoimmune disease	• Canine carcinomas and sarcomas	• Lymphoreticular neoplasms, carcinomas, lymphoma, and leukemia
DISPENSIBLE FORMS	• Tablet and injectable	• Injectable (IV)	• Tablet and injectable
PRECAUTIONS	• Use with caution in patients with liver dysfunction or currently taking allopurinol		• **Wear gloves when splitting or crushing tablets**
CONTRA-INDICATIONS	• Not recommended for treatment in cats or pregnant animals	• Not recommended for usage in cats	• Preexisting bone marrow suppression, severe hepatic/renal insufficiency, or hypersensitivity to drug
PATIENT CARE/ CLIENT EDUCATION	• **Pregnant women should not handle this medication** • **Wash hands thoroughly after handling** • Monitor leukocytes biweekly for first 8 weeks, then monthly • Monitor for leukopenia, anemia, thrombocytopenia, pancreatitis, jaundice, skin problems, and poor hair growth	• Monitor for stomatitis, diarrhea, leukopenia, thrombocytopenia, anemia, and ataxia	• Monitor for vomiting, nausea, diarrhea, leukopenia, anemia, thrombocytopenia, renal tubular necrosis, bone marrow suppression, alopecia, and gastrointestinal toxicity
NOTES	• Store at room temperature and protected from light		• Store at room temperature and protect from light

Table 9-13   Cancer/Chemotherapy Drugs: Enzyme—Vinca Alkaloid

Drug Class	Enzyme	Immunomodulating	Synthetic Hormone	Vinca Alkaloid
DRUG (TRADE NAME)	• L-asparaginase (Elspar, Oncaspar, Erwinase)	• Interferon (Interferon Alpha 2a, Roferon A)	• Danazol (Danocrine, Cyclomen)	• Vincristine (Oncovin, Vincasar)
ACTION	• Hydrolyzes asparagines into aspartic acid and ammonia	• Regulation of lymphocytes (immunomodulating) and blocks replication of viral cells (antiviral)	• Suppresses LH and FSH and estrogen synthesis and stabilizes RBCs	• Arrests cancer cell division
INDICATIONS	• Lymphoma, lymphoblastic leukemia, mast cell tumors, and idiopathic thrombocytopenia	• Feline leukemia	• Canine immune-mediated thrombocytopenia and hemolytic anemia associated with prednisolone or prednisone	• Lymphoid, hematopoietic neoplasms, feline mammary neoplasms, sarcomas, canine venereal tumors, mast cell tumors, and immune-mediated thrombocytopenia
DISPENSIBLE FORMS	• Injectable (IV, IM, SC)	• Solution	• Capsule	• Injectable (IV)
PRECAUTIONS	• Liver disease, diabetes mellitus, infection, history of urate calculi, preexisting renal, hepatic, hematologic, GI or CNS dysfunction		• Hepatopathy in dogs, severe cardiac or renal impairment, and undiagnosed abnormal vaginal bleeding	• Use with caution in patients with liver disease, leukopenia, bacterial infections, or neuromuscular disease • Can cause severe tissue irritation and necrosis if placed perivascularly. Infiltrate with sodium bicarbonate, dexamethasone, or hyaluronidase

CONTRA-INDICATIONS	• Do not use with methotrexate unless necessary, and then 48 hours between medications is recommended • Pancreatitis (current or history of having)	• Monitor for constipation, alopecia, gastrointestinal toxicity, peripheral neuropathy, perivascular slough, and leukopenia
CLIENT EDUCATION	• Monitor for hypersensitivity, vomiting, diarrhea, hypotension, pruritis, pancreatitis, pain at injection site, DIC, sensitivity to drug, and collapse	• Response time may be 2–3 months • Stored in tightly sealed containers at room temperature
NOTES	• Solution of 3 million IU/mL must be diluted into 1 liter of sterile saline, placed into appropriate aliquots, and frozen (ϕ)	• May $\downarrow$ total serum thyroxine (T_4) and $\uparrow T_3$ uptake (thyroid-binding globulin is decreased)	• Store in the refrigerator and protect from light

(ϕ) = Handbook of Veterinary Drugs, Allen.

CARDIOVASCULAR DRUGS

Table 9-14   Cardiovascular Drugs

Drug Class	Anti-anemic	
DRUG (TRADE NAME)	• Erythropoieten (Epogen, Marogen, Procrit)	• Ferrous sulfate (Fer-In-Sol, Slow-Fe)
ACTION	• Hormone that stimulates production of erythrocytes	• Supplements iron
INDICATIONS	• Anemia resulting from renal failure	• Iron-deficiency anemia
DISPENSIBLE FORMS	• Injectable (SC)	• Tablet, syrup, elixir
PRECAUTIONS	• Use with caution in animals prone to seizures	• Antacids ↓ absorption of iron
CONTRA-INDICATIONS	• Hypertension, low iron levels, or pregnant/nursing • Animal currently taking desmopression, androgens, or probenecid	• Gastrointestinal tract (GIT) ulcers, enteritis, colitis, and hemolytic anemia
PATIENT CARE. CLIENT EDUCATION	• Monitor for fever, arthralgia, rash at the injection site, and seizures (cats) • Monitor packed cell volume (PCV) while on medication	• Monitor for GI upset
NOTES		

Table 9-15   Cardiovascular Drugs: Antiarrhythmic

Drug Class	Antiarrhythmic		
	Beta-Blockers (Class II)	Calcium Channel Blockers (Class IV)	Sodium Influx Inhibitors (Class I)
DRUG (TRADE NAME)	• Atenolol (Tenormin) • Metoprolol (Lopressor) • Propranolol (Inderal)	• Amlodipine besylate (Norvasc) • Diltiazem (Cardizem) • Verapamil hydrochloride	• Lidocaine (Xylocaine) • Procainamide (Pronestyl, Procan SR) • Quinidine (Duraquin, Cardioquin, Quiniglute)
ACTION	• Blocks the sympathetic nervous system receptors (beta-1) in the heart	• Blocks calcium entry into cells via blockade of slow channel	• Inhibits the movement of sodium ions across damaged cell membranes
INDICATIONS	• Cardiac arrhythmias, hypertension, and hypertrophic cardiomyopathy	• Supraventricular tachycardia, atrial flutter, and atrial fibrillation, hypertrophic cardiomyopathy, and hypertension (cats)	• Ventricular arrhythmias and atrial fibrillation
DISPENSIBLE FORMS	• Tablet, capsule, solution, and injectable	• Tablet and injectable	• Lidocaine: injectable (IV: bolus or slow drip) Procainamide and quinidine: tablet and injectable
PRECAUTIONS	• Use with caution in diabetic animals as it ↓ insulin secretion • Hyperthyroidism ± ↓ dosages • Use with caution in patients with renal insufficiency or bronchoconstriction	• Use with caution with liver and kidney impairment and Wolff-Parkinson-White syndrome	• Do not mix lidocaine with epinephrine • Use of quinidine in combination with digoxin may increase digoxin concentrations
CONTRA-INDICATIONS	• Chronic heart failure, thromboembolic disease, 2nd- or 3rd-degree heart block, bronchoconstrictive disease, and sinus bradycardia	• Hypotension and digitalis intoxication	• Myasthenia gravis, digitalis intoxication and heart block (quinidine)
PATIENT CARE/ CLIENT EDUCATION	• Monitor dose effectiveness • Monitor for bradycardia, hypotension, bronchoconstriction, hypoglycemia, and diarrhea	• Monitor for hypotension, cardiac depression, bradycardia, AV block, pulmonary edema, fatigue, dizziness, nausea, and anorexia	• Monitor for sedation, shock, seizures, and vomiting (lidocaine) • Monitor for hypotension, vomiting, diarrhea, anorexia, weakness, and urine retention (quinidine)
NOTES	• Propranolol loses its effectiveness over extended usage period	• Diltiazem is less potent than verapamil	

Table 9-16 Cardiovascular Drugs: Anticoagulants – Calcium Supplements

Drug Class	Anticoagulants		Calcium Supplements	
DRUG (TRADE NAME)	Heparin sodium (Heparin)	Warfarin (Coumadin)	Calcium chloride	Calcium gluconate
ACTION	Potentiates anticoagulant effects of antithrombin III	Interferes with clotting and depletes vitamin K	↑ Available calcium	↑ Available calcium
INDICATIONS	Thrombosis, DIC, and burn victims	Thromboembolic disease or hypercoagulable disease	Cardiac arrest and hypocalcemia	Hypocalcemia, ventricular asystole, severe bradycardia, hyperkalemic cardiotoxicity, and eclampsia
DISPENSIBLE FORMS	Injectable	Tablet	Injectable	Injectable
PRECAUTIONS			Inject slowly to avoid an extravascular injection causing inflammation, tissue necrosis, and sloughing • Use with caution with nephrocalcinosis • ↑ Toxicity risk if used with digitalis	Inject slowly to avoid an extravascular injection causing inflammation, tissue necrosis, and sloughing • ↑ Toxicity risk if used with digitalis • Use with caution in patients receiving digitalis, with renal or cardiac insufficiency
CONTRA-INDICATIONS	Animals with coagulation disorders			Ventricular fibrillation, renal calculi, and hypercalcemia
PATIENT CARE/CLIENT EDUCATION	Monitor for bleeding and thrombocytopenia	Monitor for pale mucous membranes, weakness, or dyspnea	Monitor for bradycardia, arrhythmias, hypotension, and hypercalcemia	Monitor for constipation
NOTES	Do not use heparin flushes or heparin catheters in animals with coagulation disorders			

Table 9-17 Cardiovascular Drugs: Contractility Enhancers

Drug Class	Contractility Enhancers: Positive Inotropic Agents			
	Beta-adrenergic	Bipyridine Derivatives	Cardiac Glycosides	Catecholamines
DRUG (TRADE NAME)	• Isoproterenol (Isuprel, Iperenol)	• Amrinone (Inocor)	• Digoxin	• Dobutamine HCl • Dopamine • Epinephrine
ACTION	• ↑ AV conduction and ventricular excitability and promotes bronchodilation	• ↑ Cardiac output and ↓ pulmonary capillary pressure	• ↑ Cardiac contractility and ↓ heart rate	• Stimulates myocardium
INDICATIONS	• Short-term management of incomplete heart block, sinus bradycardia, and sick sinus syndrome	• Congestive heart failure (CHF) and cardiomyopathy	• CHF, atrial fibrillation, and supraventricular tachycardia	• CHF, atrial fibrillation, and supraventricular tachycardia
DISPENSIBLE FORMS	• Injectable and inhalation	• Injectable	• Tablet and elixir	• Injectable
PRECAUTIONS		• Use with caution in animals with liver or kidney dysfunction or aortic stenosis	• Dobermans and cats ↑ sensitivity	• Avoid alkalinizing agents when mixing dobutamine (dilute with 5% dextrose solution, e.g., 250 mg in 1 L 5% dextrose)*
CONTRAINDICATIONS				
PATIENT CARE/ CLIENT EDUCATION	• Monitor for tachycardia, tachyarrhythmias, vomiting, and weakness	• Monitor for tachycardia, arrhythmias, hypotension, anorexia, vomiting, and diarrhea	• Monitor for anorexia, vomiting, diarrhea, and arrhythmias	• Monitor for hypertension or hypotension, arrhythmias, dyspnea, anxiety, excitability, and nausea
NOTES	• Short-term use • Administered via carefully monitored constant rate of infusion		• Metabolized through the kidneys	• Administer via carefully monitored constant rate infusion

*The 5 Minute Veterinary Consult, Canine and Feline, Second Edition

Table 9-18 Cardiovascular Drugs: Diuretics

Drug Class	Diuretics	
DRUG (TRADE NAME)	• Furosemide (Lasix)	• Mannitol (Osmitrol)
ACTION	• Prevents reabsorption of sodium from the renal tubules	• Draws water into the renal tubules
INDICATIONS	• CHF with pulmonary edema (reduces preload) • Oliguria	• Prevention/treatment of oliguria • Acute glaucoma • Management of acute cerebral edema
DISPENSIBLE FORMS	• Tablet, solution, and injectable	• Injectable
PRECAUTIONS	• Use with caution in animals receiving angiotensin-converting enzyme (ACE) inhibitors to ↓ risk of azotemia • May cause ototoxicity in cats	• Use cautiously when intracranial bleeding is suspected, because it may ↑ bleeding
CONTRAINDICATIONS	• Anuria or progressive kidney disease	• Dehydrated patients
PATIENT CARE/CLIENT EDUCATION	• Monitor for leukopenia, hypokalemia, hyponatremia, hypochloremic acidosis, dehydration, vomiting, and diarrhea • PU/PD is common	• Monitor fluid and electrolyte balances • Monitor for nausea, vomiting, and dizziness
NOTES	• Prolonged use can lead to low potassium levels	

Table 9-19 Cardiovascular Drugs: Vasodilators

Drug Class	Vasodilators		
DRUG (TRADE NAME)	• Captopril (Capoten) • Enalapril (Enacard and Vasotec)	• Hydralazine (Apresoline)	• Nitroglycerin ointment (Nitrobid and Nitrol) • Prazosin (Minipress)
ACTION	• Blocks the formation of angiotensin II	• Direct relaxation of the smooth muscle cells in vessels (stimulates angiotensin II release)	• Results in dilation of venous system and "pools" blood in the peripheral tissues to reduce preload • Blocks vasoconstriction caused by the sympathetic nervous system (blocks alpha-1 receptors)
INDICATIONS	• Class II–IV heart failure (mainly dogs) and hypertension	• CHF and other cardiovascular disorders characterized by high peripheral vascular resistance	• Heart failure and in cases of pulmonary hypertension • CHF, dilated cardiomyopathy (dog), systemic hypertension, and pulmonary hypertension
DISPENSIBLE FORMS	• Tablet	• Tablet and injectable	• Injectable, ointment, and transdermal patch • Tablet and capsule
PRECAUTIONS	• Antihypertensive effectiveness may be reduced if given with NSAIDs • Use with caution with diuretics and potassium supplements or with patients with renal disease		• **Wear gloves when applying ointment**
CONTRA-INDICATIONS			
PATIENT CARE/ CLIENT EDUCATION	• Give on an empty stomach • Monitor electrolytes and kidney function 3–7 days after initiating therapy and periodically thereafter • Monitor for hypotension, azotemia, hyperkalemia, vomiting, and diarrhea	• Monitor for tachycardia, hypotension, vomiting, diarrhea, sodium and water retention	• Monitor for hypotension and a rash at the application site • Monitor for hypotension, syncope, vomiting, diarrhea, nausea, and constipation
NOTES	• Captopril is considered the better choice for patients with liver disease		• Rotate application sites • Intermittent use for optimum effect • 1 inch of ointment is ~15 mg

DERMATOLOGIC DRUGS

Table 9-20 Dermatologic Drugs

Drug Class			Antiseborrheics	
DRUG (TRADE NAME)	• Sulfur (SebaLyt Shampoo, Allerseb T Shampoo, Sebbafon)	• Salicylic acid (Allerseb T, Sebbafon)	• Coal tar	• Benzoyl peroxide (Oxy-Dex Shampoo, Ben-A-Derm, Pyoben)
ACTION	• Loosens horny layer of the epidermis, promotes normalization of keratin development and mildly antibacterial	• Promotes normalization of keratin development	• Keratolytic • Keratoplastic • Antipruritic • Vasoconstrictive	• Loosens horny layer of the epidermis and promotes normalization of keratin development
INDICATIONS	• Seborrhea, mites, lice, chiggers, fleas, dermatophytosis, pyoderma, pruritis, crusts, and scales	• Seborrhea and hyperkeratotic skin disorders	• Seborrhea and as a degreaser	• Seborrhea oleosa, hot spots, skinfold dermatitis, superficial folliculitis, schnauzer comedo syndrome, tail gland hyperplasia, and stud tail (cats)
DISPENSIBLE FORMS	• Shampoo	• Shampoo	• Shampoo	• Shampoo
PRECAUTIONS			• Stains; wear gloves	• Stains; wear gloves
CONTRA-INDICATIONS			• Cats	
PATIENT CARE/ CLIENT EDUCATION				
NOTES	• Not recommended for routine bathing	• Not recommended for routine bathing		• Not recommended for routine bathing

Table 9-21   Dermatologic Drugs: Antipruritics/Antihistamines

Drug Class	Antipruritics/Antihistamines	
DRUG (TRADE NAME)	• Chlorpheniramine maleate (Chlor-Trimeton) • Diphenhydramine (Benadryl)	• Hydroxyzine (Atarax)
ACTION	• Blocks the histamine receptor on the smooth muscle surrounding the bronchiole and decreases sinus/nasal secretions with an upper respiratory infection	• Acts at peripheral tissues and centrally in the brain
INDICATIONS	• Pruritis and allergic reactions • Relax skeletal, pharyngeal, and laryngeal muscles	• Pruritis and behavioral disorders (compulsive scratching and self-trauma)
DISPENSIBLE FORMS	• Tablet and injectable	• Tablet, solution, and injectable
PRECAUTIONS		
CONTRAINDICATIONS	• Glaucoma, urinary retention, CNS disorders, and GIT disorders • Pregnant animals	
PATIENT CARE/CLIENT EDUCATION	• Monitor for sedation, vomiting, and diarrhea	• Monitor for hypotension, drowsiness, dry mucous membranes, seizures, tremors, urinary retention, ▼ appetite, and diarrhea
NOTES		

GASTROINTESTINAL DRUGS

Table 9-22 Gastrointestinal Drugs

Drug Class	Antidiarrheals			
	Antibiotic • Tylosin (Tylan, Tylocine, Tylosin tartrate)	*Anticholinergics* • Atropine • Aminopentamide (Centrine) • Propantheline (Pro-Banthine)	• Bismuth subsalicylate (Pepto-Bismol)	*Opiates* • Diphenoxylate (Lomotil) • Loperamide (Imodium)
DRUG (TRADE NAME)				
ACTION	• Binds to ribosome and inhibits synthesis (macrolide antibiotic)	• Modifies intestinal motility by blocking the effect of acetylcholine (reduces peristalsis and GI secretions)	• Blocks hypersecretion (bismuth coats the intestinal mucosa as a protectant; salicylate inhibits the secretion of fluids) • Mild antibacterial properties	• Modifies intestinal motility by increasing segmental contractions and reducing peristaltic movements
INDICATIONS	• Colitis	• Diarrhea and vomiting	• Diarrhea	• Diarrhea
DISPENSIBLE FORMS	• Tablet and powder	• Tablet, solution, ointment, and injectable	• Tablet and solution	• Tablet, capsule, and solution
PRECAUTIONS		• May ↓ GI tract secretions and motility • May ↑ serum digitalis levels	• Use with caution in cats; salicylate is absorbed systemically. ± ↓ Absorption of tetracyclines; separate doses by at least 2 hours	
CONTRA-INDICATIONS		• Heart insufficiencies, suspected bacterial toxin, glaucoma, asthma, intestinal ileus, gastroparesis, and tachycardia		• Heart insufficiencies or septicemia • Liver disease, obstructive gastrointestinal disease, glaucoma, and obstructive uropathy (loperamide)
PATIENT CARE/ CLIENT EDUCATION	• May cause pain at site if injected	• Monitor for sinus tachycardia, dry mouth, dry eye, and urinary hesitancy		• Monitor for constipation, bloating, and sedation
NOTES	• Monitor for diarrhea and anorexia	• Discontinue if diarrhea is present >72 hours (propantheline)	• Eliminated in the feces, resulting in dark, tarry stools	• May cause stool discoloration • Discontinue loperamide if diarrhea is present >48 hours

Table 9-23 Gastrointestinal Drugs: Antiemetics

Drug Class	Antiemetics		
	Antihistamines	Motility Modifiers	Phenothiazines
DRUG (TRADE NAME)	• Meclizine (Antivert) • Promethazine (Phenergan) • Trimethobenzamide HCl (Tigan—dogs)	• Cisapride (Propulsid) • Metoclopramide (Reglan)	• Acepromazine (PromAce and Atravet) • Chlorpromazine (Thorazine) • Prochlorperazine (Compazine and Darbazine)
ACTION	• ↓ Neural impulses from the vestibular cranial nerve to the vomiting center	• Blocks the dopamine receptors at the chemoreceptor trigger zone and directly ↑ gastric emptying	• Blocks receptors at the chemoreceptor trigger zone and the vomiting center of the brain
INDICATIONS	• Gastroesophageal reflux and vomiting	• Gastroesophageal reflux, gastric motility disorders, and vomiting	• Gastroesophageal reflux and vomiting
DISPENSIBLE FORMS	• Tablet and liquids	• Tablet, syrup, and injectable	• Tablet, capsule, suppository, and injectable
PRECAUTIONS	• Produces a sedative effect • Affects allergy testing	• IV usage: administer slowly	• ± ↓ Blood pressure and seizure threshold • ± Vasodilation • Check drug's interactions with other drugs (chlorpromazine) • Use with caution in patients with liver failure
CONTRA-INDICATIONS	• Allergy testing	• Animals using atropine • GIT obstruction, perforation, or epilepsy	• Tetanus • Dehydrated patients
PATIENT CARE/ CLIENT EDUCATION	• Monitor for sedation	• Monitor for sedation or excitement (cats), dyspnea, convulsions, or diarrhea • Cisapride is typically given 15 minutes before a meal • Metoclopramide is typically given 30 minutes before a meal	• Monitor for hypotension, aggression, seizures, and constipation
NOTES		• Metoclopramide is a direct-acting agonist cholinergic	• Protect from light

Table 9-24 Gastrointestinal Drugs: Anti-ulcer

Drug Class	Anti-ulcer				
DRUG (TRADE NAME)	*Antacids, nonsystemic* • Aluminum hydroxide (Amphojel, Basaljel, Dialume, Maalox, and Mylanta) • Aluminum carbonate (Basalgel) • Calcium carbonate (Tums and Rolaids) • Magnesium hydroxide (Phillips Milk of Magnesia, Riopan, Carmilax, Magnalax, and Rulax II)	*Antacids, systemic* • Cimetidine (Tagamet) • Famotidine (Pepcid) • Ranitidine (Zantac)	• Omeprazole (Prilosec)	• Misoprostol (Cytotec)	• Sucralfate (Carafate)
ACTION	• ↑ Stomach pH to neutralize stomach acids	• Blocks the histamine receptor of the parietal cell thereby ↓ the acidity of the stomach • Neutralize stomach acids	• Directly blocks/disables parietal cell proton-pump mechanism, thereby shutting down gastric acid production	• Protects the GIT mucosa, and ↓ acid secretion	• Binds to proteins found in the active ulcers
INDICATIONS	• Gastritis and ulcers • Hyperphosphatemia caused by renal failure	• Gastritis and ulcers	• Gastrointestinal ulceration and gastrinoma (Zollinger/ Ellison syndrome)	• Ulcer preventative for patients taking NSAIDS	• Gastric mucosa ulcers
DISPENSIBLE FORMS	• Tablet, capsule, and solution	• Tablet, solution, and injectable	• Tablet	• Tablet	• Tablet and suspension

PRECAUTIONS	• May interfere with absorption of other drugs • Use with caution in patients with gastric obstruction	• Cimetidine may interfere with absorption of other drugs	• Pregnant animals	• Animals taking antacids
CONTRA-INDICATIONS	• Kidney disease (magnesium) • Alkalosis	• Patients being given acid-dependent drugs		
PATIENT CARE/ CLIENT EDUCATION	• Monitor phosphate levels • Monitor for constipation (calcium) and diarrhea (magnesium)		• Monitor for vomiting, diarrhea, flatulence, and discomfort	• Monitor for constipation
NOTES	• Poor palatability	• Ranitidine more potent than cimetidine	• Omeprazole is more potent than cimetidine	

Table 9-25 Gastrointestinal Drugs: Emetics

Drug Class	Emetics		
DRUG (TRADE NAME)	• Apomorphine (dogs)	• Syrup of Ipecac	• Hydrogen peroxide • Warm salt water • Mustard and water
ACTION	• Stimulates dopamine receptors in the chemoreceptor trigger zone	• Irritates the GIT to stimulate the vagus nerve	• Irritates the GIT to stimulate the vagus nerve
INDICATIONS	• Initiate vomiting (e.g., acute toxin ingestion)	• Initiate vomiting (e.g., acute toxin ingestion)	• Initiate vomiting (e.g., acute toxin ingestion)
DISPENSIBLE FORMS	• Tablet	• Suspension	• Solution
PRECAUTIONS	• May cause CNS depression and prolonged vomiting • Verify with DVM or poison control that the substance should be brought back up (e.g., caustic materials)	• High concentrations can lead to toxic effects on the heart • Verify with DVM or poison control that the substance should be brought back up (e.g., caustic materials)	• Avoid contact with patient's eyes and mucus membranes • Verify with DVM or poison control that the substance should be brought back up (e.g., caustic materials)
CONTRA-INDICATIONS	• Strychnine poisoning, narcosis, or unconscious patients • Patients with respiratory or CNS depression • Ingestion of sharp object	• Animals recently receiving activated charcoal • Ingestion of sharp object	• Ingestion of sharp object
PATIENT CARE/ CLIENT EDUCATION	• Monitor for bradycardia, hypotension, respiratory depression, sedation, salivation, and prolonged vomiting • If the tablet was placed in the conjunctival sac, use an eyewash to remove any remaining tablet after vomiting		
NOTES	• The tablet also may be dissolved in a syringe with saline and injected SC	• Do not exchange extract of ipecac for syrup	

Xylazine is also used as an emetic. Please refer to Chapter 2 for detailed information on this drug.

Table 9-26 Gastrointestinal Drugs: Enzyme—Lubricants

Drug Class	Enzyme	Laxatives	Lubricants
DRUG (TRADE NAME)	• Pancreatic enzyme replacement (Pancrezyme)	• Psyllium (Metamucil) • Lactulose (Chronulac) • Magnesium hydroxide (Milk of Magnesia)	• Cod liver oil • Mineral oil • White petrolatum (Laxatone, Petromalt)
ACTION	• Replaces enzymes	• Pulls water into the feces and stimulates colonic/rectal peristalsis by distension • Decreases blood ammonia by lowering pH of colon (lactulose)	• Coats the feces for easier passage
INDICATIONS	• Pancreatic exocrine insufficiency	• Hairballs, constipation (prevention), and colitis • Hepatic encephalopathy (lactulose)	• Hairballs and constipation
DISPENSIBLE FORMS	• Tablet and powder	• Tablet, powder, and solution	• Gel, liquid
PRECAUTIONS			• Long-term usage can decrease absorption of lipid-soluble vitamins (A, D, E, and K) from the bowel
CONTRA-INDICATIONS		• Cats or small dogs with kidney disease • Dehydration, pain, vomiting, or fecal impaction	• Vomiting, diarrhea, pain, obstruction, or dysphagia
PATIENT CARE/ CLIENT EDUCATION	• Mix powder thoroughly with moistened food; tablets are given before feeding • Monitor for nausea, cramping, diarrhea, skin and nasal irritation • Used in conjuction with a bland, easily digestible diet with low levels of fat	• Monitor for dehydration, cramping, flatulence, and bloating (psyllium and lactulose) • Monitor for hypotension, depression, loss of deep tendon reflexes, and weakness (magnesium) • Water should be available to the patient • May be unpalatable	• Store in a cool place
NOTES	• Cimetidine may improve efficacy	• May take 12–24 hours for effectiveness	• May take 6–12 hours for effectiveness

Table 9-27   Gastrointestinal Drugs: Protectant—Stool Softeners

Drug Class	Protectants	Stool Softener
DRUG (TRADE NAME)	• Activated charcoal (Superchar and Tox-iban)	• Docusate sodium succinate (Colace, Docusate solution, Disposaject) • Docusate calcium (Surfak)
ACTION	• Adsorbent that binds with enterotoxins	• Reduces surface tension of feces to permit water to penetrate the dry stool
INDICATIONS	• Poisoning (acetaminophen, atropine, digitalis, glycosides, phenytoin, mercuric chloride, morphine sulfate, and ethylene glycol)	• Constipation
DISPENSIBLE FORMS	• Solution	• Tablet, capsule, solution, syrup, and enema
PRECAUTIONS	• Do not use with Syrup of Ipecac because it negates adsorbent qualities of charcoal	• Do not use with mineral oil unless separating administration by 2 hours
CONTRA-INDICATIONS		
PATIENT CARE/CLIENT EDUCATION	• Monitor for vomiting, diarrhea, and constipation • Stools often will have altered color	• Monitor for dehydration, cramping, nausea, vomiting, diarrhea, and throat irritation
NOTES	• Not effective against cyanide, mineral acids, caustic alkalis, organic solvents, ethanol, lead, iron, and methanol	

(Stool Softener column — PRECAUTIONS row continued:) • Do not use 2 hours before or 3 hours after administration of antimicrobial drugs or digoxin

(Stool Softener column — PATIENT CARE/CLIENT EDUCATION row:) • Monitor for vomiting, diarrhea, and constipation

METABOLIC DRUGS

Table 9-28 Metabolic Drugs

Drug Class	Adrenal Cortex			
DRUG (TRADE NAME)	• Desoxycorticosterone acetate—DOCA (Percoten acetate) • Desoxycorticosterone pivalate—DOCP (Percorten pivalate)	• Fludrocortisone (Florinef)	• Mitotane (Lysodren)	• Selegiline–l-deprenyl (Anipryl, Eldepryl)
ACTION	• Replaces aldosterone in the body	• Promotes sodium retention and urinary potassium excretion	• Suppresses adrenal cortex	• Restores brain dopamine
INDICATIONS	• Hypoadrenocorticism (replacement therapy)	• Hypoadrenocorticism (replacement therapy)	• Pituitary-dependent hyperadrenocorticism in dogs and adrenal tumors	• Uncomplicated pituitary-dependent hyperadrenocorticism in dogs • Canine cognitive dysfunction syndrome
DISPENSIBLE FORMS	• Injectable (IM)	• Tablet	• Tablet	• Tablet
PRECAUTIONS			• Use with caution in patients with liver disease • May ↓ insulin requirements in diabetic patients	
CONTRA-INDICATIONS				• Animal on Amitraz or phenylpropanolamine (discontinue 2 weeks before starting Anipryl)
PATIENT CARE/CLIENT EDUCATION	• Monitor for edema, hypotension, hypokalemia, hypernatremia, and weakness • Monitor electrolyte status of patients at 14 and 25 day intervals to determine dosing	• Monitor for edema, hypotension, hypokalemia, PU/PD, and weakness • Monitor electrolyte status of patients • If discontinuing medication, taper off dose gradually over a few days	• Administer with food to ↑ absorption • Monitor for vomiting, diarrhea, lethargy, weakness, and anorexia	• Monitor for vomiting, diarrhea, and listlessness • If discontinuing therapy, allow 14 days before initiation of a tricyclic antidepressant
NOTES				

Table 9-29 Metabolic Drugs: Pancreatic: Insulin

Drug Class	Pancreatic: Insulin		
DRUG (TRADE NAME)	*Short-acting Insulin* • Regular (R) • Semi-Lente	*Intermediate-acting Insulin* • NPH • Lente	*Long-acting Insulin* • Protamine Zinc (PZI) • Ultralente
ACTION	• Enhances distribution of glucose to tissues and organs, thereby ↓ blood glucose levels	• Enhances distribution of glucose to tissues and organs, thereby ↓ blood glucose levels	• Enhances distribution of glucose to tissues and organs, thereby ↓ blood glucose levels
INDICATIONS	• Diabetes ketoacidosis	• Diabetes mellitus, uncomplicated (dogs/cats)	• Diabetes mellitus, uncomplicated (cats)
DISPENSIBLE FORMS	• Injectable (IV, SC)	• Injectable (SC)	• Injectable (SC)
PRECAUTIONS	• Inaccurate dosing may lead to hypoglycemia	• Inaccurate dosing may lead to hypoglycemia	• Inaccurate dosing may lead to hypoglycemia
CONTRA-INDICATIONS	• Hypoglycemia	• Hypoglycemia	• Hypoglycemia
PATIENT CARE/ CLIENT EDUCATION	• Feed several small-portion meals throughout the day (3–4) • Monitor for weakness, ataxia, shaking, and seizures (signs of iatrogenic hypoglycemia) • Serum fructosamine levels (every 4–12 months) and serial blood glucose curves (1–2 times a year) are recommended	• Feed several small-portion meals throughout the day (3–4) • Monitor for weakness, ataxia, shaking, and seizures (signs of iatrogenic hypoglycemia) • Serum fructosamine levels (every 4–12 months) and serial blood glucose curves (1–2 times a year) are recommended	• Feed several small-portion meals throughout the day (3–4) • Monitor for weakness, ataxia, shaking, and seizures (signs of iatrogenic hypoglycemia) • Serum fructosamine levels (every 4–12 months) and serial blood glucose curves (1–2 times a year) are recommended
NOTES	• For insulin administration, see Chapter 6, Skill Box 6-5 and 6-6 Client Education—Insulin Administration • Refrigerate insulin	• For insulin administration, see Chapter 6, Skill Box 6-5 and 6-6 Client Education—Insulin Administration • Refrigerate insulin	• For insulin administration see Chapter 6, Skill Box 6-5 and 6-6 Client Education—Insulin Administration • Refrigerate insulin

Table 9-30 Metabolic Drugs: Pancreatic

Drug Class		Pancreatic
DRUG (TRADE NAME)	• Desmopressin acetate (DDAVP)	• Vasopressin (Pitressin)
ACTION	• Stimulates the release of preformed factor VIII from storage sites	• Stimulates the release of preformed factor VIII from storage sites
INDICATIONS	• Central diabetes insipidus • von Willebrand's type I (presurgery)	• Diabetes insipidus
DISPENSIBLE FORMS	• Injectable (IV, IM) and nasal drops	• Injectable (IV, IM)
PRECAUTIONS	• Perform a response test in vWF dogs • Buccal mucosal bleeding time test and plasma vWF pre and post administration of DDAVP and presurgery is recommended	• Use with caution with heart failure or asthma patients
CONTRAINDICATIONS		• Cardiorenal disease, hypertension, or epilepsy
PATIENT CARE/CLIENT EDUCATION	• Monitor for hypotension, tachycardia, and fluid retention	• Monitor for nausea, vomiting, and fluid retention
NOTES		

Table 9-31 Metabolic Drugs: Parathyroid - Thyroid

Drug Class	Parathyroid	Thyroid
DRUG (TRADE NAME)	• Calcitriol (Rocaltrol, Calcijex)	• Levothyroxine sodium (L-Thyroxine, Soloxine, Thyro-tabs, Synthroid, Eltroxin)	• Methimazole (Tapazole)
ACTION	• Increases calcium absorption in the intestines	• Converted to active T_3 form	• Prevents the production of normal thyroid hormones
INDICATIONS	• Hypocalcemia or secondary hyperparathyroidism with chronic renal failure	• Hypothyroidism (via supplementation), von Willebrand's disease and platelet dysfunction	• Hyperthyroidism
DISPENSIBLE FORMS	• Capsule and injectable	• Tablet	• Tablet
PRECAUTIONS	• Use with caution on animals taking digitalis or calcium carbonate		
CONTRA-INDICATIONS		• Cardiac insufficiency, primary hypertension, diabetes, or hypoadrenocorticism	
PATIENT CARE/CLIENT EDUCATION	• Monitor calcium plasma concentration for hypercalcemia (PU/PD, vomiting, depression, anorexia, trembling, and muscle weakness)	• Monitor serum thyroid levels every 6–12 months • Monitor for tachycardia, panting, abnormal papillary reflexes, nervousness, polyphagia, PU/PD, weight loss, vomiting, and diarrhea	• Monitor serum thyroid levels (every 6–12 months), weight, and blood pressure every 3–6 months • Monitor for anorexia, vomiting, skin eruptions, and lethargy
NOTES		• Protect from light • Blood work should be checked 4–6 hours after last dose (check with your local laboratory facility on special drawing/handling instructions)	• May need to increase dosage as thyroid grows • Blood work should be checked 4–6 hours after medication • Can cause bone marrow disease

MUSCULOSKELETAL DRUGS
Anti-Inflammatory Drugs

Potential side effects of corticosteroids: Most common side effects are polyphagia, PU/PD, panting, weakness, bilateral alopecia, and HPA-axis suppression. Other possible side effects are GI ulceration, anorexia, diarrhea, melena, hepatopathy, diabetes mellitus, hyperlipidemia, immunosuppression, ↓ thyroid hormone, protein synthesis, and wound healing. Overuse of glucocorticoids can lead to hyperadrenocorticism.

General Notes: Corticosteroids **will** affect blood values as well as intradermal allergy skin testing, so perform testing before administration. These medications are not recommended during the healing phase of fractures, in young animals, or in pregnant animals. Caution should be used in animals with CHF, diabetes mellitus, and renal disease.

Table 9-32 Musculoskeletal Drugs

Drug Class	Anti-Inflammatory: Corticosteroids		
	Short Acting (<12 hours)	Intermediate Acting (12–36 hours)	Long Acting (>48 hours)
DRUG (TRADE NAME)	• Cortisone acetate • Hydrocortisone • Hydrocortisone sodium succinate (Solu-Cortef)	• Methylprednisolone (Medrol, Depo-Medrol) • Prednisone (Deltasone) • Prednisolone (Delta-cortef) • Prednisolone sodium succinate (Solu-Delta-Cortef) • Triamcinolone (Vetalog, Trimtabs, Aristocort)	• Betamethasone (Betasone, Betavet solus-pan) • Dexamethasone (Azium, Azium SP) • Flumethasone (Flucort) • Paramethasone
ACTION	• Inhibits phospholipase	• Inhibits phospholipase	• Inhibits phospholipase
INDICATIONS	• Anti-inflammatory, replacement therapy, shock, asthma (cat) and acute hypoadrenocortical crisis	• Anti-inflammatory, replacement therapy, immunosuppression, shock, and CNS trauma	• Anti-inflammatory, immunosuppression, and CNS inflammation
DISPENSIBLE FORMS	• Tablet, topical, and injectable	• Tablet, topical, and injectable	• Tablet, topical, and injectable
PRECAUTIONS	*See paragraph above for side effects and precautions*	*See paragraph above for side effects and precautions*	• May ↓ sperm viability in stud dogs (betamethasone)
CONTRA-INDICATIONS	*See paragraph above for side effects and precautions*	*See paragraph above for side effects and precautions*	
PATIENT CARE/ CLIENT EDUCATION	• When reducing dosages, taper gradually as recommended per veterinarian (abrupt cessation from long-term administration may result in Addison's disease) • Monitor for PU/PD, polyphagia, panting, lethargy, weakness, and bilateral alopecia • Provide lots of fresh water and continuous access to litter box or outdoors	• When reducing dosages, taper gradually as recommended per veterinarian (abrupt cessation from long-term administration may result in Addison's disease) • Monitor for PU/PD, polyphagia, panting, lethargy, weakness, and bilateral alopecia • Provide lots of fresh water and continuous access to litter box or outdoors	• When reducing dosages, taper gradually as recommended per veterinarian (abrupt cessation from long-term administration may result in Addison's disease) • Monitor for PU/PD, polyphagia, panting, lethargy, weakness, and bilateral alopecia • Provide lots of fresh water and continuous access to litter box or outdoors
NOTES		• Prednisone is 4× more potent than cortisol • Methylprednisolone and Triamcinolone is 1.25× more potent than prednisone • Cats typically require higher doses than dogs, but usually suffer fewer side effects	• Dexamethasone is used in testing for hyperadrenocorticism • Betamethasone, dexamethasone is 30× more potent than cortisol • Flumethasone is 15× more potent than cortisol

Table 9-33 Musculoskeletal Drugs: NSAIDS

Drug Class	Nonsteroidal Anti-inflammatory Drugs (NSAIDs)		
DRUG (TRADE NAME)	• Acetylsalicylic acid (Aspirin)	• Carprofen (Rimadyl)	• Etodalac (Etogesic)
ACTION	• Inhibits cyclooxygenase and antithrombotic	• Inhibits cyclooxygenase (predominantly cox-2)	• Inhibits cyclooxygenase (predominantly cox-2)
INDICATIONS	• Pain, inflammation, fever, cardiomyopathy (cat), endotoxic shock • Used in conjunction with postadulticide heartworm treatment	• Pain, inflammation, and fever	• Pain and inflammation
DISPENSIBLE FORMS	• Tablet	• Tablet	• Tablet
PRECAUTIONS	• Use cautiously in coagulopathic deficient patients • Administer no less than every 3 days to cats, because of salicylate intoxication (cats are very slow to metabolize)	• Possible adverse effects on kidney function	• May cause ↓ platelet function and kidney injury
CONTRA-INDICATIONS	• Pregnant animals	• Cats • Animals taking glucocorticoids	• Cats
PATIENT CARE/ CLIENT EDUCATION	• Monitor for ulceration, bleeding, and vomiting • Administer with food	• Monitor for ulceration, bleeding, vomiting, and aggression • Chemistry profile screening should be done before and during chronic therapy • Administer with food	• Monitor for weight loss, vomiting, and diarrhea • Administer with food • Chemistry profile screening should be done before and during chronic therapy
NOTES	• Use of the enteric-coated brands is not typically recommended • Metabolized by the liver • 1 gr "baby" aspirin = 65 mg 1.25 gr "baby" aspirin = 81 mg	• Idiosyncratic acute hepatic toxicity (2–3 weeks after beginning treatment	

Table 9-34　Musculoskeletal Drugs: NSAIDs continued

Drug Class	Anti-Inflammatory: Nonsteroidal Anti-inflammatory Drugs (NSAIDs)		
DRUG (TRADE NAME)	• Flunixin meglumine (Banamine)	• Phenylbutazone (Butazolidin)	Piroxicam (Feldene)
ACTION	• Inhibits cyclooxygenase	• Inhibits cyclooxygenase	• Inhibits cyclooxygenase
INDICATIONS	• Short-term treatment of moderate pain and inflammation • Intestinal endotoxemia (e.g., Parvovirus)	• Arthritis and musculoskeletal pain and inflammation	• Degenerative joint disease
DISPENSIBLE FORMS	• Granules, ophthalmic, and injectable	• Tablet and injectable	• Capsule
PRECAUTIONS	• Ulcerogenic effects are potentiated when administered with corticosteroids	• May cause bone marrow suppression and kidney necrosis	• Use with caution in patients with renal or cardiac dysfunction, hypertension, and coagulopathy disorders
CONTRA-INDICATIONS			• Hemophilia, GI ulcers, or bleeding
PATIENT CARE/ CLIENT EDUCATION	• Monitor for ulceration, bleeding, and vomiting • Administer with food	• Monitor for ulceration, bleeding, vomiting, and water retention	• Monitor for anorexia, vomiting, and anemia
NOTES	• IM injection may cause irritation • Only used for 3–4 days • More potent analgesic than other NSAIDS	• IM and SC injections may cause irritation • Metabolized by the liver	• Also used in the management of pain from transitional cell carcinoma of the bladder and inducing partial remission of squamous cell carcinoma in canines

Table 9-35   Musculoskeletal Drugs: Protectant - Supplement

Drug Class	Protectant	Muscle Relaxer	Supplement
DRUG (TRADE NAME)	• Polysulfated glycosamino-glycans—PSGAG (Adequan IM)	• Methocarbamol (Robaxin, Robaxin-V)	• Glucosamine + chondroitin sulfate (Cosequin)
ACTION	• Stimulates the synthesis of glycosamino-glycans, inhibits collagen and proteoglycan catabolism, and inhibits neutrophil migration into synovial fluid	• Depresses polysynaptic reflexes	• Stimulates synthesis of snyovial fluid and inhibits degradation of articular cartilage
INDICATIONS	• Osteoarthritis	• Muscular spasm	• Degenerative joint disease
DISPENSIBLE FORMS	• Capsule and injectable	• Tablet and injectable	• Tablet and capsule
PRECAUTIONS			
CONTRA-INDICATIONS	• Dogs with bleeding disorders	• Renal disease or pregnant animals	
PATIENT CARE/ CLIENT EDUCATION	• Monitor for allergic reactions	• Monitor for sedation, vomiting, weakness, and ataxia	• Results are typically seen by the seventh week
NOTES			

NEUROLOGIC DRUGS

A listing of anesthetic drugs can be found in Chapter 2: Anesthesiology

Table 9-36 Neurologic Drugs

Drug Class	Appetite Stimulator	Cholinergics
DRUG (TRADE NAME)	• Cyproheptadine HCl (Periactin)	*Indirect acting agonists:* • Edrophonium chloride (Tensilon) • Neostigmine bromide (Prostigmine) • Physostigmine (Antilirium)
ACTION	• Competes with histamine for H-1 receptor sites	• Inhibits acetylcholine breakdown, thereby prolonging postsynaptic stimulation
INDICATIONS	• Feline appetite stimulant	• Aid in diagnosing myasthenia gravis and treatment of curare poisoning (edrophonium) • Myasthenia gravis (neostigmine, physostigmine) • Antidote for neuromuscular blockers (neostigmine)
DISPENSIBLE FORMS		• Tablet, solutions, and injectable
PRECAUTIONS	• Use with caution on patients with prostatic hypertrophy, angle-closure glaucoma, pyloric or duodenal obstruction, urinary retention, acute asthma, and severe cardiac disease • May cause aggression or exitability in cats	• Use with caution with asthma or cardiac arrhythmias
CONTRAINDICATIONS		
PATIENT CARE/CLIENT EDUCATION	• Monitor for polyphagia, sedation, and CNS depression	• Monitor for bradycardia, hypotension, heart block, lacrimation, papillary constriction, laryngospasm, nausea, diarrhea, vomiting, ↑ intestinal activity or rupture, and muscle weakness
NOTES		• Atropine can be used to counteract effects of neostigmine and physostigmine • Physostigmine crosses blood–brain barrier
	• Also used as a bronchospasm manager	

Table 9-37 Neurologic Drugs: Autonomic Nervous System

Drug Class	Autonomic Nervous System	
	Adrenergic Agents: ALPHA Stimulators	
DRUG (TRADE NAME)	• Methoxamine (Vasoxyl)	• Ephedrine (Vatronol)
ACTION	• Peripheral vasoconstriction	• Alpha receptor stimulant
INDICATIONS	• Anesthetic hypotension	• ↑ Blood pressure, bronchodilator, nasal decongestant, and to control urinary incontinence by increased smooth muscle sphincter tone in urethra
DISPENSIBLE FORMS	• Injectable (IM, IV)	• Capsule, injectable
PRECAUTIONS		• Use caution with patients currently taking sodium bicarbonate or amitriptyline
CONTRAINDICATIONS		
PATIENT CARE/CLIENT EDUCATION	• Monitor for tachycardia, hypertension, nervousness, and cardiac dysrhythmias	• Monitor for tachycardia, hypertension, excitability, and urine retention
NOTES		

Table 9-38 Neurologic Drugs: CNS

Drug Class	Central Nervous System Anticonvulsants			
DRUG (TRADE NAME)	• Diazepam (Valium and Valrelease)	• Pentobarbital (Nembutal)	• Phenobarbital (Luminal)	• Potassium Bromide (KBr)
ACTION	• Potentiates inhibitory actions of GABA	• Potentiates inhibitory actions of GABA	• Potentiates inhibitory actions of GABA	• Stabilized neuronal cell membranes
INDICATIONS	• Appetite stimulant, behavioral issues, or urethral obstruction • Poisoning (chocolate, nicotine, amphetamine, strychnine, or salicylate) • Seizuring animals	• Seizuring animals	• Seizuring animals	• Seizuring animals
DISPENSIBLE FORMS	• Tablet, solution, and injectable	• Injectable	• Tablet, capsule, powder, elixir, and injectable	• Solution
PRECAUTIONS			• Use with caution with hepatic disease • If given with erythromycin, ketoconazole, or propanolol, excessive sedation may occur	

CONTRA-INDICATIONS				
PATIENT CARE	• Monitor for sedation, cardiac or respiratory depression, anxiety, incoordination, agitation, polyphagia, aggression, PU/PD, and lethargy	• Monitor for respiratory depression	• Monitor for sedation, cardiac or respiratory depression, and polyphagia • Monitor serum phenobarbital levels every 6 months (collect a trough sample just before the next dose)	• Monitor for sedation, cardiac or respiratory depression, dehydration, vomiting, diarrhea, and ataxia • Monitor serum KBr levels every 6 months
NOTES	• Not recommended for use for more than 2 days as an appetite stimulant • A controlled substance • Seizure control duration of 3–4 hours	• Short-acting barbiturate • A controlled substance • Pentobarbital—seizure control duration of 1–3 hours	• Long-acting barbiturate • Phenobarbital causes ↑ metabolism of phenylbutazone, glucocorticoids, estrogens, and methylxanthines, because it is a hepatic enzyme inducer • If using with chloramphenicol, ↓ the dosage of phenobarbital • A controlled substance	• Diets with a high chloride content may require a higher dosaging of KBr. (e.g., Hill's S/D or I/D) • KBr is used with phenobarbital when phenobarbital is not totally effective alone

Table 9-39   Neurologic Drugs: Euthanasia Agents—Muscle Relaxers

Drug Class	Euthanasia Agents	Muscle Relaxers
DRUG (TRADE NAME)	• Pentobarbital sodium (Sleepaway, Beuthanasia-D, Euthanasia-6, Fatal-Plus)	• Methocarbamol (Robaxin, Robaxin-V)
ACTION	• Produces unconsciousness and cessation of all vital functions	• Depresses polysynaptic reflexes
INDICATIONS	• Euthanize	• Muscular spasm
DISPENSIBLE FORMS	• Solution and powder	• Tablet and injectable
PRECAUTIONS	• Handle with care and avoid contact with open wounds	
CONTRAINDICATIONS		• Renal disease or pregnant animals
PATIENT CARE/CLIENT EDUCATION		• Monitor for sedation, vomiting, weakness, and ataxia
NOTES	• Pentobarbital sodium products are controlled substances • Medications must be given as prescribed to be effective	

OPHTHALMIC DRUGS

Table 9-40   Ophthalmic Drugs

Drug Class	Adrenergic Agonist	Carbonic Anhydrase Inhibitors	Immunosuppressant
DRUG (TRADE NAME)	• Epinephrine (Adrenalin)	• Acetazolamide (Acetazolam, Diamox) • Dichlorphenamide (Daranide)	• Cyclosporine (Optimmune, Sandimmune)
ACTION	• Reduces intraocular pressure	• Reduces the production of the aqueous humor at cellular pump level	• Inhibits B- and T- lymphocyte activation
INDICATIONS	• Intraocular pressure • Diagnose Horner's syndrome	• Glaucoma	• Chronic keratoconjunctivitis sicca
DISPENSIBLE FORMS	• Injectable	• Tablet	• Ointment
PRECAUTIONS	• Potentially toxic effects when used with sympathomimetic agents	• Use with caution in animals sensitive to sulfonamides	• Cimetidine, erythromycin, and ketoconazole ↑ cyclosporine concentration
CONTRA-INDICATIONS	• Closed-angle glaucoma (mydriasis can exacerbate glaucoma)	• Obstructive pulmonary disease, hyponatremia, hypokalemia, hyperchloremic acidosis, liver or renal disease, or adrenocortical insufficency	• IV injection may cause acute anaphylactoid reactions in dogs
PATIENT CARE/ CLIENT EDUCATION	• Monitor for local irritation	• Monitor for hypokalemia, weakness, polyuria, dysuria, vomiting, diarrhea, panting, and skin rash • Chronic users should monitor serum potassium levels	• Monitor for vomiting, diarrhea, anorexia, gingival hyperplasia, pyoderma, and papillomatosis
NOTES			• May also be used in management of autoimmune disease, perianal fistulae, and organ/tissue rejection

Table 9-41   Ophthalmic Drugs: Miotics—Stains

Drug Class	Miotics	Mydriatics and Cycloplegics	Topical Anesthetics	Stains
DRUG (TRADE NAME)	• Carbachol (Carbacel, Carbamylcholine chloride)	• Atropine sulfate	• Proparacaine hydrochloride (Ophthaine, AK-Taine, Alcaine, Kainair, Ocu-Caine, and Ophthetic)	• Fluorescein strips (Fluorets)
ACTION	• Increases outflow of aqueous humor by miosis	• Dilation of the pupils and paralyzation of the ciliary body muscle	• Desensitizes cornea and conjunctiva	• Adheres to corneal stroma, not intact epithelium
INDICATIONS	• Reduces intraocular pressure, stimulates tear production, chronic open-angle glaucoma, and closed-angle glaucoma	• Acute inflammatory conditions	• Anesthesize the cornea for examination	• Diagnose anterior and posterior segments and in the patency of the nasolacrimal system
DISPENSIBLE FORMS	• Solution and injectable	• Ointment and injectable	• Drops	• Paper strips
PRECAUTIONS			• Use cautiously in animals with allergies, cardiac disease, and hyperthyroidism • Wear gloves when dispensing	• Fluorescein will stain the patient's fur
CONTRA-INDICATIONS	• Cardiac or respiratory disease, GIT obstruction, and aged animals • Pregnant animals	• Glaucoma, KCS, asthma, paralytic ileus, and adhesions between the iris and lens		
PATIENT CARE/ CLIENT EDUCATION	• Monitor for hypotension and bronchoconstriction	• Monitor for salivation	• Monitor for local irritation	
NOTES				• Store open bottles in the refrigerator • Discard any discolored solutions • Not meant for long-term usage

OTIC DRUGS

Table 9-42 Otic Drugs

Drug Class	Topical Anti-Infective			
DRUG (TRADE NAME)	• Chloramphenicol with prednisolone, tetracaine, and cerumene (Liquichlor)	• Dimethyl sulfoxide with fluocinolone acetonide (Synotic)	• Gentamicin sulfate with betamethasone valerate and clotrimazole (Gentocin Otic Solution, Otomax)	• Thiabendazole, neomycin, and dexamethasone (Tresaderm)
ACTION	• Bactericidal, anti-inflammatory, and anesthetic	• Bacteriostatic, fungicidal	• Bactericidal, fungicidal, and anti-inflammatory	• Bactericidal and anti-inflammatory
INDICATIONS	• Acute otitis externa and pyoderma	• Acute/chronic otitis and pruritis	• Otitis (dogs) and superficial infected lesions (cats)	• Otitis externa and inflammatory dermatoses
DISPENSIBLE FORMS	• Solution	• Liquid	• Ointment and solution	• Solution
PRECAUTIONS	• Wear gloves when administering	• Wear gloves when administering	• Remove any debris before administration	• Remove any debris before administration
CONTRA-INDICATIONS		• Pregnant animals • Ocular, renal, or liver disease • Animals < 4.5 kg	• Ruptured eardrums • Pregnant animals	• Ruptured eardrums
PATIENT CARE/ CLIENT EDUCATION	• Monitor for PU/PD and weight gain	• Monitor for erythema, pruritis, or pain	• Monitor for ototoxicity, emesis, PU/PD, diarrhea, erythema, stinging, blistering, peeling edema, pruritis, and urticaria	• Monitor for tachycardia, ototoxity, erythema, increased thirst, weakness, lethargy, oliguria, vomiting, and diarrhea
NOTES		• May result in oyster-like breath • Inactive in purulent exudates	• Monitor for Cushing's with prolonged usage	• Store in the refrigerator • Do not use for more than 1 week

RENAL/URINARY DRUGS

Table 9-43 Renal/Urinary Drugs

Drug Class	Acidifiers		Adrenergic Agent: Beta Inhibitor	Alpha-Adrenergic Agent: Alpha Blocker
DRUG (TRADE NAME)	• Ammonium chloride	• dl-methionine (Racemethione, Uroeze, Methio-Tabs)	• Phenylpropanolamine (Proin, Propagest)	• Phenoxybenzamine (Dibenzyline)
ACTION	• Acidifies urine	• Acidifies urine	• ↑ Smooth muscle sphincter tone in urethra	• Binds with alpha −1 receptor on smooth muscles
INDICATIONS	• Metabolic acidosis, urinary tract infection, struvite urolithiasis	• Struvite urolithiasis	• Urinary incontinence	• Vasodilator, urethral obstruction to reduce urethral sphincter tone (cats)
DISPENSIBLE FORMS	• Tablet and granule	• Tablet, powder, and gel	• Tablet, capsule, and drops	• Capsule
PRECAUTIONS			• Use caution in patients on NSAIDs or animals wearing tick preventive collars (amitraz)	
CONTRA-INDICATIONS	• Severe hepatic disease, renal failure, and pregnant animals	• Metabolic acidosis, renal/hepatic function impairment, pancreatic disease, and kittens	• Patients currently on Anipryl (l-deprenyl) • Heart disease, hypertension, glaucoma, diabetes mellitus, and hyperthyroid	• Cardiovascular disease
PATIENT CARE/CLIENT EDUCATION	• Monitor for nausea and vomiting			• Monitor for hypotension, tachycardia, muscle tremors, seizures, ↑ intraocular pressure, nausea, and vomiting
NOTES	• Poor palatability		• May be used in conjunction with DES if it is ineffective alone	

Table 9-44 Renal/Urinary Drugs: Anabolic Steroid—Tricyclic Antidepressant

Drug Class	Anabolic Steroid	Cholinergic: Direct acting agonists	Enzyme Inhibitor	Tricyclic Antidepressant
DRUG (TRADE NAME)	• Nandrolone deconate (Deca-Durabolin) • Stanozolol (Winstrol-V)	• Bethanechol chloride (Urecholine and Duvoid)	• Allopurinol (Zyloprim, Lopurin)	• Amitriptyline (Elavil)
ACTION	• Reverses catabolic conditions	• Mimics the action of acetylcholine	• Inhibits xanthine oxidase enzyme and blocks the formation of uric acid	• Inhibits uptake of serotonin
INDICATIONS	• Chronic renal failure	• ↑ Contraction of urinary bladder	• Canine urolithiasis or canine leishmaniasis	• Inappropriate feline urination
DISPENSIBLE FORMS	• Tablet and injectable (IM)	• Tablet, solution, and injectable	• Tablet	• Tablet and syrup
PRECAUTIONS	• May ↑ the effects of anticoagulants	• Administer SC only (bethanechol)	• Use with caution if animal has renal disease or is using azathioprine	• ECG screening is recommended before administration • Use with caution in animals with diabetes mellitus, hyperthyroid, and renal/hepatic disease
CONTRA-INDICATIONS	• Cardiac/renal insufficiency, hypercalcemia, neoplastic disease, and pregnant animals	• Obstructive pulmonary disease, bronchial asthma, epilepsy, hyperthyroidism, cystitis, and urethral obstruction • Patient currently being administered neostigmine		• Cardiac disease, diabetic animals, urinary retention, seizure history (drug ↓ seizure threshold) • Animals on Anipryl (monoamine oxidase inhibitor) • Pregnant animals
PATIENT CARE	• Monitor for hepatotoxicity • Monitor blood glucose	• Monitor for arrhythmias, hypotension, and bronchospasm	• Administer after a meal • Monitor for skin reactions	• Monitor for hyperexcitability, vomiting, constipation, arrhythmias, dry mouth, ataxia, and sedation • Periodic liver enzyme analysis recommended (metabolized by the liver)
NOTES				• Also used for excessive grooming or separation anxiety in dogs and cats

REPRODUCTIVE SYSTEM DRUGS

Table 9-45   Reproductive System Drugs

Drug Class	Androgens	Estrogens	Gonadotropins
DRUG (TRADE NAME)	• Methyltestosterone (Android) • Testosterone cypionate (DEPO-Testosterone) • Testosterone enanthate (Malogex) • Testosterone propionate (Testex)	• Mibolerone (Cheque drops) • Diethylstilbestrol (DES)	• Gonadorelin (Cystorelin and Factrel)
ACTION	• Releases free testosterone	• Blocks release of LH (luteinizing hormone) • Stimulates and maintains normal female physiologic reproductive processes and enhances sphincter tone	• Stimulates release of LH and follicle-stimulating hormone (FSH)
INDICATIONS	• Testosterone replacement therapy	• Prevent estrus and treat pseudocyesis and galactorrhea • Abortion • Previously used to treat estrogen-responsive incontinence (DES)	• Diagnose reproductive failure, identify intact animals, and induce estrus
DISPENSIBLE FORMS	• Tablet and injectable	• Solution • Tablet and injectable	• Injectable

PRECAUTIONS	• Use with caution with hepatic, renal, and cardiac disease • May ↓ blood glucose concentrations
CONTRA-INDICATIONS	• Prostatic carcinoma • Cats and Bedlington terriers • Perianal adenoma, perianal adenocarcinoma, liver and renal disease • Pregnant animals
PATIENT CARE/ CLIENT EDUCATION	• Monitor for prostatic hyperplasia (male dogs), masculinization (female dogs), and hepatopathy • Monitor immature females for premature epiphyseal closure and vaginitis • Monitor mature females for vulvovaginitis, clitoral hypertrophy, mounting behavior, seizures, and ↑ body odor • Monitor for endometrial hyperplasia, pyometra, leukopenia, thrombocytopenia, and fatal aplastic anemia
NOTES	• Testosterones are administered IM • Methyltestosterone is administered orally

Table 9-46 Reproductive System Drugs: Oxytocin—Prostaglandin

Drug Class	Oxytocin	Progestins	Prostaglandin
DRUG (TRADE NAME)	• Oxytocin (Pitocin and Syntocinon)	• Megestrol acetate (Ovaban, Megace) • Medroxyprogesterone acetate (Depo-Provera, Provera)	• Prostaglandin F-2α (Lutalyse)
ACTION	• Stimulates uterine muscle contraction	• Suppresses secretion of FSH and LH	• Contracts the myometrium and relaxes the cervix
INDICATIONS	• Induce or continue labor and stimulate milk letdown	• Control estrus cycle, behavior management, dermatologic disorders, and benign prostatic hyperplasia	• Open pyometra and abortion
DISPENSIBLE FORMS	• Injectable and intranasal solution	• Tablet and injectable	• Injectable
PRECAUTIONS			
CONTRA-INDICATIONS	• Dystocia or closed cervix	• Reproductive problems or mammary tumors • Pregnant animals	
PATIENT CARE/CLIENT EDUCATION	• Monitor for fetal stress and progression of labor, listlessness, depression, seizure	• Monitor for PU/PD, adrenal suppression, diabetes, weight gain, immunosuppression, pyometra, diarrhea, and neoplasia	• Monitor for tachycardia, vocalization, panting, fever, vomiting, diarrhea, and abdominal discomfort
NOTES		• Inguinal area is recommended site of injection (medroxyprogesterone)	• Walking the animal for 20–40 minutes after administration tends to → side effects (1)

(1)Handbook of Veterinary Drugs, Dana Allen.

RESPIRATORY DRUGS

Table 9-47 Respiratory Drugs

Drug Class	Antitussives		
DRUG (TRADE NAME)	• Codeine phosphate (Methylmorphine)	• Dextromethorphan (Benylin)	• Hydrocodone (Hycodan and Tussigon)
ACTION	• Suppresses the cough center in the brainstem	• Suppresses the cough center in the brainstem	• Suppresses the cough center in the brainstem
INDICATIONS	• Nonproductive cough (dog)	• Nonproductive cough (dog)	• Nonproductive cough (dog)
DISPENSIBLE FORMS	• Tablet, syrup, and solution	• Tablet, syrup, and solution	• Tablet and syrup
PRECAUTIONS	• Use with caution in seizure and cardiac patients		• Use with caution in aged patients, liver and kidney impairment, hypothyroidism, Addison's, and narrow-angle glaucoma
CONTRA-INDICATIONS	• Liver disease and GIT dysfunction		
PATIENT CARE/CLIENT EDUCATION	• Monitor for sedation and constipation	• Monitor for sedation and constipation	• Monitor for sedation and constipation
NOTES		• 15–20 times less potent than butorphanol	

Table 9-48 Respiratory Drugs: Bronchodilators—Mucolytics

Drug Class	Bronchodilators	Mucolytics
DRUG (TRADE NAME)	*Beta-adrenergic agonists:* • Albuterol (Ventolin, Proventil) • Epinephrine (Adrenalin) • Terbutaline (Brethine, Bricanyl) *Methylxanthines:* • Aminophylline (Phylloconton) • Theophylline (Theo-Dur, Theolair, Quibron-T/SR, Slo-Bid)	• Acetylcysteine (Mucomyst)
ACTION	• Stimulates sympathetic nervous system receptors involved in bronchodilation and inhibits histamine release • Inhibits phosphodiesterase	• ↓ Viscosity of secretions
INDICATIONS	• Bronchospasm	• Bronchial nebulizing • Acetaminophen toxicity
DISPENSIBLE FORMS	• Tablet and solution • Tablet, caplet, and injectable	• Solution
PRECAUTIONS	• Do not use terbutaline within 14 days of an MAO inhibitor • Barbiturates ↑ metabolism (methylxanthines)	• Oral administration can cause nausea or vomiting • Use with caution in patients with asthma
CONTRA-INDICATIONS	• Cardiovascular disease, hyperthyroid, and diabetes mellitus • Pregnant animals • Cardiovascular disease, hyperthyroid, diabetes mellitus, glaucoma, gastric ulcers, liver and kidney disease • Pregnant animals	
PATIENT CARE	• Monitor for tachycardia, hypertension, muscle tremors, nervousness, fear, depression, vomiting, urine retention, site irritation, and panting • Monitor serum levels 29–30 hours (dogs) and 40 hours (for cats) after therapy initiation and just before the next dose (theophylline) • Monitor for tachycardia, hypertension, hyperglycemia, muscle tremors, nervousness, fear, depression, vomiting, polyphagia, and panting	• Monitor for nausea and vomiting
NOTES	• Onset of action is 15–30 minutes; duration ≤ 8 hours • Metabolized by the liver • Do not inject air into aminophylline vials to avoid precipitation • Onset of action is 15–30 min; duration ≤ 8 hours (extended release: ≥ 12 hours) • Check drug interactions when combining with other drugs • Metabolized by the liver	• Drug has a bad taste

Table 9-49   Respiratory Drugs: Stimulants

Drug Class	Stimulants		
DRUG (TRADE NAME)	Doxapram HCl (Dopram)	Naloxone (Narcan)	Yohimbine (Yobine, Antagonil)
ACTION	Stimulates the respiratory center of the brainstem	↑ Cardiac output, ↑ arterial blood pressure, ↓ hemoconcentration, ↓ metabolic acidosis, and helps prevent hypoglycemia	α_2-Adrenergic blocking agent
INDICATIONS	Depressed anesthetic respiration and neonate resuscitation	Narcotic-induced respiratory depression	Xylazine overdose
DISPENSIBLE FORMS	Injectable	Injectable	Injectable
PRECAUTIONS	Do not mix with alkaline solutions		
CONTRA-INDICATIONS			
PATIENT CARE/ CLIENT EDUCATION	Monitor for hypertension, arrhythmias, coughing, dyspnea, hyperventilation, laryngospasm, muscle tremors, seizures, vomiting, and diarrhea	Monitor for seizures if high dosaging is used	
NOTES			

TOXICOLOGIC DRUGS

Table 9-50 Toxicologic Drugs

Drug Class	Chelating	Chelating	Synthetic alcohol dehydrogenase inhibitor
DRUG (TRADE NAME)	• Dimercaprol (BAL)	• d-Penicillamine (Cuprimine, Depen)	• 4-Methylpyrazole, (Fomepizole, Antizol-Vet)
ACTION	• Chelates arsenic, lead, mercury, and gold	• Chelates cystine, lead, copper, and promotes excretion	• Inhibits dehydrogenase enzyme
INDICATIONS	• Arsenic, lead, mercury or gold poisoning	• Copper or lead toxicity • Hepatitis due to copper • Cystine urolithiasis	• Ethylene glycol toxicity
DISPENSIBLE FORMS	• Injectable	• Tablet and capsule	• Injectable (IV)
PRECAUTIONS		• Use with caution in patients who are renal impaired	
CONTRA-INDICATIONS	• Hepatic insufficiency	• Pregnant animals	
PATIENT CARE	• Monitor for vomiting, tachycardia, tremors, seizures, and coma	• Administer on an empty stomach (1–2 hours before a meal) • Monitor for vomiting	• Monitor for CNS depression, decrease appetite, weight loss, and sweet breath
NOTES	• IM injection is painful • Can form toxic compounds with iron, selenium, uranium, and cadmium		• Not as effective as ethanol in cats • Should be administered within 8 hours of ingestion

Chapter **10**

Radiography

RADIOLOGY

Radiographs are an extremely useful diagnostic tool for the veterinarian. However, to be diagnostic, the radiograph must reflect proper measurement and positioning of the patient. Veterinary technicians are a valuable resource in the production of these radiographs. An understanding of the anatomic layout of the species and the manner in which a radiograph is taken is of great assistance to the production of a diagnostic radiograph. This chapter deals with basic review information of radiographic equipment, imaging factors, positioning information, and contrast radiography.

Table 10-1   Radiographic Equipment

Equipment	Description	Maintenance
Processing Tanks	• Develops the film • May be manual or automatic	• Clean routinely, and replenish liquids as needed • Clean thoroughly every 2–3 months • Check manufacturer's guidelines for your specific machine
Film	• Imprints the image (various types)	• Handle carefully • Store in a vertical position in a cool, dry, dark place
Cassettes	• Houses the film and intensifying screens	• Do not drop or allow leaking liquids into the cassette • Clean the exterior regularly with mild soap and water • Clean the intensifying screens routinely with a commercial solution, mild soap and water, or dilute ethyl alcohol • Leave the cassette open and propped in a vertical position to dry • Store in a vertical position when loaded with film
Protective Apparel	• Aprons • Thyroid shields • Gloves • Dosimeter	• Hang aprons vertically or lay flat • Gloves should be placed on vertical holders or over bottomless soup cans to allow airflow and avoid cracks in the lead lining • Radiograph all apparel quarterly to assess protectiveness of shield and check for cracks, tears, or other irregularities

Table 10-2   Radiographic Exposure and Image Factors

Factor	Definition	Application
Contrast	• The difference between the lightest and darkest part of the film, reflecting two adjacent radiographic densities	• High kVp (low contrast) for tissue • Low kVp (high contrast) for bone
Density	• The degree of "blackness" of a film	• To produce a darker film ↑ mA, kVp, or exposure time
Detail	• The "clarity" of the image on the film	• For better detail: use longer source–image distance (SID), have the patient closer to the film, and a shorter exposure time
Distortion	• The alteration of the original image	• For less distortion: use short SID, have the patient closer to the film, and less angulation of the film or patient
Exposure Time (s)	• Measures the length of time electrons are allowed to flow across the tube	• Longer exposure time = production of more X-rays • **mA-s** is the product of milliamperage and the exposure time. It indicates the number of X-rays being produced during an exposure • Using a high mA setting allows for the use of shorter exposure times
Grid Factor	• The increase in exposure to compensate absorption by the grid device	• Used in the formation of a technique chart (part of Santes' Rule)
Kilovoltage peak (**kVp**)	• Measurement of the electric potential difference between the cathode and anode in the X-ray tube	• Higher kVp = greater penetration • Directly proportional to film density and inversely proportional to film contrast
Milliamperage (**mA**)	• Measurement of the number of electrons that flow across the tube from cathode to anode	• Higher mA = production of more X-rays • Directly proportional to film density
Source image distance (**SID**); previously known as Focal spot to film distance (**FFD**)	• The distance between the focal spot on the target anode and the radiographic film	• ↑ SID= a ↓ in the number of X-rays reaching the film

TECHNIQUE CHARTS

Every clinic with an X-ray machine should have a technique chart that has been assessed by the local radiologist to fit your particular machine. These charts significantly decrease the time involved in the calculation of the machine settings and thereby reduce the time spent on taking each radiograph. The chart also ensures consistency among the personnel using the machine. Factors involved in a technique chart are the species, the anatomic region, the X-ray machine, screen type, and the film type. The basic steps to set up a technique chart are:

1. Choose an animal of respective size to reflect its species (i.e., canine—an animal around 50 pounds; feline—an animal around 9 pounds).

2. Measure the animal laterally around the thickest part of the thorax. Set standard SID as a constant (40).

3. Calculate the kVp requirement using Santes' Rule:

   (2 × tissue thickness in cm) + SID + Grid Factor = kVp

   Example.: (2 ×15 cm) + 40 (SID) + 8 (Grid Factor) = 78 kVp

4. Determine mA-s requirement based on the following chart:

Fast/Hi-speed Screens	Average Dog	Medium/Par Speed Screens
mA-s	Anatomical Region	mA-s
2.5	Extremity	5.0
5.0	Thorax	7.5
7.5	Abdomen	10.0
10.0	Pelvis	12.5

Average Cat: mA-s is recommended at 1.5

5. Determine the mA and exposure time with emphasis on the highest mA possible. Divide mA by mA-s to get exposure time (seconds).

   Example: 300 divided by 5.0 = 1/60

6. Take a trial radiograph of the animal, using the calculated factors and assess its quality. Modify the mA-s by 30%–50% in the appropriate direction and retake the radiograph.

7. Once a diagnostic radiograph is produced, use these factor numbers to start your chart. This will need to be repeated for the various areas of the body and for each species. See guidelines below for the chart making:

For each cm change, add or subtract 2 kVp, up to 80 kVp
For each cm change, add or subtract 3 kVp, from 80–100 kVp
For each cm change, add or subtract 4 kVp, above 100 kVp

8. Modifications to this method would include:

   a. Pleural fluid or ascites or obvious organ enlargement (e.g., cardiomegaly) (↑ mA-s 50%)

   b. Obesity, heavily muscled dogs, or contrast studies (↑ mA-s 50%)

   c. Excessively thin animals or puppies/kittens (↓ mA-s by 50%)

The following charts reflect two different styles of a technique chart. It is helpful to have your chart reviewed by your area radiologist.

EXAMPLE 1: VETERINARY X-RAY TECHNIQUE GUIDE

The following is for use with: QUANTA 3 screens　　SID is 40"　　Grid ratio is 8:1
CRONEX 7 film
Kodak LANEX REGULAR
Kodak TMG-1 film.

	mA	Time	mA-s	kVp
SKULL				
Small Dogs and Cats	300		3.3	$(2 \times cm) + 55$ kVp
Medium and Large Dogs	300	1/60	5	$(2 \times cm) + 55$ kVp
CERVICAL				
Small Dogs and Cats	300	1/60	5	$(2 \times cm) + 50$ kVp
Medium and Large Dogs	300	1/30	10	$(2 \times cm) + 48$ kVp
THORAX				
Small Dogs and Cats	300		3.3	$(2 \times cm) + 43$ kVp
Medium and Large Dogs	300	1/60	5	$(2 \times cm) + 43$ kVp
ABDOMEN & THORACIC SPINE				
Small Dogs and Cats	300	1/60	5	$(2 \times cm) + 45$ kVp
Medium and Large Dogs	300	1/30	10	$(2 \times cm) + 50$ kVp
PELVIS				
Small Dogs and Cats	300	1/60	5	$(2 \times cm) + 52$ kVp
Medium and Large Dogs	300	1/30	10	$(2 \times cm) + 52$ kVp
Extra-Large Dogs	300	1/30	10	$(2 \times cm) + 60$ kVp
EXTREMITIES: Femur & Humerus				
Small Dogs and Cats	300	1/45	6.6	$(2 \times cm) + 45$ kVp
Medium and Large Dogs	300	1/30	10	$(2 \times cm) + 45$ kVp
EXTREMITIES: Radius & Ulna				
Small Dogs and Cats	300	1/45	6.6	$(2 \times cm) + 45$ kVp
Medium and Large Dogs	300	1/30	10	$(2 \times cm) + 45$ kVp

EXAMPLE 2: VETERINARY X-RAY TECHNIQUE CHART

Cm	BONE 300 mA				CHEST 300 mA				ABDOMEN 300 mA			
	Time	Table kVp		Grid kVp	Time	Table kVp		Grid kVp	Time	Table kVp		Grid kVp
4	1/30	42		-	1/60	44		-	1/30	-		-
5	"			-	"	46		-	"	-		-
6	"	45		-	"	48		-	"	-		-
7	"			55	"	50		-	"	-		-
8	"			57	"	52		-	1/15	-		51
9	"	46		59	"	54		-	"	-		53
10	"	-		61	"	56		-	"	-		55
11	"	-		63	"	58		-	"	-		57
12	"	-		65	"	60		74	"	-		59
13	"	-		67	"	62		76	"	-		61
14	"	-		69	"	64		78	"	-		63
15	"	-		71	"	66		80	"	-		65
16	"	-		73	"	68		82	"	-		67
17	"	-		75	"	-		85	"	-		69
18	"	-		77	"	-		88	"	-		71
19	"	-		79	"	-		91	"	-		73
20	"	-		81	"	-		95	"	-		75
21	"	-		84	"	-		99	"	-		77
22	"	-		87	"	-		103	"	-		79
23	"	-		90	"	-		103	"	-		82
24	"	-		94	1/30	-		96	"	-		85
25	"	-		96	"	-		100	"	-		88
26	"	-		103	"	-		105	"	-		91
27	"	-		108	"	-		110	"	-		95

ARTIFACTS

Table 10-3 Artifacts on Radiographs

Problems Seen on Radiograph	Artifact	Solution
Blurred images	• Motion • Double exposure	• Proper positioning and handling of animal • Double-check cassette tray for foreign objects
Clear areas on the sides of the radiograph	• Film fog • Mislocation of beam to film	• Proper handling of film • Verification that the beam and cassette are aligned
Dark line with mirror image of object	• Film folded on itself	• Proper loading of cassette
Dark semicircle impression	• Finger pressure mark	• Proper handling of film
Dark striations (sea lichen or dotted)	• Static electricity	• Proper handling of film
Gray streaks	• Wet animal fur	• Clean off and dry animal before radiographing
Lines or objects visualized outside/inside the animal's body that are unexplainable	• Foreign objects in or on the cassette (hair, paper, etc.)	• Proper cleaning of cassette • Proper handling of film
White lines across the film	• Scratches on the film	• Proper handling of film

RADIOGRAPHIC POSITIONING

The most important factor in positioning a patient for radiographs is to have a mental vision of the part of the body to be radiographed and a good understanding of its anatomic placement. A second important factor is to use supports to ensure that the patient is aligned properly and to decrease the operator's exposure. These supports can include sandbags, non-radiopaque wedges, non-radiopaque "V" troughs, gauze, and tape. Depending on the species, size, and condition of the animal being radiographed, the following positioning guidelines may need to be adjusted accordingly.

SOFT TISSUES

Table 10-4   Soft Tissues

Anatomic Area	Pharynx	Thorax			Abdomen	
VIEW	Lateral	Lateral	V/D	D/V	Lateral	V/D
POSITIONING	• Lateral recumbency • Forelimbs flexed caudally • Head should be parallel to the table (may require support) and neck extended	• Lateral recumbency • Forelimbs and head extended cranially • Rear limbs extended caudally (When assessing: *Lungs = Left* side down; *Heart = Right* side down; but may need both sides taken)	• Dorsal recumbency • Forelimbs extended cranially • Rear limbs flexed	• Sternal recumbency • Forelimbs extended caudally and elbows abducted • Head lies low between forelimbs • Rear limbs in crouching position	• Right lateral recumbency • Forelimbs extended cranially • Hindlimbs extended caudally	• Dorsal recumbency • Forelimbs extended cranially and parallel • Hindlimbs extended caudally and parallel
MEASUREMENT	• Base of the skull	• Widest area of ribcage	• Widest area of ribcage	• Widest area of ribcage	• Caudal aspect of the 13th rib or widest area	• Caudal aspect of the 13th rib or widest area
BEAM CENTER	• Just caudal the base of the skull	• Caudal border of scapula	• Caudal border of scapula (6th rib)	• Caudal border of scapula (6th rib)	• Caudal aspect of the 13th rib	• Caudal aspect of the 13th rib
FIELD OF VIEW	• Lateral canthus to C3	• Thoracic inlet to the last rib	• Thoracic inlet to the last rib	• Thoracic inlet to the last rib	• 2–3 inches cranial to xyphoid process of sternum to the femoral head	• 2–3 inches cranial to xyphoid process of sternum to the femoral head

Table 10-4 **Soft Tissues (Continued)**

Anatomic Area	Pharynx		Thorax			Abdomen	
VIEW	Lateral		Lateral	V/D	D/V	Lateral	V/D
SPECIAL ADJUSTMENTS	• None		• *Pneumothorax/emphysema*: ↓ exposure • *Pulmonary edema/hemorrhage/severe cardiomyopathy/diaphragmatic hernia*: ↑ exposure			• *Fat/obese*: ↑ exposure • *Young or malnutritioned*: ↓ exposure	
NOTES	• On image, the wings of atlas (C2) should be superimposed (minimize cervical rotation)		• Taken on peak inspiration • If pneumothorax is suspected, expiratory radiographs may also be required • May require support (wedges) to keep sternum in line with thoracic vertebrae	• Taken on peak inspiration • If pneumothorax is suspected, expiratory radiographs also may be required • Restraining the animal at the scapula/armpits results in a straighter thorax	• Taken on peak inspiration • If pneumothorax is suspected, expiratory radiographs also may be required • Preferred view for cardiac evaluation or for animal in respiratory distress	• Taken on expiratory pause • A left lateral may also be requested • Two films may be needed with large dogs	• Taken on expiratory pause • Two films may be needed with large dogs

HEAD

Ensuring that the skull is level to the cassette is extremely important in producing a diagnostic radiograph. Supports strategically placed under the muzzle, neck, or cranium will assist in this endeavor.

Table 10-5 Head: Skull

Anatomic Area	Skull		
VIEW	Lateral	D/V	V/D	Cranium—Rostrocaudal
POSITIONING	• Lateral recumbency • Foam wedge placed under the mandible to make muzzle parallel • Nasal septum parallel to cassette • Forelimbs extended caudally	• Sternal recumbency • Head is parallel to the cassette • Forelimbs are relaxed with carpus flexed and out of the beam	• Dorsal recumbency • Head is extended on cassette with support under the mid-cervical region to keep proper alignment • Nose is parallel to cassette • Skull is level on the cassette • Forelimbs extended caudally	• Dorsal recumbency • Base of skull is resting on cassette with neck in a flexed position and the chin pulled toward the thorax with tape or gauze • Forelimbs extended caudally
MEASUREMENT	• Highest point of zygomatic arch	• Widest point of cranium	• Lateral canthus of eye	• Frontal sinuses
BEAM CENTER	• Lateral canthus of eye	• Lateral canthus of eye	• Lateral canthus of eye	• Between the eyes
FIELD OF VIEW	• Tip of nose to base of skull	• Tip of nose to base of skull	• Tip of nose to base of skull	• Entire cranium
NOTES	• May require heavy sedation or general anesthesia	• May require heavy sedation or general anesthesia	• May require heavy sedation or general anesthesia	• May require heavy sedation or general anesthesia • Monitor for crimping if endotracheal tube is in place

Table 10-6 Head: Zygomatic Arch

Anatomic Area	Zygomatic Arch				
VIEW	Lateral	D/V	Frontal	Lateral oblique	V/D-open mouth
POSITIONING	• Lateral recumbency • Foam wedge placed under mandible • Nasal septum parallel to cassette • Forelimbs extended caudally	• Sternal recumbency • Head is resting on the cassette • Forelimbs are relaxed with carpus flexed and out of the beam	• Dorsal recumbency • Head is resting on cassette with neck in a relaxed flexed position • Nose is slightly off perpendicular to X-ray beam • Skull is level on the cassette • Forelimbs extended caudally	• Lateral recumbency • Cranium supported with wedge to achieve the oblique angle of the arch • Nasal septum perpendicular to cassette	• Dorsal recumbency • Head is extended with support under the mid-cervical region • Mandible supported open using gauze • Skull is level on the cassette • Forelimbs extended caudally
MEASUREMENT	• Highest point of zygomatic arch	• Highest point of cranium	• Lateral canthus of eye	• Highest point of cranium	• Lateral canthus of eye
BEAM CENTER	• Lateral canthus of eye	• Lateral canthus of eye	• Lateral canthus of eye	• Slight off center from mid-cranium	• At a 45 degree angle to the maxilla between the upper 3rd and 4th premolars
FIELD OF VIEW	• Tip of nose to base of skull	• Tip of nose to base of skull	• Tip of nose to base of skull	• Tip of nose to base of skull	• Nasal cavities to cranial temporal skull
NOTES	• May require heavy sedation or general anesthesia	• May require heavy sedation or general anesthesia	• May require heavy sedation or general anesthesia	• May require heavy sedation or general anesthesia	• Monitor for crimping if endotracheal tube is in place

Table 10-7 Head: Tympanic bullae

Anatomic Area		Tympanic bullae	
VIEW	D/V	Lateral oblique	Rostrocaudal—open mouth
POSITIONING	• Sternal recumbency • Head is resting on the cassette • Forelimbs are relaxed with carpus flexed and out of the beam	• Lateral recumbency • *Unaffected bullae* toward the cassette • Skull slightly oblique • Forelimbs slightly extended caudally	• Dorsal recumbency • Nose is perpendicular to cassette with maxilla and mandible supported open • Base of skull is level on the cassette • Forelimbs extended caudally
MEASUREMENT	• Highest point of cranium	• Level of tympanic bullae	• Level of commissure of lips
BEAM CENTER	• Center of tympanic bullae	• Center of tympanic bullae	• Center of mouth and between commissure of lips
FIELD OF VIEW	• Lateral canthus of eye to base of skull	• Lateral canthus of eye to base of skull	• Entire nasopharyngeal area
NOTES	• Superimposition of cranium makes view of bullae less than ideal; however, it permits comparison of L and R bullae in one view		

Table 10-8 Head: Temporomandibular Joint

Anatomic Area	Temporomandibular Joint	
VIEW	D/V	V/D oblique (Sagittal oblique)
POSITIONING	• Sternal recumbency • Head is resting on the cassette • Forelimbs are relaxed with carpus flexed and out of the beam	• Lateral recumbency • Cranium rotated 20 degrees toward the cassette (with support under mandible)
MEASUREMENT	• Highest point of cranium	• Lateral canthus of eye
BEAM CENTER	• Lateral canthus of eye	• Temporomandibular Joint
FIELD OF VIEW	• Base of the nose to the base of the skull	• Medial canthus of eye to base of skull
NOTES		

Table 10-9 Head: Nasal cavities/sinuses

Anatomical Area	Nasal cavities/sinuses					
VIEW	Lateral	D/V	D/V—occlusal	V/D—open mouth	Lateral oblique	Frontal or rostro-caudal
POSITIONING	• Lateral recumbency • Foam wedge placed under mandible to keep muzzle parallel to cassette • Nasal septum parallel to cassette • Forelimbs extended caudally	• Sternal recumbency • Head is resting on the cassette • Forelimbs are relaxed with carpus flexed and out of the beam	• Sternal recumbency • Head is resting on the cassette • Film is between maxilla and mandible • Forelimbs are relaxed with carpus flexed and out of the beam	• Dorsal recumbency • Forelimbs extended caudally • Head is extended on cassette with support under the mid-cervical region • Nose is parallel to cassette with mandible extended caudally with supports • Maxilla may be taped into position if necessary • Skull is level on the cassette	• Lateral recumbency • Head supported with wedge • Nasal septum perpendicular to cassette	• Dorsal recumbency • Forelimbs extended caudally • Head is resting on cassette with neck in a relaxed flexed position and muzzle pointing up at the tube • Nose is slightly off perpendicular to cassette (10 degrees) • Skull is level on the cassette

Table 10-9 Head: Nasal cavities/sinuses (Continued)

Anatomical Area	Nasal cavities/sinuses					
VIEW	Lateral	D/V	D/V—occlusal	V/D—open mouth	Lateral Oblique	Frontal or rostrocaudal
MEASUREMENT	• Highest point of zygomatic arch	• Highest point of cranium	• Caudal portion of maxilla	• 3rd upper premolar	• Highest point of cranium	• Most caudal aspect of muzzle
BEAM CENTER	• Lateral canthus of eye	• Lateral canthus of eye	• Caudal portion of maxilla	• 15 degrees from vertical with the beam angled into the open mouth between the upper 3rd and 4th premolars	• Lateral canthus of eye	• Between the eyes
FIELD OF VIEW	• Tip of nose to base of skull	• Tip of nose to commissure of lips	• Tip of nose to orbital bones	• Tip of nose to pharyngeal area	• Tip of nose to base of skull	• Tip of nose to base of skull
NOTES			• Best to use "cassette-less" film (e.g., mammography film)	• Remove or tie endotracheal tube to mandible		• Same technique could be used to radiograph the foramen magnum • Remove or tie endotracheal tube to mandible

SPINE

The spine must be kept level as films are taken. A misaligned spine will result in distortion on the radiograph and therefore possibly a nondiagnostic radiograph. Levelness can be accomplished with supports under the mandible, neck, thorax, or between the limbs. A "V" trough or wedges are recommended on all ventrodorsal views to stabilize the body of the animal. Always collimate down to exclude the soft tissues. Most of these positions will require some form of sedation or general anesthesia. Abbreviations have been used to conserve space and are as follows:

O = occipital, A = atlantal, C = cervical vertebra, T = thoracic vertebra, TL = thoracolumbar vertebra, L = lumbar vertebra, S = sacral vertebra

Table 10-10 Spine

Anatomic Area		Cervical			
VIEW	Lateral	V/D	Extended lateral	Flexed lateral	Oblique lateral
POSITIONING	• Lateral recumbency • Forelimbs retracted caudally • O-A joint is flexed at a 45-degree angle • Elevate the mandible to be parallel to table with support • Gauze may be needed around the mouth to keep head pulled slightly forward	• Dorsal recumbency • Forelimbs extended caudally alongside the body • Spine parallel to cassette • Support under the neck can minimize distortion caused by a misaligned vertebra	• Lateral recumbency • Forelimbs extended caudally • Extend the neck dorsally until resistance is met; gauze may be placed around the muzzle • Place support under the mandible and neck to maintain a level spine (especially with long-necked dogs)	• Lateral recumbency • Forelimbs extended caudally • O-A is flexed at a 90-degree angle • Elevate the neck if necessary to keep it level with the spine (wedges) • Pull the lower mandible open with gauze to maintain the 90-degree angle	• Lateral recumbency • Elevate the mandible to be parallel to table with support (wedges) • Elevate the sternum 20-degrees above vertebral level/plane with support (wedges)
MEASUREMENT	• Over C7	• C5/C6	• Thoracic inlet (C7)	• Thoracic inlet (C7)	• Thoracic inlet (C7)
BEAM CENTER	• C4/C5 and vertebral column	• C4/C5 and vertebral column	• C4/C5 and vertebral column	• C4/C5 and vertebral column	• C4/C5 and vertebral column
FIELD OF VIEW	• Caudal skull to T1	• Caudal skull to T1/T2	• Caudal skull to T1/T2	• Caudal skull to T1/T2	• Caudal skull to T1/T2
NOTES	• Two films are recommended for large dogs	• Two films are recommended for large dogs		• Be careful not to over flex the neck, because damage to the trachea can occur	

Table 10-11 Spine: Thoracic–Lumbar

Anatomic Area	Thoracic		Thoracolumbar		Lumbar	
VIEW	Lateral	V/D	Lateral	V/D	Lateral	V/D
POSITIONING	• Lateral recumbency • Forelimbs extended cranially • Hindlimbs extended caudally • Elevate sternum to thoracic vertebrae level to reduce rotational artifact	• Dorsal recumbency • Forelimbs extended cranially • Hindlimbs are in a relaxed position	• Lateral recumbency • Forelimbs slightly extended cranially • Hindlimbs slightly extended caudally	• Dorsal recumbency • Forelimbs extended cranially • Hindlimbs are in a relaxed position	• Lateral recumbency • Forelimbs are in a relaxed position • Hindlimbs are extended caudally with support between them to keep hips parallel to the table	• Dorsal recumbency • Forelimbs extended cranially • Hindlimbs are in a relaxed position
MEASUREMENT	• 7th–8th rib	• Highest point of the sternum	• TL junction	• TL junction	• Thickest area (L1)	• Thickest area (L1)
BEAM CENTER	• T6/T7	• T6/T7 (caudal border of scapula)	• TL junction	• TL junction	• L4	• L4
FIELD OF VIEW	• C7 to L1	• C7 to L1	• T8 to L5	• T8 to L5	• T13 to S1	• T13 to S1
NOTES			• May require support under sternum and mid-lumbar region for prevention of axial rotation artifact		• May require support under sternum and mid-lumbar region for proper alignment and prevention of axial rotation artifact (especially in chondrodystrophic dogs with elongated backs)	

Table 10-12 Spine: Sacrum—Caudal

Anatomic Area	Sacrum			Caudal	
VIEW	Lateral	V/D	Lateral	V/D	
POSITIONING	• Lateral recumbency • Hindlimbs are slightly apart and relaxed with a support between them • Tail is extended caudally, not supported	• Dorsal recumbency • Hindlimbs are relaxed in semiflexion	• Lateral recumbency • Tail is extended caudally and supported as needed to prevent excessive sagging or lateral flexion	• Dorsal recumbency • Hindlimbs are relaxed in semiflexion • Tail is extended straight caudally and supported as needed to prevent excessive sagging or lateral flexion	
MEASUREMENT	• Trochanters	• Mid-sacrum	• Area of concern	• Area of concern	
BEAM CENTER	• Greater femoral trochanter	• At 30-degrees toward pubis	• Area of concern	• Area of concern	
FIELD OF VIEW	• Pelvis to proximal caudal vertebral segments	• L6 to proximal caudal vertebra	• Includes area of concern plus several vertebra on either side	• Includes area of concern plus several vertebra on either side	
NOTES					

SHOULDER AND FORELIMBS

Table 10-13   Shoulder and Forelimbs: Scapula–Shoulder

Anatomic Area	Scapula			Shoulder	
VIEW	Lateral—with tension	Lateral—without tension	Caudocranial	Lateral	Caudocranial
POSITIONING	• Lateral recumbency • Affected forelimb is flexed at the elbow 90-degrees and pulled caudally until the humerus is parallel to the spine and radius/ulna are perpendicular to spine • Unaffected forelimb is extended caudally	• Lateral recumbency • Affected forelimb is extended caudally • Unaffected forelimb is extended cranially	• Dorsal recumbency • Forelimbs are extended cranially • Sternum is rotated slightly away from the scapula of interest (just opposite midline)	• Lateral recumbency • Affected forelimb is extended cranially • Unaffected forelimb is flexed caudodorsally, parallel to the thorax • Head is extended cranially	• Dorsal recumbency • Forelimbs are extended cranially
MEASUREMENT	• Thickest area of shoulder/cranial thorax	• Thickest area of shoulder/cranial thorax	• Thickest area of shoulder	• Over manubrium	• Thickest area of shoulder
BEAM CENTER	• Mid-scapula	• Mid-scapula	• Mid-scapula	• Shoulder joint	• Shoulder joint
FIELD OF VIEW	• Cranial aspect of the shoulder joint to the caudal scapular crest	• Cranial aspect of the shoulder joint to the caudal scapular crest	• Shoulder joint to T6	• Mid-scapula to mid-humerus	• Mid-humerus to mid-scapula
NOTES		• Used when patient is injured or in pain	• Best method for viewing acromial process of scapular spine	• Ensure that the manubrium and cranial sternebrae do not overlap shoulder joint	• Be aware of any rotation in the humerus that would result in an oblique view

Table 10-14 Shoulder and Forelimbs: Humerus–Elbow

Anatomic Area	Humerus			Elbow		
VIEW	Lateral	Caudocranial	Craniocaudal	Lateral	Flexed Lateral	Craniocaudal
POSITIONING	• Lateral recumbency • Affected forelimb is extended cranioventrally • Unaffected forelimb is extended caudodorsally • Head is extended dorsally	• Dorsal recumbency • Forelimbs extended cranially • Affected forelimb is parallel to cassette	• Dorsal recumbency • Affected forelimb extended caudally alongside the body but just clear of the thorax	• Lateral recumbency • Affected limb extended slightly cranioventrally with elbow slightly flexed • Unaffected limb extended caudodorsally • Head is extended dorsally	• Lateral recumbency • Affected limb flexed at the elbow joint with carpus pulled toward neck • Unaffected limb extended caudoventrally • Head is extended dorsally	• Sternal recumbency • Affected limb extended cranially • Unaffected limb acts as a support for the animal's head • Head is placed resting over unaffected limb
MEASUREMENT	• Thickest area of shoulder	• Thickest area of shoulder	• Thickest area of shoulder	• Thickest part of elbow joint	• Thickest part of elbow joint during flexion	• Thickest part of elbow joint
BEAM CENTER	• Mid-humerus	• Mid-humerus	• Mid-humerus	• Elbow joint	• Elbow joint	• Elbow joint
FIELD OF VIEW	• Shoulder joint to elbow joint	• Shoulder joint to elbow joint	• Shoulder joint to elbow joint	• Mid-humerus to mid-radius/ulna	• Mid-humerus to mid-radius/ulna	• Mid-humerus to mid-radius/ulna
NOTES						• Make sure that, when pulling the carpus, the elbow does not rotate • This view is best for screening for elbow dysplasia (especially lesions of anconeal process of ulna) • A hyperflexed view also may be needed for diagnostic analysis

Table 10-15   Shoulder and Forelimbs: Radius/Ulna–Metacarpus/Phalanges

Anatomic Area	Radius and Ulna		Carpus		Metacarpus and Phalanges	
VIEW	Lateral	Craniocaudal	Lateral	Dorsopalmar	Lateral	Dorsopalmar
POSITIONING	• Lateral recumbency • Affected limb extended cranially and slightly flexed at the elbow • Unaffected limb extended caudally • Head is extended dorsally away from cassette	• Sternal recumbency • Affected limb extended cranially • Unaffected limb is extended cranially • Head is placed resting over unaffected limb	• Lateral recumbency • Affected limb extended cranially • Unaffected limb extended ventrally and relaxed • Head is extended dorsally away from cassette	• Sternal recumbency • Affected limb extended cranially • Unaffected limb is extended cranially • Head is placed resting over unaffected limb	• Lateral recumbency • Affected limb extended cranially • Affected phalange is isolated with gauze or tape and pulled dorsally • Unaffected limb extended caudally and relaxed • Head is extended dorsally away from cassette	• Sternal recumbency • Affected limb extended cranially • Unaffected limb is extended cranially • Head is placed resting over unaffected limb
MEASUREMENT	• Elbow joint	• Thickest area of elbow joint	• Distal carpus	• Mid-carpus	• Middle phalanx	• Mid-metacarpal

558   VETERINARY TECHNICIAN'S DAILY REFERENCE GUIDE: CANINE AND FELINE

Table 10-15 Shoulder and Forelimbs: Radius/Ulna–Metacarpus/Phalanges (Continued)

Anatomic Area	Radius and Ulna		Carpus		Metacarpus and Phalanges	
VIEW	Lateral	Craniocaudal	Lateral	Dorsopalmar	Lateral	Dorsopalmar
BEAM CENTER	• Mid-radius/ulna	• Mid-radius/ulna	• Mid-carpus	• Mid-carpus	• Middle phalanges or affected phalanx	• Mid-metacarpal
FIELD OF VIEW	• Distal humerus to mid-metacarpals	• Distal humerus to mid-metacarpals	• Distal radius/ulna to distal metacarpals	• Distal radius/ulna to distal metacarpals	• Distal radius/ulna to distal digits	• Distal radius/ulna to distal digits
NOTES	• Avoid rotation of radius/ulna in cats		• Support under the elbow may assist in maintaining proper carpal positioning • Stressed views under sedation or general anesthesia may be needed to show presence of ligament laxity	• Support under the elbow may assist in maintaining proper carpal positioning • Oblique view at a 45-degree angle also may be required	• Support under the elbow may assist in maintaining proper carpal positioning • Oblique view(s) may be needed in some cases	• Support under the elbow may assist in maintaining proper carpal positioning • Oblique view at 45-degree angle also may be required

Pelvis and Hindlimbs

Table 10-16   Pelvis and Hindlimbs: Pelvis

Anatomic Area	Pelvis			
VIEW	Lateral	Lateral-oblique	V/D—Frog leg	V/D—extended
POSITIONING	• Lateral recumbency • Hindlimbs are extended down ventrally, slightly apart with the affected limb slightly cranial to unaffected limb, separated with a support to avoid spine rotation	• Lateral recumbency • Affected hindlimb is extended down ventrally and slightly cranially • Unaffected hindlimb is elevated to a 20-degree angle dorsally	• Dorsal recumbency • Hindlimbs should be abducted and flexed at a 45-degree angle to spine; positioned identically	• Dorsal recumbency • Pelvis flat on table • Hindlimbs start in a "flexed frog leg position." Hocks (or just above the hocks) are grasped and limbs are rotated medially so stifles come within 1–2 inches of each other, then extended caudally over the pubis region and ending in a full straight extension of the hindlimbs with patella centered over the femurs
MEASUREMENT	• Greater trochanter	• Greater trochanter	• Acetabulum (groin)	• Acetabulum (groin)
BEAM CENTER	• Greater trochanter	• Greater trochanter	• Pubis/acetabulum	• Pubis/acetabulum
FIELD OF VIEW	• Mid-lumbar spine to mid-femurs	• Mid-lumbar spine to mid-femurs	• Mid-lumbar spine to mid-caudal vertebrae	• Mid-lumbar spine to distal stifle
NOTES	• Best view for L-S bony changes if cauda equina pain suspected • Requires high mAs to penetrate large dog's pelvic bones		• Used if trauma to the pelvis is suspected • Sandbags and V tray will assist in proper positioning	• Sedation is necessary • Standard for assessment of hips • Correct positioning will result in parallel femurs; patellae centered between femoral condyles; left and right pelvis should be displayed as a mirror image • If hip laxity is in question, sometimes the Penn-HIP method is also recommended, which requires special certification of the veterinarian

Table 10-17 Pelvis and Hindlimbs: Femur–Tibia/Fibula

Anatomic Area	Femur		Stifles		Tibia/Fibula	
VIEW	Lateral	Craniocaudal	Lateral	Caudocranial	Lateral	Caudocranial
POSITIONING	• Lateral recumbency • Affected limb joints slightly flexed and relaxed • Unaffected limb extended dorsally or abducted out of the beam	• Dorsal recumbency • Affected limb extended caudally with slight abduction • Unaffected limb is flexed and relaxed • Tail (if long) gently laid under unaffected limb	• Lateral recumbency • Affected limb slightly flexed and relaxed, with support under the hock if necessary to keep knee from rotating • Unaffected limb extended dorsally out of the beam	• Sternal recumbency • Affected limb extended caudally • Unaffected limb is flexed, relaxed and supported	• Lateral recumbency • Affected limb slightly flexed and relaxed, with support under tarsus to keep tibia from rotating • Unaffected limb extended cranially	• Sternal recumbency • Affected limb extended caudally • Unaffected limb is flexed, relaxed and supported
MEASUREMENT	• Mid-femur	• Mid-femur	• Thickest part of stifle	• Thickest part of stifle	• Mid-tibia/fibula	• Mid-tibia/fibula
BEAM CENTER	• Mid-femur	• Mid-femur	• Mid-stifle joint	• Mid-stifle joint	• Mid-tibia/fibula	• Mid-tibia/fibula
FIELD OF VIEW	• Hip joint to proximal tibia/fibula	• Hip joint to proximal tibia/fibula	• Mid-femur to mid-tibia/fibula	• Mid-femur to mid-tibia/fibula	• Stifle joint to distal tarsus joint	• Stifle joint to distal tarsus joint
NOTES	• Best view for bony neoplasia of femur					• Depending on size of animal, elevation of the pelvic area will alleviate weight off the stifle

Table 10-18 Pelvis and Hindlimbs: Tarsus–Metatarsals

Anatomic Area	Tarsus			Metatarsals		
VIEW	Lateral	Plantarodorsal	Dorsoplantar	Lateral	Plantarodorsal	Dorsoplantar
POSITIONING	• Lateral recumbency • Affected limb slightly flexed and relaxed with support under tarsus • Unaffected limb extended cranially	• Sternal recumbency • Affected limb extended caudally with support under the stifle • Unaffected limb is flexed, relaxed, and supported	• Sternal recumbency • Affected limb extended cranially with support under the stifle	• Lateral recumbency • Affected limb slightly flexed at stifle and tarsus with support under stifle • Unaffected limb extended cranially	• Sternal recumbency • Affected limb extended caudally with support under the stifle • Unaffected limb is flexed, relaxed, and supported	• Sternal recumbency • Affected limb extended cranially with support under the stifle and stifle rotated laterally
MEASUREMENT	• Thickest area of tarsus	• Thickest area of tarsus	• Thickest area of tarsus	• Distal tarsal joint	• Distal tarsal joint	• Distal tarsal joint
BEAM CENTER	• Mid-tarsus	• Mid-tarsus	• Mid-tarsus	• Mid-metatarsals	• Mid-metatarsals	• Mid-metatarsals
FIELD OF VIEW	• Mid-tibia/fibula to mid-metatarsals	• Mid-tibia/fibula to mid-metatarsals	• Mid-tibia/fibula to mid-metatarsals	• Distal tibia/fibula to distal digits	• Distal tibia/fibula to distal digits	• Distal tibia/fibula to distal digits
NOTES						

RADIOGRAPHIC CONTRAST STUDIES

Contrast studies are done in cases in which the area of concern cannot be viewed diagnostically from the survey radiographs. The contrast provides the veterinarian with a more thorough observation of the affected area. Many of the procedures listed in the following tables are to be performed by a veterinarian only. However, the tables are provided so the technician can be ready for the procedure and efficiently assist the veterinarian throughout the procedure. Patient preparation is of extreme importance, and the animal should always be clean and dry for these procedures. In some cases, an enema and fasting may be required so that the gastrointestinal tract is clear of food or feces that could superimpose or distort the anatomic images. The technician should be aware of the possible side effects from the contrast medium and be prepared for appropriate emergency procedures. Preparation for these procedures as well as the dosage of the contrast medium should always be reviewed with the veterinarian before the procedure.

TYPES OF CONTRAST MEDIA

Table 10-19 Types of Contrast Media

Contrast Media	Positive Insoluble	Positive Soluble Iodine Containing		Negative
		Ionic (Salt Preparation)	Nonionic (Low osmolar)	
CLASSIFICATION	• Barium sulfate (micro-pulverized suspension)	• Ionic (Salt Preparation)	• Nonionic (Low osmolar)	• Gases
TRADE NAME	• Microtrast, Esophotrast, E-Z Past, Novopaque, Barotrast, Polibar	• Conray & Conray 43, Hypaque, Renografin 76 (IV, intraurethral, fistulas, intraperitoneal) • Gastrografin (oral only)	• Optiray 240, 320, and 350, Isovue (iopamidol), Omnipaque (iohexol), Visipaque (iodixanol) • Given IV, intraurethrally, into fistulas, intraperitoneally	• Carbon dioxide, nitrous oxide, oxygen, and room air
INDICATIONS	• Visualization of esophagus, stomach, small and large bowel, bronchography, and rhinography	• Intravascular usage	• Intravascular and myelographic studies	• Visualization of the bladder, peritoneum, pericardium, and brain
CONTRA-INDICATIONS	• Perforations or ruptures suspected	• Myelography and arthrography • Congestive heart failure (CHF), dehydration, and renal failure	• CHF and renal failure	
SIDE EFFECTS	• *Results in granulomas/lesions if leaks outside GI tract* • Has excellent mucosal-coating properties, but can mask foreign bodies	• *Acute renal failure, transient pulmonary edema, diarrhea, dehydration, and vomiting (bitter tasting to cats; use gastric tube to administer)*	• Less frequently noted	• *Gases may result in an embolism; possibly fatal if they access the vascular system*
MONITORING	• Vomiting and apnea	• Nausea, vomiting, skin erythema, facial swelling, pulmonary edema (respiration), dehydration, hypotension, hypovolemia (pulse, CRT, MM, and temperature)		
NOTES	• Radiopaque—shows white on radiograph	• Radiopaque—shows white on radiograph • Patient must be well hydrated for any ionic contrast medium		• Radiolucent—shows up black on radiograph

ABDOMINAL CONTRAST STUDIES

Table 10-20   Abdominal Contrast Studies

Procedure	Peritoneography (Celiography) Positive Contrast
AREA OF STUDY	• Peritoneal cavity (diaphragm, abdominal wall, and serosal surfaces of abdominal viscera)
INDICATIONS	• Suspected presence of diaphragmatic hernia
CONTRAINDICATIONS	
CONTRAST MEDIA	• Positive (iodinated)
EQUIPMENT	• ± Catheter/needle
PATIENT PREPARATION	• Sedation or general anesthesia • Empty patient's bladder • Abdominal survey radiographs
TECHNIQUE	*Performed by a DVM only* 1. Needle or catheter placement into the peritoneal cavity (lateral to midline and caudal to umbilicus) 2. Aspiration test performed (injection into the umbilical fat will invalidate the study) 3. Infusion of nonionic iodinated contrast media and animal rolled carefully 4. Radiograph
RADIOGRAPIC VIEWS	• Right and Left LAT + VD + DV
NOTES	

FISTULOGRAPHY

Table 10-21   Fistulography

Procedure	Fistulography
AREA OF STUDY	• Fistulous tracts and draining wounds
INDICATIONS	• Nonresponsive draining wound
CONTRAINDICATIONS	
CONTRAST MEDIA	• Positive, negative or double
EQUIPMENT	• Balloon-tip catheter
PATIENT PREP	• Sedation • Survey radiographs
TECHNIQUE	1. Place catheter into the sinus or fistula 2. Inject ionic or nonionic iodinated contrast media to fill the cavity 3. Leave catheter in place and radiograph
RADIOGRAPIC VIEWS	• LAT + VD ± Oblique
NOTES	

GASTROINTESTINAL TRACT CONTRAST STUDIES

Table 10-22 Gastrointestinal Tract Contrast Studies

Procedure	Esophagography	Gastrography		
		Positive Contrast Study	Negative Contrast Study (Pneumogastrogram)	Double-Contrast Study
AREA OF STUDY	• Esophageal location and morphology	• Gastric morphology	• Gastric morphology	• Gastric morphology
INDICATIONS	• Vomiting of undigested food, gagging, or dysphagia	• Gastric masses/foreign body, or vomiting	• Gastric masses/foreign body, or vomiting	• Gastric masses/foreign body, or vomiting
CONTRA-INDICATIONS	• Inability to swallow, bronchoesophageal, rupture/perforation, or dyspnea	• Parasitic infection	• Presence of ingesta or fluid	• Diabetes mellitus (if glucagon will be used)
CONTRAST MEDIA	• Barium sulfate or if perforation is suspected iodinated contrast	• Barium sulfate 30%–50% OR • Organic iodide (diatrizoate solution 10%)	• Carbon dioxide, nitrous oxide, or oxygen	• Barium sulfate 30%–50% and a negative contrast gas
EQUIPMENT	• Large syringe • Wet towels	• Orogastric tube • Large syringe • Wet towels • Bite block	• Orogastric tube (only if gas is to be used) • Large syringe • 3-way valve • Bite block	• Orogastric tube • Large syringe • Wet towels • 3-way valve • Bite block
PATIENT PREPARATION TECHNIQUE RADIOGRAPIC	• Fasting: 12 hours • Survey radiographs • Conscious patient	• Fasting: 12–24 hours • Large bowel evacuation or enema • No sedation for functional study • Survey radiographs • Conscious patient	• Fasting: 12–24 hours • No sedation for functional study • Survey radiographs • Conscious patient	• Fasting: 12–24 hours • No sedation for functional study • Survey radiographs • Conscious patient

TECHNIQUE	*Technique I:* *Mucosal assessment:* 1. Administer barium sulfate paste or thick liquid at a concentration of 80%–100% as per veterinarian's dosage into the buccal pouch 2. Let animal swallow 2–3 times. -OR- *Technique II:* *Stricture:* 1. Feed varying sizes of barium-filled gelatin capsules, or barium-injected marshmallows, or mix with food	1. Insert an orogastric tube into the stomach; verify placement 2. Infuse barium sulfate as per veterinarian's dosage recommendation	1. Insert an orogastric tube into the stomach; verify placement 2. Infuse gas per veterinarian's dosage recommendation 3. Remove orogastric tube and hold muzzle closed during radiographing	1. Insert an orogastric tube into the stomach; verify placement 2. Infuse barium sulfate 30%–50% per veterinarian's dosage recommendation 3. Infuse gas for a tympanic stomach and then gently roll the animal, to coat stomach.
RADIOGRAPIC VIEWS	• Right LAT + Right VD OBL of neck and thorax	• Right and left LAT + DV + VD	• Right and left LAT + DV + VD	• Right and left LAT + DV + VD
NOTES	• Monitor for aspiration of contrast • Fluoroscopy may aid in evaluation of motility and function • Iodinated contrast materials are bitter tasting and may result in vomiting. They are also hypertonic (if inhaled, could result in pulmonary edema). • General anesthesia is not recommended because of the risk of aspiration after vomiting	• Monitor for aspiration of contrast • General anesthesia is not recommended because of inhibition of GI motility and risk of aspiration after vomiting	• Monitor for aspiration of contrast • General anesthesia is not recommended because of inhibition of GI motility and risk of aspiration after vomiting	• Monitor for aspiration of contrast • Fluoroscopy may aid gastric lesion evaluation • General anesthesia is not recommended because of inhibition of GI motility and risk of aspiration after vomiting

Table 10-23   Gastrointestinal Tract Contrast Studies: UGI-LGI

Procedure	Upper Gastrointestinal Study (UGI)—Barium	Upper Gastrointestinal Study (UGI)—Iodinated Contrast	Lower Gastrointestinal Study—(LGI) Double-Contrast Barium Enema
AREA OF STUDY	• Small intestine morphology and functionality	• Small intestine morphology and functionality	• Large bowel morphology
INDICATIONS	• Vomiting, diarrhea, neoplasias, or obstructions	• Bloody diarrhea	• Large bowel obstruction, or bloody diarrhea
CONTRA-INDICATIONS	• Perforated esophagus or stomach • Lower bowel obstruction	• Dehydrated patient • Hypertonic mediums should not be used in hypovolemic patients (e.g., Gastrografin)	• Rupture/perforation
CONTRAST MEDIA	• Barium sulfate 30%	• Ionic or nonionic iodinated contrast	• Barium sulfate diluted (10%–20%)
EQUIPMENT	• Orogastric tube • Wet towels • Large syringe • Bite block	• Orogastric tube • Wet towels • Large syringe • Bite block	• Examination gloves • Warmed barium sulfate • Enema syringe • Lubricant • Foley catheter • 3-way stopcock • Compression paddle • Wet towels
PATIENT PREPARATION	• Fasting: 24 hours • Tepid saline enema 4–12 hours before • Chemical restraint may be necessary; however, do not use parasympatholytic agents • Conscious patient • Survey radiographs	• Fasting: 24 hours • Tepid saline enema 4–12 hours before • Chemical restraint may be necessary; however, do not use parasympatholytic agents • Conscious patient • Survey radiographs	• Fasting: 24 hours • Oral laxative and tepid water (or isotonic saline) enema • General anesthesia • Survey radiographs

TECHNIQUE	1. Insert orogastric tube into the stomach 2. Slowly infuse barium sulfate as per veterinarian's dosage recommendation	1. Insert orogastric tube into the stomach 2. Infuse iodinated contrast as per veterinarian's dosage recommendation	1. Insert the balloon catheter in the anus and completely occlude the anal canal, but do not overinflate the cuff. 2. Place the animal in **right lateral recumbency** and slowly infuse the diluted barium sulfate mixture into the large bowel and cecum as per veterinarian's dosage recommendation. 3. Radiograph 4. After these radiographs have been completed, ***evacuate the barium***, *place the animal in* **left lateral recumbency** *and infuse gas to redistend the colon and take a second set of radiographs.*
RADIOGRAPHIC VIEWS	• LAT (Right and Left) + VD immediately, then Right LAT + VD at 5–15, 30, ± 45, 60 minutes and then hourly until contrast is in the large intestine • Considered complete when stomach is empty	• LAT + VD every 10–30 minutes until the contrast is in the large intestine	• VD + Right LAT abdominal after barium infusion and then again after gas infusion
NOTES	• Care must be taken on choice of anesthesia/sedation so as not to impede the motility of the GI tract.	• Care must be taken on choice of anesthesia/sedation so as not to impede the motility of the GI tract	• If study is for diagnosis of obstruction or intussusception, no fecal evacuation is necessary • Elevation of the cranial two thirds of the body may assist removal of the contrast media

HEAD CONTRAST STUDIES

Table 10-24 Head Contrast Studies

Procedure	Dacryocystorhinography	Rhinography	Sialography
AREA OF STUDY	• Nasolacrimal duct	• Nasal cavity	• Salivary ducts and glands
CONTRAST MEDIA	• Positive iodinated	• Positive (barium sulfate 20%–30% or iodinated media)	• Positive iodinated
INDICATIONS	• Conjunctivitis, dacryocystitis, or neoplasia	• Suspected obstruction	• Mucoceles, swelling, abscesses, or neoplasias
CONTRA-INDICATIONS			
EQUIPMENT	• Cannula • 23–27-gauge lacrimal needle • Syringe	• Syringe	• Cannula • Syringe
PATIENT PREPARATION	• General anesthesia • Nasal survey radiographs	• General anesthesia • Nasal survey radiographs including lateral and open mouth VD views	• General anesthesia • Skull/neck survey radiographs
TECHNIQUE	*Performed by a DVM only* 1. Cannulation of the superior or inferior lacrimal puncta 2. Injection of iodinated contrast as per veterinarian's dosage recommendation until several drops are seen in the external nares	*Performed by a DVM only* 1. Infusion of positive contrast as per veterinarian's dosage recommendation into the ventral nasal meatus 2. With the infused side dependent, elevate the nose approximately 15-degrees	*Performed by a DVM only* 1. Cannulation of the salivary duct 2. Injection of iodinated contrast as per veterinarian's dosage recommendation
RADIOGRAPIC VIEWS	• LAT + DV	• LAT + OPEN MOUTH VD	• LAT + DV
NOTES			

SPINAL AND JOINT CONTRAST STUDIES

Table 10-25 Spinal and Joint Contrast Studies

Procedure	Myelography	Epidurography	Discography	Arthrography
AREA OF STUDY	• Spinal cord	• Epidural space	• Central portion of invertebral disk	• Joint evaluation (shoulder and stifle)
CONTRAST MEDIA	• Positive **nonionic** media only (e.g., iopamidol, iohexol)	• Positive **nonionic** media only (e.g., iopamidol, iohexol)	• Positive **nonionic** media only (e.g., iopamidol, iohexol)	• Positive iodinated diluted to DVM's recommendation
INDICATIONS	• Clinical transverse myelopathies	• Disk protrusion/extrusion, suspected lesion, or tumor	• Hernia or rupture	• Articular defects or joint capsule abnormalities
CONTRA-INDICATIONS	• Disseminated myelopathy, meningopathy, cerebrospinal fluid (CSF) infection			
EQUIPMENT	• 20–22-gauge spinal needle in various sizes: $1\frac{1}{2}$, $2\frac{1}{2}$, and $3\frac{1}{2}$	• Spinal needle	• Spinal needle • Sterile gloves • Slides • Culture	• Sterile gloves • 22-gauge needle • Slides
PATIENT PREPARATION	• General anesthesia • Spinal survey radiographs • Aseptic preparation of appropriate spinal location	• General anesthesia • Spinal survey radiographs • Aseptic preparation of lumbosacral or coccygeal interarcuate space	• Spinal needle • Sterile gloves • General anesthesia • Spinal survey radiographs • Aseptic preparation of appropriate disk space	• General anesthesia • Joint survey radiographs • Prepare area around joint of interest

Table 10-25 Spinal and Joint Contrast Studies (continued)

Procedure	Myelography	Epidurography	Discography	Arthrography
TECHNIQUE	*Performed by a DVM only:* 1. Aseptic spinal puncture of subarachnoid space at either cisterna magna or an interarcuate space of caudal lumbar spine (L5–L6) 2. Nonionic contrast media is injected slowly to fill the subarachnoid space. The needle may be removed or left in place for the radiographs	*Performed by a DVM only:* 1. Place animal in sternal or lateral recumbency 2. Aseptic placement of spinal needle into the floor of the spinal canal at the lumbosacral or coccygeal interarcuate space 3. Nonionic contrast media is injected to fill the space 4. The needle is removed	*Performed by a DVM only:* 1. Place animal in lateral recumbency 2. Aseptic placement of spinal needle through the interarcurate ligament and spinal canal into the disk of interest 3. Nonionic contrast media is injected into the space	*Performed by a DVM only:* 1. Aseptic articular puncture 2. Removal of small amount of joint fluid for analysis 3. Diluted nonionic contrast media is injected, dependent on animal size as per veterinarian's recommended dosage 4. Needle is removed 5. Joint is manipulated
RADIOGRAPIC VIEWS	• VD + LAT ± DV + OBL + Extended/Flexed LAT	• LAT + Flexed LAT + Extended LAT + VD or DV	• Neutral LAT + hyperflexed LAT + DV or VD	• Caudocranial + LAT OBL • Radiographs should be taken as soon as contrast is injected
NOTES	• Tilting of the body may be necessary to assist in the coating of the contrast media • Elevate head during recovery • Monitor for apnea and seizures			• Positive contrast study provides more information • Double-contrast study is not recommended

URETHRA AND VAGINAL STUDIES

Table 10-26 Urethra and Vaginal Studies

Procedure	Urethrography			Vaginography
	Male dog	Female dog	Male and Female Cats	Retrograde Vaginourethrography
AREA OF STUDY	• Urethra location and morphology	• Urethra location and morphology	• Urethra location and morphology	• Vagina, cervix, and urethra morphology
CONTRAST MEDIA	• Iodinated contrast medium (1 part iodine to 2 parts water; 10%–15% solution)	• Iodinated contrast medium (1 part iodine to 2 parts water; 10%–15% solution)	• Iodinated contrast medium (1 part iodine to 2 parts water; 10%–15% solution)	• Iodinated contrast medium (1 part iodine to 2 parts water; 10%–15% solution)
INDICATIONS	• Stranguria, hematuria, dysuria, suspected masses or lesions	• Stranguria, hematuria, dysuria, suspected masses or lesions	• Stranguria, hematuria, dysuria, suspected masses or lesions	• Masses, suspected ectopic ureter
CONTRA-INDICATIONS	• Uncontrolled hematuria	• Uncontrolled hematuria	• Uncontrolled hematuria	
EQUIPMENT	• Urinary catheter (Foley, soft polyethylene male catheter) prefilled with contrast media • Large syringe • 3-way stopcock • Sterile saline • Lubricant • Wet towels • Bowl • Lidocaine	• Urinary catheter (Foley, Swan-Ganz, soft polyethylene male catheter) prefilled with contrast media • Large syringe • 3-way stopcock • Sterile saline • Lubricant • Wet towels • Bowl • Radiolucent paddle or wooden spoon	• Urinary catheter (Tomcat catheter for males) prefilled with contrast media • Large syringe • 3-way stopcock • Sterile saline • Lubricant • Wet towels • Bowl • Lidocaine	• Urinary catheter (Foley, soft polyethylene male catheter) prefilled with contrast media • 2 syringes (20–60 mL) • 3-way stopcock • Sterile saline • Lubricant • Wet towels • Bowl • Suture or Babcock forceps
PATIENT PREPARATION	• Fasting: 24 hours • Enema 4 hours before • Sedation • Survey radiographs: Male dog: Additional lateral of perineal and penile regions with hindlimbs extended cranially	• Fasting: 24 hours • Enema 4 hours before • Sedation • Survey radiographs	• Fasting: 24 hours • Enema 4 hours before • Sedation • Survey radiographs	• Fasting: 24 hours • Enema 4 hours before • General anesthesia • Survey radiographs

Table 10-26   Urethra and Vaginal Studies (Continued)

Procedure	Urethrography			Vaginography
	Male dog	Female dog	Male and Female Cats	Retrograde Vaginourethrography
TECHNIQUE	***Typically performed by a DVM only:*** 1. Aseptic placement of a urinary catheter to distal urethra (or distal pelvic urethra for prostatic assessment) 2. Infuse undiluted contrast (5–15 mL) to fill urethra	***Typically performed by a DVM only:*** Technique I: *Voiding urethrogram after cystogram* 1. With paddle or wooden spoon, empty the bladder Technique II: *Retrograde urethrogram after positive contrast cystogram:* 1. Inject undiluted contrast through catheter while extracting it from the urethra. Radiograph should be taken during contrast infusion. Technique III: 1. Place a balloon-tip catheter into the distal urethra 2. Inflate the balloon 3. Inject 5–10 mL contrast media. 4. Radiograph should be taken at the end of infusion. Repeat infusion for additional radiographs.	***Typically performed by a DVM only:*** 1. Voiding urethrogram after cystogram with paddle or wooden spoon.	***Typically performed by a DVM only:*** 1. Placement of catheter in vestibule and inflated 2. Pursestring suture or a Babcock forceps is used to keep the vulvar lips closed and the Foley catheter in place during the procedure 3. Infuse with undiluted iodinated contrast media to overdistend the vagina 4. Radiograph as the infusion is administered, and the vagina is overdistended
RADIOGRAPIC VIEWS	• LAT (including perineal area). Can be performed after cystogram. Repeat infusion for any additional radiographs	• LAT + VD	• LAT ± OBL	• LAT of pelvis and caudal abdomen ± VD
NOTES	• Can be performed after cystogram			• Overdistention of the vagina forces the contrast medium up the urethra and into the bladder

URINARY TRACT CONTRAST STUDIES

Preparation of the patient is extremely important in producing quality contrast radiographs of the urinary tract. An enema should always be done before the procedure, because fecal compression on the ureters or the dorsal bladder wall can ruin a study. The enema should be a warmed isotonic saline enema. Hydration should be assessed and stabilized before beginning any of these procedures. The technician should note the special precautions and monitoring needed when doing an IVU/EU/IVP. Although rare, when complications do occur, they can be fatal, and being prepared for the possible emergency situation can make a difference.

Table 10-27 Urinary Tract Contrast Studies

Procedure	Intravenous Urography (IVU) Excecretory Urography (EU) Intravenous Pyelography (IVP)	Cystography		
		Positive Contrast	Negative Contrast (Pneumocystography)	Double Contrast
AREA OF STUDY	• Urinary system: kidneys, ureters, and urinary bladder	• Urinary bladder wall integrity and position	• Urinary bladder	• Urinary bladder mucosal detail
CONTRAST MEDIA	• Iodinated contrast for intravascular injection; warmed	• Iodinated contrast (1 part contrast to 3 parts water)	• Gas (carbon dioxide, nitrous oxide, oxygen)	• Negative and postive iodinated contrast media
INDICATIONS	• Pyuria, hematuria, masses, tender abdomen, abnormal renal size, incontinence, trauma, or suspected ectopic ureters	• Trauma, hematuria, or straining	• Trauma, hematuria, or straining	• Trauma, hematuria, or straining
CONTRA-INDICATIONS	• Hypovolemia • Creatinine > 3–3.5 mg/dL • Dehydration • No compression if abdominal masses or enlarged or cystic kidneys are suspected	• Enlarged bladder	• Enlarged bladder	• Enlarged bladder
EQUIPMENT PATIENT PREPARATION	• IV catheter; large bore, short (contrast is viscous) • Syringe • 22-gauge—1-inch needle • Iodinated contrast • Compression bandage • Fluids ready to use • Resuscitation kit (epinephrine, AMBU bag, oxygen ready)	• Urinary catheter (Foley, tomcat, or soft flexible male catheter) • Large syringe • 3-way stopcock • Sterile saline • Lubricant • Wet towels • Bowl • 5–10 mL 2% lidocaine (to decrease spasticity)	• Urinary catheter (Foley, tomcat, or soft flexible male catheter) • Large syringe • 3-way stopcock • Sterile saline • Lubricant • Wet towels • Bowl • 5–10 mL 2% lidocaine (to decrease spasticity)	• Urinary catheter (Foley, tomcat, or soft flexible male catheter) • Large syringe • 3-way stopcock • Sterile saline • Lubricant • Wet towels • Bowl • 5–10 mL 2% lidocaine (to decrease spasticity)

PATIENT PREPARATION	• 24-hour fast but have water available • Enema—4 hours before • Hydration assessed, stabilized, and monitored • Urine sample obtained prior to procedure • IV catheter • Sedation or general anesthesia • Abdominal survey radiographs	• 24-hour fast • Enema—4 hours before • Urine sample obtained before procedure • Sedation or general anesthesia • Survey radiographs	• 24-hour fast • Enema—4 hours before • Urine sample obtained before procedure • Sedation or general anesthesia • Survey radiographs	• 24-hour fast • Enema—4 hours before • Urine sample obtained before procedure • Sedation or general anesthesia • Survey radiographs
TECHNIQUE	*Performed by a DVM only:* 1. Rapid intravenous infusion of a warmed iodinated contrast media as per veterinarian's dosage recommendations; radiograph immediately 2. Compression may be needed as long as no abdominal masses are noted to view ureters (take VD radiograph at 10 minutes) 3. On removal of compression, take LAT + VD immediately	*Performed by a DVM only:* 1. Aseptic placement of a urinary catheter to the bladder neck 2. Empty the bladder and flush 3. Infuse *diluted contrast* as per veterinarian's dosage recommendations to distend the bladder 4. Palpate bladder and proceed with radiographs	*Performed by a DVM only:* 1. Aseptic placement of a urinary catheter to the bladder neck 2. Empty the bladder and flush 3. Infuse *gas* as per veterinarian's dosage recommendations to distend the bladder 4. Palpate bladder and proceed with radiographs	*Performed by a DVM only:* 1. Aseptic placement of a urinary catheter to the bladder neck 2. Empty the bladder and flush 3. Infuse *gas* as per veterinarian's dosage recommendations to distend the bladder 4. Palpate bladder and then inject small amount of *iodinated contrast* as per veterinarian's dosage recommendations into bladder. Do NOT occlude urethra. 5. Roll animal to coat bladder wall and proceed with radiographs

Table 10-27 Urinary Tract Contrast Studies (Continued)

Procedure	Intravenous Urography (IVU) Excretory Urography (EU) Intravenous Pyelography (IVP)	Cystography		
		Positive Contrast	Negative Contrast (Pneumocystography)	Double Contrast
RADIOGRAPHIC VIEWS	Minute Exposure 0 VD + LAT 3–5 VD ± LAT ± VD OBL± R-LAT OBL 10–15 VD + LAT ± LAT OBL 30–120 VD + LAT ± LAT OBL	• LAT + VD OBL If further radiographs are necessary, inject additional contrast media	• LAT + VD ± OBL If further radiographs are necessary, inject additional contrast media	• LAT + VD OBL
NOTES	• Monitor for hypotension, vomiting, arrhythmia, cardiovascular collapse, anaphylaxsis, and CMIARF (contrast medium-induced acute renal failure) • Abdominal compression may be used to visualize the renal collecting system and proximal ureters • Oblique radiographs may be required to visualize the distal ureters • Do not use soapy enemas • Contrast media may cause vasodilation and may sting • Three stages include nephrogram, pyelogram, and cystogram	• Complications may include: trauma due to improper catheterization, iatrogenic infection, or chemical cystitis	• Room air may cause an air embolus; carbon dioxide is recommended • Complications may include trauma caused by improper catheterization, iatrogenic infection, or air emboli	• Room air may cause an air embolus; carbon dioxide is recommended • Complications may include trauma caused by improper catheterization, iatrogenic infection, air emboli, or chemical cystitis

Chapter 11

Specialized and Ancillary Procedures

CAVM: COMPLEMENTARY AND ALTERNATIVE VETERINARY MEDICINE

Complementary and Alternative Veterinary Medicine (CAVM) or Holistic Veterinary Medicine: Medical treatment of the whole body and mind in the context of the environment

This section provides a brief survey of various types of CAVM. It is meant to introduce the technician to other options that might complement an existing medical plan or be used as an alternative.

The philosophies and techniques should only be performed by a licensed DVM with additional training and degrees in these particular areas.

Table 11-1 CAVM: Ayurveda, Chiropractic, and Flower Essences

Procedure	Ayurveda	Chiropractic	Flower Essences
DEFINITION	• The use of diet, massage, herbal supplements, and exercise to create balance among the three elements of nature and provide a gradual process of healing • The three elements of nature or Doshas (Vata, Pitta, and Kapha) constitute the body	• Realignment of misaligned vertebrae to treat disease caused by an interference with nerve function • Subtle vertebral misalignments can block the essential flow of energy passing through the spinal column	• Flower essences are used to treat the mental and emotional states of a patient on a level of vibrational healing • The mental healing often provides physical improvements as well • Their use is usually complementary to other treatments versus an alternative
DIAGNOSTICS	To determine the physical constitution type and mental status of the patient (Dosha) through: • A thorough history and physical examination • Pulse strength and rate • Gross examination of urine, tongue, skin, and nails	• Thorough history and physical examination of the patient	• Thorough history to evaluate the personality, feelings, and mood of a patient
TECHNIQUE	*Prevention therapy:* • Prophylaxis therapy: specific combination of diet, lifestyle, herbal medicine, and therapeutic purification exercises to strengthen or weaken specific Doshas to establish balance among all three Doshas *Disease therapy:* • Purification therapy: combination of vomiting, enemas, smoke inhalation, and blood letting • Alleviation therapy: combination of basic foods	• Tension is applied to the misaligned vertebrae, and a quick controlled thrust is applied along the plane of motion to a controlled depth, speed, and amplitude	• Single or a combination of essences based on the above findings *Dosages:* • Dilute 2 drops of each essence into 1 oz of mineral water and give 1–4 times daily • Full-strength essences dropped onto the tongue, rubbed behind the ears, or dropped onto the lips • To avoid the 20% alcohol content, the essences can be applied externally or dropped into hot water to allow the alcohol to evaporate

INDICATIONS	• Any alteration from normal and disease prevention	• Lameness, gait changes, inability to sit for long periods, refusing to jump, head tilting, and muscle atrophy	• Altered mental and emotional health
SPECIALIZED EQUIPMENT	• None	• ± Activator—small impacting device used to make indirect adjustments	• None
PRECAUTIONS	• Disease therapy should only be used on patients strong enough to withstand the intense process	• Patients should also be evaluated by using other diagnostic aids such as radiography, blood work, and electrocardiogram (ECG) • Incorrect adjustment may lead to severe outcomes (e.g., paralysis)	• Patients may initially experience a few hours of exaggerated symptoms or development of suppressed symptoms as the healing process begins; however, alterations may be needed to alleviate these symptoms if they do not subside on their own
NOTES	• Considered a medical procedure by the AVMA to be performed only by a licensed DVM with postgraduate training in ayurvedic medicine	• Chiropractic medicine is meant as an adjunct to other forms of veterinary medicine, not as a replacement • Considered a medical procedure by the AVMA and should only be performed by a licensed DVM with postgraduate training in chiropractic care	• There is no documentation or standardized preparations available for veterinary medicine • If an incorrect remedy is chosen, there are no side effects, but no effect is seen • If no results are seen after a few weeks, reevaluate the combination selected

Table 11-2 CAVM: Homeopathy, Magnetic Field Therapy, and Western Herbal Medicine

Procedure	Homeopathy	Magnetic Field Therapy	Western Herbal Medicine
DEFINITION	• The treatment of clinical signs with incredibly small doses of a certain preparation (e.g., herbal, mineral, and animal products) • The chosen preparation may actually cause the clinical sign at pharmaceutical or high doses or if given repeatedly to a healthy animal	• Magnet lines of force permeate the area of injury and stimulate healing • Pulsed electromagnetic field therapy (PEMF) is pulsating a magnetic field by means of a pulsing current moving through a coil of wire	• A complex combination of whole medicinal plants and other products that are commonly found in the United States and Europe • Administered as teas, powders in capsules, tablets, extracts, poultices, ointments, and in bulk
DIAGNOSTICS	• Evaluation of the mental, emotional, and physical state of the patient	• Physical examination	• Thorough history and physical examination
TECHNIQUE	• An appropriate remedy or combination of remedies is chosen • Pellets or tablets are poured into the back of the animal's mouth from either a folded piece of paper or from a hollowed-out cap of the bottle • Liquid preparations may be dropped into the animal's mouth or added to a water bowl	• Placement of magnets either in the cage with the animal or taped to the affected area on the animal for minutes, hours, or days • (PEMF) Coils are placed over the area to be treated for 30–60 minutes, as often as daily	• Fresh or dried herbs may be boiled and steeped overnight or mixed directly into the animal's food
INDICATIONS	• Any alteration from normal and disease prevention	• Bone and wound healing, epilepsy, and pain caused by arthritis • (PEMF) nonunion fractures, acute and chronic injury and chronic musculoskeletal conditions	• Stimulation of digestion and various organs and glands in the body

SPECIALIZED EQUIPMENT	• None	• Magnets of different strengths and sizes (PEMF) Battery-powered therapy devices consisting of several coils of wire, a control box with varying pulse settings, and a power source	• None
PRECAUTIONS	• Do not touch the remedy • Incorrect potencies may have no effect if too low, or aggravate the condition if too high	• Magnet strength and size needed for each animal are highly variable • Magnet therapy should begin with lower strengths and for short periods and then ↑ if well tolerated • Worsening conditions (e.g., ↑ seizures and lethargy)	• A selection of herbs are not interchangeable between humans, dogs, and cats (e.g., marigold, nutmeg, cocoa, and mistletoe) • No dosages exist for herbs, and it can often be through trial and error that the correct amount is discovered • Healing effects may take longer than with medical drugs because of ↓ concentrations • Gastrointestinal disturbances, restlessness, and itchy skin
NOTES	• Considered a medical procedure by the AVMA and should only be performed by a licensed DVM with postgraduate training in homeopathy • Homeopathic remedies should be stored away from sunlight, odors, moisture, and computers • It is thought by some that all other forms of vibrational or energy medicine (e.g., acupuncture, flower essences, and certain foods) are contraindicated in combination with homeopathy • If the incorrect remedy is chosen, there are no side effects, but no effect is seen	• Because there is no current research regarding the use of magnets with animals, testimony makes up the background for their use • The composition and size of the magnetic affect its strength and intensity • The size and shape of a magnet are related to the depth of penetration	• Often requires large amounts of herbs, frequently over a long period • Herbs are relatively safe when compared with medical drugs, but they can still be deadly • Herbs are classified as food supplements and are not subjected to the same research on purity, quality, and usage as medical drugs • Store dried herbs in a cool, dark place for ≤ 1 year

Table 11-3 Traditional Chinese Medicine (TCM)

TCM can be used as a complement to Western medicine and as an alternative treatment. Traditional Chinese medicine encompasses four aspects: acupuncture, herbal medicine, therapeutic massage, and nutrition. Acupuncture and Chinese herbal medicine are the most commonly used portions of this medical system. Acupuncture itself can have many different techniques: dry-needle acupuncture, acupressure, aquapuncture, electroacupuncture, sonapuncture, laserpuncture, and implantation. The needles themselves also may be stimulated in different ways: electroacupuncture, moxibustion, and manually.

The goal is not always to heal the patient; it can also be used to allow the body to be better able to deal with disease conditions. Animals treated with acupuncture may reach death more peacefully and with less suffering.

Procedure	Acupuncture	Chinese Herbal Medicine (CHM, Phytotherapy)
DEFINITION	• The adjustment of energy, known as "Qi," to provide homeostasis and promote healing	• A complex combination of selected parts of medicinal plants and other products used to help improve and restore internal organ function and balance energy, "Qi"
DIAGNOSTICS	To discover the "Qi" imbalance: • Thorough history • Pulse strength and rate • Tongue appearance	To discover the "Qi" imbalance: • Thorough history • Pulse strength and rate • Tongue appearance
TECHNIQUE	• Insertion of fine-gauge needles into specific sites along the body to regulate bodily function • The depth of the needle, the type of stimulation applied to the needle, and the duration of the treatment are determined by the condition being treated and constitution of the patient ± Moxibustion uses a source of external heat over the acupuncture site or the acupuncture needle itself	• After the diagnosis of an imbalance (excesses or deficiencies), specific herbs are chosen to restore balance
INDICATIONS	• Any alteration from normal • Long-term chronic degenerative conditions (e.g., arthritis, liver or kidney failure, and autoimmune problems) • Short-term after illness (e.g., chemotherapy and radiation therapy) • Preventatively to strengthen the body	• Any alteration from normal • Long-term chronic degenerative conditions (e.g., arthritis, liver or kidney failure, and autoimmune problems) • Short-term after illness (e.g., chemotherapy and radiation therapy) • Antiviral • Preventatively to strengthen the body • Drug sensitivity • Vague symptoms with no Western diagnosis

SPECIALIZED EQUIPMENT	• Sterile, disposable acupuncture needles • Moxa stick	• None
PRECAUTIONS	• Incorrect points may lead to worsening condition (e.g., ↑ tumor growth) • Do not perform acupuncture on fatigued animals, after a heavy meal, in animals that are emotional, pregnant, recently bathed, soon to be bathed, or after injections of certain drugs (e.g., atropine and narcotics)	• Herbs may cause gastrointestinal disturbances, restlessness, and itchy skin as minor side effects, and severe side effects can be deadly
NOTES	• Considered a medical procedure by the AVMA and should only be performed by a licensed DVM with postgraduate training in acupuncture	• Considered a medical procedure by the AVMA and should only be performed by a licensed DVM with postgraduate training in CHM • Some herb formulas can be used for extended periods with little or no side effects

DIAGNOSTIC IMAGING MODALITIES

In addition to radiographs, the following modalities can be used to assist in the diagnosis of a patient's medical problem. Survey radiographs should always be evaluated before any of these modalities. All of these procedures are performed by a DVM.

Table 11-4　Diagnostic Imaging Modalities: Computed Tomography, Echocardiography, and Endoscopy

Procedure	Computed Tomography (CT, CAT scan)	Echocardiography	Endoscopy
DEFINITION	• A cross-sectional view of a patient's body, using x-rays and a computer	• Noninvasive study of the heart and its structures (aorta, ventricles, atria, auricular appendages, and all the cardiac valves), using ultrasonography	• The study of the internal structures of the patient through a natural or surgical opening with a rigid or flexible tube and optical system
TECHNIQUE	• A thin X-ray beam passes through the patient transaxially from many directions (as the tube rotates), and a view of the area of interest is reconstructed by a computer using the transmitted data (the amount of transmitted X-rays through a particular tissue) onto a video screen	• The ultrasound transducer is placed on a clipped and cleaned area with ultrasound gel. M-mode is used to view the cardiac structures and produce the image. The animal may be in lateral or dorsal recumbency or standing if necessary.	• Rigid endoscopic procedures include: arthroscopy, cystoscopy, laparoscopy, otoscopy, rhinoscopy, thoracoscopy, urethrocystoscopy, vaginoscopy • Flexible endoscopic procedures include: rhinoscopy and bronchoscopy
INDICATIONS	• Confirmation or further evaluation of radiographic results • Intracranial disease, musculoskeletal, spinal, thoracic, and abdominal disorders	• Visualize internal cardiac structures • Evaluate function and size of the heart • Evaluate defects of the heart: valvular lesions, shunts, myocardial abnormalities, masses, effusions, or stenotic lesions	• Endoscopes are used when a closer look at the internal structures are needed to provide a definitive diagnosis and in some cases to retrieve foreign objects or biopsies of the area of interest

SPECIALIZED EQUIPMENT	• Computerized Tomography Unit	• Ultrasound machine, transducers, Doppler (permits detection and analysis of blood cells in transit), ultrasound gel	• Endoscope and variety of telescopes
PRECAUTIONS	• None	• None	• None
SIDE EFFECTS	• None	• None	• None
NOTES	• Two studies are usually required (one without and one with contrast media)	• None	• Extremely important to follow manufacturer's instructions on handling and cleaning • Train all personnel that may be involved with the endoscope regarding handling, setup, and cleaning/maintenance • Always pick up the rigid endoscopes by the ocular (eyepiece) • Avoid overflexion of the endoscope during the procedure

Table 11-5 Diagnostic Imaging Modalities: Fluoroscopy, Magnetic Resonance Imaging, and Nuclear Medicine

Procedure	Fluoroscopy	Magnetic Resonance Imaging (MRI)	Nuclear Medicine (Scintigraphy)
DEFINITION	• Real-time radiographic viewing of moving anatomic parts, using an X-ray machine and a fluoroscopic screen with an image intensifier	• A cross-sectional view of a patient's body, using magnetic fields and radio waves	• The use of radiopharmaceutical drugs to ascertain the functional status of an organ or body part of a patient
TECHNIQUE	• X-rays pass through the patient's body to the image intensifier tube	• A magnet surrounds a patient's body, and the magnetic field reacts with the protons in the patient's body, which is reconstructed by a computer onto a video screen	• A radionuclide is administered intravenously to the patient. Travel throughout the area is captured on X-ray film, using a gamma scintillation camera
INDICATIONS	• Used in assessing the motility and function of the pharynx, esophagus, stomach, and bowel • Evaluation of respiratory and cardiac function	• Confirmation of further evaluation of radiographic results • When soft tissue contrast is required for diagnostic assessment	• Specific areas requiring more information on functionality of specific organs for diagnostic assessment (e.g. hyperthyroidism, lameness, and liver dysfunction)
SPECIALIZED EQUIPMENT	• Fluoroscopic X-ray tube • Image intensifier tube • Mirror imaging or television viewing system • Radiopaque contrast medium • Protective apparel	• Magnetic resonance imaging unit (MRI) • Special room/building for unit • Nonferrous contrast media	• Radiopharmaceutical drugs • Gamma scintillation camera • Radiographic film • Protective lab coat • Latex gloves • Specialized training in handling drug, patient, and patient's excretions
PRECAUTIONS	• Radiation exposure	• Patient and operator must be free of any metallic devices (pacemakers), metallic foreign bodies (bullets, shrapnel, skin staples, etc.), or ferromagnetic implants • Operator is in a separate area from the patient	• Requires special handling of animal's excretion and restricted contact time with patient
NOTES	• None	• None	• Specific drugs are used to analyze various areas: • ^{99m}TC technetium sodium pertechnetate for thyroid, salivary glands, stomach, and kidney evaluation • ^{99m}TC sulfur colloid for reticuloendothelial system of liver, spleen, and bone marrow • ^{99m}TC methylene diphosphonate (MDP) for bone imaging • ^{99m}TC macroaggregated albumin (MAA) for pulmonary thromboembolism

Table 11-6   Diagnostic Imaging Modalities: Ultrasonography

Procedure	Ultrasonography
DEFINITION	• The production of an image based on the emission and return of soundwaves from the ultrasound transducer into an animal's body
TECHNIQUE	• Ultrasound transducing gel is placed on the clipped and cleaned area of interest. A transducer probe is placed on the gel. B-mode is used to view the abdominal structures. Sound waves are emitted through the transducer into the body, and echoes are received back from the structures the sound waves strike and are reproduced as a gray scale image on the screen.
INDICATIONS	• Confirmation needed or further evaluation of anomalies found on radiographs in the thorax or abdomen or palpable masses
SPECIALIZED EQUIPMENT	• Ultrasound machine, appropriate transducers, ultrasound gel • General anesthesia will be necessary if a biopsy is to be performed
PRECAUTIONS	• N/A
SIDE EFFECTS	• N/A
NOTES	• When doing abdominal studies, the animal should be fasted (water is okay) • Owners should be made aware that a large area of fur may be clipped • Wipe probe clean of gel as soon as possible • Wash transducer probe with cold water (do not immerse) and dry with a soft towel

LASER SURGERY

Laser surgery is more commonly found in nonspecialized clinics as the equipment becomes more available and affordable. This procedure, however, does require additional training and practice to be a useful surgical option. There are a large number of risks to both the patient and those performing the procedure that need to be thoroughly addressed.

Table 11-7 Laser Surgery

Procedure	Laser Surgery (Light Amplification by the Stimulation *Emission of Radiation*)
DEFINITION	• Laser surgery consists of the light interaction with tissue, causing certain effects • The amount of light transmitted maybe reflected, absorbed, scattered, or transmitted through the tissue
TECHNIQUE	• Variable depending on desired outcome (e.g., focused laser location for drilling a hole)
INDICATIONS	• Surgery requiring precise dissection and hemostasis • Lithotripsy and angioplasty • Soft tissue dental procedures
EQUIPMENT	• Several different lasers exist with varying wavelengths, delivery, and application techniques
PRECAUTIONS	• Human exposure risk (e.g., ocular damage and burns) • Red rubber endotracheal tubes wrapped in metal tape or aluminum foil should be used to avoid melting of the tube and subsequent explosion of the flowing oxygen • A bucket of water and CO_2 fire extinguisher should be within reach to distinguish any fires • Proper evacuation of noxious smoke should be in place • Use moistened gauze sponges around surgical area and blackened or pitted instruments to absorb stray or reflected light • Patient should have eyes covered, endotracheal tube protected, and rectum packed
SIDE EFFECTS	• ± ↑ Healing time
NOTES	• → Amount of postoperative edema, drainage, and pain • Laser surgery continues to increase in its indications as new techniques are discovered and perfected

RADIATION THERAPY

Radiation therapy is meant to supply enough radiation to a specific site to cause abnormal cell death while minimizing the amount of surrounding tissue damage. This form of neoplastic treatment is gaining popularity and access as the equipment becomes more available. Its uses and positive outcomes are endless and showing great promise to the treatment of varying types of tumors.

Table 11-8   Radiation Therapy: Teletherapy, Brachytherapy, and Systemic Therapy

Procedure	Teletherapy (External Beam)	Brachytherapy (Interstitial)	Systemic Therapy
DEFINITION	• Radiation therapy delivered from an external source to a specific tissue/tumor site	• Radiation therapy delivered from an external source to a radioactive implant placed within the tumor site	• Systemically injecting radioactive material to target specific tissues/tumor sites
TECHNIQUE	• Patient must be positioned in exactly the same position for each treatment • Tattoos or other marking methods may be used to ensure proper positioning • General anesthesia is often required	• Patient must be positioned in exactly the same position for each treatment • Tattoos or other marking methods may be used to ensure proper positioning • Short-acting anesthesia is often required • Radiation is often administered in one prolonged dose over minutes, hours, or days	• Administration of radionuclides orally, IV, or by peritoneal or pleural space injection
INDICATIONS	• Oral, nasal, rectal, perianal, and anal tumors • Soft-tissue sarcomas, mast cell tumors, osteosarcoma, malignant melanoma, lymphoproliferative disorders, and CNS tumors	• Oral, nasal, rectal, perianal and anal tumors • Soft-tissue sarcomas, mast cell tumors, osteosarcoma, malignant melanoma, lymphoproliferative disorders, and CNS tumors	*131I treatment* • Hyperthyroidism • Metastatic thyroid carcinoma
SPECIALIZED EQUIPMENT	• Megavoltage machine—suited for deep-seated tumors • Orthovoltage machine—suited for superficial tumors	• Megavoltage machine—suited for deep-seated tumors • Orthovoltage machine—suited for superficial tumors	• Isolation ward • 131I is the most currently used radionuclide

Table 11-8   Radiation Therapy: Teletherapy, Brachytherapy, and Systemic Therapy (Continued)

Procedure	Teletherapy (External Beam)	Brachytherapy (Interstitial)	Systemic Therapy
PRECAUTIONS	• Human exposure risk	• Human exposure risk	• Human exposure risk
SIDE EFFECTS	• Dependent on site being treated • Patient becomes radioactive with ± environmental contamination • Often seen near the end of treatment or 6 months to 1 year after treatment • Typically limited to the treatment site	• Dependent on site being treated • Patient becomes radioactive with ± environmental contamination	• Dependent on site being treated • Patient becomes radioactive with ± environmental contamination
NOTES	• Cells, both normal and abnormal, can repair themselves within a few hours of irradiation • Hypoxic cells are radioresistant—certain drugs ↑ oxygenation, which ↑ radiation effects	• High doses of radiation to a very localized area with tissue damage only to the tissue surrounding the tumor site	

TEMPERATURE THERAPY

The use of temperature has remained a popular complement or alternative to the treatment of neoplastic conditions. This technique has the ease of local treatment with only a few side effects, even though its scope of use is limited to mostly small tumors.

Table 11-9   Temperature Therapies: Hyperthermia and Cryotherapy

Procedure	Hyperthermia	Cryotherapy
DEFINITION	• Destruction of tissue by ↑ the temperature of the lesion and surrounding tissues to >104° F externally or internally	• Destruction of tissue by ↓ the temperature of the lesion and surrounding tissues to <−4° F
TECHNIQUE	• Local anesthesia is injected around the treatment site and a biopsy is taken • Tips are placed on either side of the lesion or if >0.2 cm deep, inserted down the sides of the lesion and then heated twice	• The area is shaved, cleaned, local anesthesia is injected and a biopsy is taken • Blood flow should be restricted to the site to prevent warming and to ↑ freezing • The lesion is rapidly frozen until it has reached <−4° F, slowly thaw and then is refrozen 1–2 more times
INDICATIONS	• Lesions <1 cm in diameter and up to 14 cm deep • Oral and facial sarcomas, squamous cell carcinoma, and hemangiopericytoma	• Lesions <1 cm in diameter • Skin and other external areas • Cataract surgery
EQUIPMENT	• Handheld radiofrequency, microwave, or ultrasound device	• Liquid nitrogen units • Nitrous oxide tanks
PRECAUTIONS		• Exhaust or runoff of liquid nitrogen spray may lead to inadvertent freezing of normal tissue on the animal or surgical team • Freezing of mast cell tumors may lead to ↑ erythema and sloughing because of local release of histamine and heparin • Not to be used when there is bone involvement because of its poor freezing ability and subsequent weakening of bone
SIDE EFFECTS	• Pain after treatment for 1–2 days • Burns • Loss of hair or change in color of skin pigment or fur at treatment site	• Burns • Loss of hair or change in color of skin pigment or fur at treatment site • Swelling, with resolution within 48 hours • Excessive bleeding because of subsequent vasodilation after biopsy and freezing • Odor from accumulated exudate and necrotic tissue
NOTES	• Whole-body hyperthermia is performed at only a few research institutions • Hyperthermia and radiation therapy are often combined because of their synergistic effects	• Liquid nitrogen is available in cans with spray nozzles, allowing treatment of larger lesions • Sedation might be required because of the pain involved in the freezing and the startling hissing noise of the unit • Cryosurgery has often been replaced by radiation therapy and laser surgery

12

Surgical Nursing

Many of the listed surgical procedures may not be performed in the average clinical setting. However, at one point or another, technicians will be faced with having to explain a particular procedure to a client.

These descriptions are not meant as directions on how to perform the procedure, but rather a quick synopsis that will allow the technician to prepare for the procedure, manage patient care, and clearly explain the procedure and aftercare to a client whose pet may be undergoing these procedures.

With every surgical procedure, pain management needs to be addressed and handled. Refer to Chapter 8, Pain Management, for more information.

INSTRUMENT PACKS

These packs are examples of the instruments included in basic surgical packs. Each clinic will need to organize packs that best fit their surgery type and surgeon. Each surgeon has preferences on individual types of instruments for different surgeries. Each pack may include gauze, laparotomy pads, towels, saline bowl, needles, sutures, and scalpel blades, or they may be prepared separately.

Basic Surgical Packs
Abdominal Pack
  Abdominal forceps
  Abdominal retractors
  Balfour retractor
General Surgical Pack
  Grooved director
  Hemostats
  Needle holders
  Retractors
  Scalpel handle
  Scissors
  Spay hook
  Thumb forceps
  Tissue forceps
  Towel clamps
Laceration Pack
  Hemostats
  Needle holder
  Scalpel handle
  Scissors
  Thumb forceps
Ophthalmic Pack
  Eyelid Forceps
  Eyelid Retractor
  Hemostats
  Lacrimal cannulas
  Needle holders
  Scalpel handle
  Scissors
  Thumb forceps

Orthopedic Pack

    Bone drill

    Bone chuck and key

    Bone-cutting forceps

    Bone-holding forceps

    Bone rasps and files

    Gigli handles and wire

    Mallet

    Osteotome

    Orthopedic wire

    Periosteal elevator

    Pin cutter

    Retractors

      Senn retractor

      Volkmann retractor

    Rongeurs

    Wire-cutting scissors

Thoracic pack

    General surgical pack instruments with long handles

    Rib retractors

      Wilson rib spreader

    Bone-cutting forceps

    Right-angle forceps

    Vessel clamps

      Bulldog clamp

Specialized Surgical Packs

Many instruments may be used only on occasion and should be set aside in separate packs. Instruments weaken with constant scrubbing and autoclaving and should therefore not be subjected to unnecessary sterilization. The instrument type and number included in each of these packs will depend on surgeon preference.

Biopsy/Trephine Pack

Curette pack

Hemostat pack

Implant set

Periosteal elevator pack

Pin set

Retractor pack

Screw set

Suction tips and tubing pack

POSTOPERATIVE CARE

The success of each surgical procedure often lies in the patient care that follows the procedure. This often ends with the client to continue at home care. Clear and concise instructions are critical to enable this transition to occur successfully. Clients should be strongly encouraged to phone if any questions or concerns arise. Follow-up phone calls 1–2 days after a surgical procedure by the staff will also encourage client communication.

Skill Box 12-1 / Standard Postoperative Care Instructions

Feed only half of the normal food and water the first evening after surgery

Check incision daily for redness, swelling, discharge, or odor

Prevent licking, chewing, or rubbing at incision line or sutures

Keep the animal and/or bandages dry and clean

Avoid bathing or swimming until suture removal or for 5–7 days with SC sutures

Phone the doctor if any of the following occur:

> Repeated vomiting
>
> Extreme listlessness
>
> Bleeding or discharge
>
> Loss of appetite for >24 hours
>
> Opened incision lines

Skill Box 12-2 / Preventing Licking, Chewing, or Rubbing at Incision Site or Sutures

1. Use an Elizabethan collar (e-collar, neck brace, etc.) at all times
2. Apply a bandage (e.g., soft padded bandage, hobbles, or Schroeder-Thomas splint with sheet aluminum)
3. Foul-tasting substance (e.g., bitter apple, atropine, Tabasco, or thumb-sucking preparations)
4. Cover the area with a sock, baby t-shirt, or stockinette
5. Body brace, side bar, or tail-tip protector

ABDOMINAL SURGERY

Table 12-1 Abdominal Surgery

Procedure	Abdominal Surgery
DEFINITION	• See particular surgery
INDICATIONS	• See particular surgery
INSTRUMENTS	• Abdominal pack • Electrocautery • Gauze sponges/laparotomy pads • General surgical pack • Retractor pack • Saline bowl • Saline, warmed • Suction tips and tubing pack
PATIENT	• See particular surgery
SURGICAL TECHNIQUE	• The organ or area to be examined should be exteriorized and packed with saline moistened gauze sponges • All tissues must be kept consistently moist with warm saline • Handling of the internal organs must be done carefully to avoid further damage, but secure enough to not allow leakage of the bowel contents into the surgery site • Provide clean, sterile drapes, towels, gloves, and instruments for abdominal closure • Patient should be monitored for excessive blood loss, contamination of peritoneal cavity, and an ↑ tendency to vomit with organ manipulation

PREPARATION

COMPLICATIONS

PROCEDURAL

- Abscess
- Dehiscence
- Gastric or intestinal perforation
- Hemorrhage (e.g., poor hemostasis and inadvertent injury to vascular organs)
- Ileus
- Intestinal stricture
- Pancreatitis
- Peritonitis/sepsis (e.g., contamination with gastrointestinal tract (GIT) contents)
- Pleural effusion
- Failure of intended surgery
- Adhesions between visceral surfaces

PATIENT

- Hyperthermia with prolonged procedures
- Abdominal pain
- Fecal incontinence
- Fever
- Tenesmus/constipation/dyschezia
- Vomiting

FOLLOW-UP

PATIENT CARE

- ± NPO for 12–24 hours
- Analgesia postoperatively
- Monitor ability, frequency, and appearance of defecation
- Standard postoperative care
- Confine and restrict activity until suture/staple removal or as directed by DVM

CLIENT EDUCATION

- Recheck/Suture removal in _____ days
- Medication:
- Lab results in _____ days

Table 12-2 Abdominal Surgery (Continued)

Procedure	Abdominal Hernia	Anal Sacculectomy	Colotomy
DEFINITION	• Repair of a hole in the abdominal wall that is allowing an organ or part of an organ to protrude	• Removal of 1 or both anal sacs and associated anal sac duct	• Incision made into the colon
INDICATIONS	• Intestinal obstruction and/or strangulation damage	• Correction of long-term anal sac infection and neoplasia	• Full-thickness biopsy and foreign body removal
PATIENT PREPARATION	• Dorsal recumbency • Prepare 3" on either side of the hernia	• Ventral recumbency with rear legs draped over end of table and tail secured cranially • Prepare a 4" radius around anus • Express anal sacs, evacuate as much of the feces from the colon as possible, and pack rectum with sponges • *Closed:* instill self-hardening gel or resin into sac(s) to be removed	• ± Multiple enemas to ↓ risk of infection and to ↑ visibility • Dorsal recumbency • Prepare entire ventral abdomen
SURGICAL TECHNIQUE	• An incision is made over the hernia and dissected down to the hernia orifice. Any adhesions are removed and the organs and/or viscera are returned to the peritoneal cavity. The edges of the hernial orifice are sharply freshened and sutured closed. Routine closure of the abdomen is performed.	• *Closed:* the hardened sac is isolated, and an incision is made over the sac. The surrounding tissue is gently dissected away from the sac, and the sac and duct are removed. The area is lavaged with warmed saline, and the remaining tissue is closed in a routine closure. • *Open:* The anal sac orifice is visualized and a grooved director is placed into the sac orifice to the most ventral aspect. An incision is made along the grooved director, and the entire sac and duct are dissected out. The area is lavaged with warmed saline, and the remaining tissue is closed in a routine closure.	• A caudal midline abdominal incision is made. The affected area is exteriorized and packed with saline-moistened gauze sponges. Stay sutures are placed, and the colonic contents are milked away from the intended incision site. An incision is made into the colon, and the foreign body is removed or biopsy specimens taken. The colotomy is closed, and the abdomen is flushed with warm saline. The colotomy is covered and tacked with a piece of omentum, and routine closure of the abdomen is performed.
NOTES	• *Client Education:* Chronic hernias may not require surgical intervention	• *Instruments:* *Closed:* self-hardening gel or resin and administration equipment *Open:* grooved director • *Surgery:* careful, atraumatic dissection with minimal muscle damage is essential to preserve nerve and sphincter function • *Patient care:* hot pack the surgical site immediately after surgery and antibiotics for 7–10 days postoperatively • *Client Education:* hot pack incision twice daily until suture removal	• *Surgery:* stay sutures may not be necessary, especially if surgical assistant is present • *Patient care:* antibiotics during surgery and postoperatively (only if contamination is suspected)

Table 12-3 Abdominal Surgery (Continued)

Procedure	Enterotomy	Gastric-Dilatation Volvulus (GDV) *See Chapter 5, Emergency Care*	Gastrotomy
DEFINITION	• Incision made into the small intestines	• To reposition the stomach and the spleen in their correct location and restore their blood circulation • Fix the stomach to the abdominal wall to prevent further torsion	• Incision made into the stomach
INDICATIONS	• Examination for ulcers, strictures, or neoplasia, full-thickness biopsy, and foreign body (FB) removal	• A stomach that dilates and twists around its central axis	• Full-thickness biopsy and foreign body (FB) removal
PATIENT PREPARATION	• Dorsal recumbency • Prepare entire abdomen	• Orogastric decompression or needle trocarization • Dorsal recumbency • Prepare midsternum to 2–3 inches below the umbilicus	• Dorsal recumbency • Prepare bottom third of the sternum to 2–3 inches below the umbilicus
SURGICAL TECHNIQUE	• A midline abdominal incision is made. The affected area is exteriorized and packed with saline-moistened gauze sponges. Stay sutures are placed, and the bowel contents are milked away from the intended incision site. An incision is made into the intestines, and the FB is removed or biopsy specimens taken. The intestines are examined for viability and resection, and anastomosis is performed if necessary. The enterotomy is closed, and the abdomen is flushed with warm saline. The enterotomy is covered with a piece of omentum and tacked, and routine closure of the abdomen is performed.	• A midline abdominal incision is made. Further orogastric decompression is performed if necessary via an orogastric tube or suction. The stomach is rotated back to its normal position, assessed for necrotic tissue, and a partial gastrectomy is performed if necessary. The spleen is evaluated for rotation and necrosis. A splenectomy is performed if there is splenic necrosis. Gastropexy is then performed on the right side of the dog by one of many methods. The abdomen is then closed with routine closure.	• A cranial midline abdominal incision is made. The stomach is exteriorized and packed with saline moistened gauze sponges. Stay sutures are placed. The stomach is excised into and suctioned free of liquid contents. The FB is removed or biopsy specimens taken. The stomach is closed in a multi-layer fashion, lavaged with warmed saline, and possibly covered with omentum. The abdomen is closed routinely.
NOTES	• *Surgery:* Stay sutures may not be necessary, especially if a surgical assistant is present • *Surgery:* Enterotomy incisions are usually made in tissue adjacent to the FB rather than directly over it for better incision healing	• *Instruments:* Orogastric tube • *Patient Care:* Monitor electrolytes, blood gases, hematocrit (Hct), total protein (TP), urinary output, electrocardiogram (ECG), and central venous pressure (CVP) as necessary, and keep NPO for 24–48 hours • *Client Education:* Feed small meals 3–4 times daily, and avoid exercise after each meal	• None

Table 12-4 Abdominal Surgery (Continued)

Procedure	Intestinal Resection and Anastomosis	Hepatectomy, partial
DEFINITION	• Removal of a diseased or nonviable section of the intestines and repair to the bowel with end-to-end bowel reattachment	• Removal of <80% of the liver
INDICATIONS	• A nonfunctioning section of bowel possibly caused by foreign body, neoplasia, intussusception, bowel necrosis, fecal infiltrative bowel disease, or volvulus	• Biopsy, neoplasia, necrosis, abscess, or hemorrhage
PATIENT PREPARATION	• Dorsal recumbency • Prepare the caudal end of the sternum to the pubis	• Coagulation tests and thrombocyte count • Dorsal recumbency • Prepare entire abdomen and caudal third of sternum
SURGICAL TECHNIQUE	• A ventral midline abdominal incision is made. The area of the intestines to be resected is exteriorized, packed with saline moistened gauze sponges, and major vessels are ligated. The bowel contents are milked away from the site, and abdominal forceps are placed. The diseased portion is removed, and one of many types of suture patterns may be used to allow complete closure of the intestines. Bowel contents are milked back into the anastomosis site to assure no leakage. The entire abdomen is flushed with warmed saline if contamination is suspected. The site of anastomosis is then flushed with saline and an antimicrobial solution and covered with a piece of omentum. Routine closure of the abdominal wall is performed.	• A ventral midline abdominal incision is made. Gauze sponges are placed between the liver and diaphragm for better visualization. The liver is examined for biopsy areas or portions to be removed. The associated vessels are securely ligated, and the partial hepatectomy is performed. The area is observed for confirmation of adequate hemostasis, and routine closure of the abdominal wall is performed.
NOTES	• None	• *Client Education:* Liver mass is restored to normal in a matter of weeks by compensatory hypertrophy of the remaining tissue*

*Current Techniques in Small Animal Surgery, M. Joseph Bojrab

AURAL

Table 12-5 Aural Surgery

Procedure	Aural Surgery
PREPARATION	
DEFINITION	• See particular surgery
INDICATIONS	• See particular surgery
INSTRUMENTS	• Buttons or Silastic tubing • Cartilage scissors • Electrocautery • Laceration pack or general surgical pack
PATIENT	• See particular surgery
SURGICAL TECHNIQUE	• Electrocautery is an important part of ear surgery because of the highly vascular tissue and degree of hemorrhage
COMPLICATIONS	
PROCEDURAL	• Hematoma formation
PATIENT	• Head shaking or scratching
FOLLOW-UP	
PATIENT CARE	• ± Bandage of ear against head and wrapped/secured with stockinette • Standard postoperative care • Analgesia postoperatively • Confine and restrict activity until suture/staple removal or as directed by DVM
CLIENT EDUCATION	• Recheck/Suture removal in _____ days • Bandage removal in _____ days • Medication: _____ • Lab results in _____ days

Table 12-6 Aural Surgery (Continued)

Procedure	Aural Hematoma	Lateral Ear Canal Resection
DEFINITION	• Drainage and apposition of the cartilage surfaces to allow healing and prevent reoccurrence of hematoma	• Removal of the lateral ear wall to allow proper drainage and exposure of the horizontal canal • Must be performed early in course of chronic otitis externa if success is to be achieved
INDICATIONS	• Irritations causing head shaking or scratching at ears	• Chronic infections, trauma, or neoplasia • Anatomic due to breed (e.g., Shar pei)
PATIENT PREPARATION	• Lateral recumbency • Place 1–2 cotton balls in ear canal to prevent fluid accumulation in deep canal • Prepare the entire pinna on both sides	• Lateral recumbency • Clean the ear canal of all waxy material and debris • Prepare entire pinna and the external ear canal region
SURGICAL TECHNIQUE	• An incision is made down the long axis of the pinna. The pinna is probed for and removed of fibrin tags and blood clots and flushed with saline. A mattress pattern of sutures (± incorporating buttons and Silastic tubing) is placed along the surface of the pinna to remove any dead space and allow complete apposition of both sides of the ear cartilage.	• Two incisions are made parallel to the vertical ear canal margins and a transverse incision joining them. The skin and SC tissue are reflected, and two incisions are made through the cartilage to expose the inside of the vertical canal. The reflected flap of cartilage is trimmed and sutured to the skin to make a drainboard ventrally.
NOTES	• *Client Education:* Strict confinement is necessary to allow pinna to heal properly • *Client Education:* Even with appropriate treatment, disfiguration (cauliflower appearance) of the pinna may occur	• *Client Education:* Do not use any foreign object (e.g., cotton balls, cotton-tipped applicators) in the shortened ear canal, to avoid damage to the tympanic membrane

INTEGUMENT

Table 12-7   Integument Surgery

Procedure		Integument Surgery
PREPARATION	**DEFINITION**	• See particular surgery
	INDICATIONS	• See particular surgery
	INSTRUMENTS	• Laceration pack or general surgical pack • ± Penrose drain
	PATIENT	• See particular surgery
	SURGICAL TECHNIQUE	• See particular surgery
COMPLICATIONS	**PROCEDURAL**	• Dehiscence, skin necrosis, and slough • Failure of intended surgery • Sepsis • Seroma
	PATIENT	• Fever • Pain or swelling from infection or SC seroma
FOLLOW-UP	**PATIENT CARE**	• Monitor for pain or swelling • Monitor appearance of drain material when a Penrose drain is placed • Analgesia postoperatively • Standard postoperative care • Confine and restrict activity until suture/staple removal or as directed by DVM
	CLIENT EDUCATION	• Hot compress drain sites twice daily for _____ to maintain open drain holes when a Penrose drain is in place • Recheck/suture removal in _____ days • Medication: • Laboratory results in _____ days

Table 12-8 Integument Surgery (Continued)

Procedure	Abscess, superficial	Laceration, superficial
DEFINITION	• Accumulation of pus, forming an isolated cavity in body tissue because of a pathogen	• A full-thickness disruption through the dermis and exposing the SC
INDICATIONS	• Swelling and painful location that is not draining and is disrupting the normal function of the animal • Sepsis	• To restore skin integrity and allow for reepithelialization by primary intention healing
PATIENT PREPARATION	• Positioned to allow access to the affected site • Prepare the site to include the location of swelling with an additional 1–2″ margin	• Positioned to allow access to the affected site • Prepare the site to include the location of injury with an additional 1–2″ margin • Clipped hair must not enter the laceration site, a vacuum, sterile lubricant, or gauze sponge may be used
SURGICAL TECHNIQUE	• A sharp object is used to make an opening into the abscess, and accumulated pus and fluid is allowed to drain out. The area is flushed with a solution (chlorhexidine, diluted hydrogen peroxide, saline, etc.) to remove any additional contaminated fluid, bacteria, or debris. Any devitalized tissue is removed, and an additional hole is made for the drain. The drain is placed through both holes and sutured into place for 3–5 days.	• The area is clipped and cleaned, and any foreign material is removed. Devitalized tissue is removed via debridement. The area is flushed with a solution (chlorhexidine, diluted hydrogen peroxide, saline, etc.) to remove any additional contaminated fluid, bacteria, or debris. A drain may be placed, and the area is closed by using sutures or staples.
NOTES	• *Surgical:* Abscesses should not be opened in sterile operating rooms to avoid contamination • *Patient care:* Systemic antibiotics postoperatively for ≥ 1 week	• *Surgical:* Flushing fluids should not contain sugars, because that provides nutrients for the pathogens, and eliminating skin tension at suture line is imperative for healing • *Postoperatively:* ± Bandage and immobilize for ↑ healing and to ↓ swelling

Table 12-9 Integument Surgery (Continued)

Procedure	Mass Removal	Onychectomy (Declaw)*
DEFINITION	• Removal of a tumor, mass, growth, or cyst	• Removal of the nail and entire third phalanx
INDICATIONS	• Obstruction with function, neoplasia, or cosmetic	• Trauma, infection, or neoplasia
PATIENT PREPARATION	• Positioned to allow access to the affected site • Prepare the site to include the tumor location with an additional 1–2" margin • Larger margins when neoplasia is suspected or confirmed as malignant	• Analgesics are administered before the procedure • Lateral recumbency • Paws are clipped if long hair is present, washed, and sprayed with an antiseptic
SURGICAL TECHNIQUE	• *Varying techniques are employed for the varying sizes and shapes of specific tumors* An elliptical incision is made around the tumor, and it is dissected out. Adequate hemostasis is applied. The dead space is closed via sutures, and a drain may be placed. The skin edges are apposed and sutured closed.	• The blood is milked proximally, and a tourniquet is placed proximal to the elbow. Nail trimmers are used to amputate each toe. The toes are then closed with suture or tissue glue. A secure bandage is placed to prevent hemorrhage.
NOTES	• *Patient Care:* ± bandage	• *Instruments:* Tourniquet, skin glue, and sterile nail trimmers • *Surgical Complications:* The third phalanx must be removed from each toe to avoid additional pain and nail regrowth, infection, "phantom" pain sensation, and/or occasional limping • *Patient Complications:* Patient biting as a substitute for clawing • *Client Education:* pain medication: _____

*The authors strongly believe this procedure should only be done as medical treatment and not as behavioral modification.

OPHTHALMIC

Table 12-10 Ophthalmic Surgery

Procedure	Ophthalmic Surgery
PREPARATION	
DEFINITION	• See particular surgery
INDICATIONS	• See particular surgery
INSTRUMENTS	• Ophthalmic surgical pack • Eyelid speculum
PATIENT	• Ventral recumbency with the head propped up on a towel or cushion • Place a sterile ophthalmic ointment in the eye to protect from clipped hair and cleaning solutions • Prepare area immediately around eye
SURGICAL TECHNIQUE	• See particular surgery
COMPLICATIONS	
PROCEDURAL	• Failure of intended surgery • Infection • Tissue necrosis • Keratitis secondary to corneal drying and/or trauma
PATIENT	• Swelling • Pain
FOLLOW-UP	
PATIENT CARE	• Analgesia postoperatively • Standard postoperative care • Confine and restrict activity until suture/staple removal or as directed by DVM
CLIENT EDUCATION	• Recheck/suture removal in _____ days • Medication: • Lab results in _____ days

Table 12-11 Ophthalmic Surgery (Continued)

Procedure	Cataracts	Entropion (Ventral, Dorsal, Lateral or Medial)	Enucleation
DEFINITION	• Removal of the anterior lens through surgical removal or physical dissolution	• Removal of a section of eyelid skin, depending on the type of entropion	• Removal of the eye (globe)
INDICATIONS	• Opacity of the lens, which could lead to uveitis, glaucoma, visual deficits, or retinal detachment	• Inward rolling of the eyelid, resulting in keratitis, corneal ulceration, and pain	• Glaucoma, trauma, neoplasia, or ocular diseases
SURGICAL TECHNIQUE	• *Extracapsular extraction:* A corneal or corneoscleral incision is made, and the anterior lens capsule is removed • *Phacofragmentation:* An ultrasound-driven needle is used to emulsify and remove the affected lens simultaneously • An intraocular lens is often placed to further ↑ vision	• An elliptical or V-shaped area of skin is removed, depending on the location of the entropion. The area is then sutured closed with a nonabsorbable suture, allowing the lid to remain in a normal anatomic position.	• *Transconjunctival:* An incision is made at the lateral canthus, and the eye is stabilized. • The eye is dissected through the muscle attachments, optic nerve, and blood vessels and then removed. The tissues are then sutured in a layered fashion. *Transpalpebral:* The eyelids are sutured closed, and an elliptical incision is made 5–6 mm from the eyelid margin. • See above
NOTES	• *Indications:* must be distinguished from nuclear sclerosis • *Patient care:* inflammation must be controlled for success	• *Surgical:* everting sutures may be used temporarily in young dogs for correction without excision of any eyelid skin	• *Complications:* hemorrhage (e.g., angularis oculi vein is severed)

Table 12-12 Ophthalmic Surgery (Continued)

Procedure	Glaucoma	Nictitating Membrane Flap Replacement	Prolapse of the Gland of the Third Eyelid (Cherry eye)
DEFINITION	• To ↓ the production and ↑ outflow of aqueous humor and to ↓ ocular pressure	• Temporary attachment of the nictitating membrane to the upper palpebra for corneal support	• Repositioning of the third eyelid gland and anchoring in a more normal position
INDICATIONS	• To retain vision and normal intraocular pressure and ↓ pain	• Deep corneal ulcers, trauma, or corneal diseases as a temporary bandage during healing	• Hypertrophy and prolapse of the third eyelid gland
SURGICAL TECHNIQUE	• *Laser Cyclophotocoagulation:* killing small areas of the ciliary body via a laser • *Cyclocryotherapy:* freezing the ciliary body in multiple sites (4-8) with liquid nitrogen administered via a cyroprobe • *Anterior Chamber Shunts:* implantation of a tube to allow continuous drainage of aqueous fluid	• The nictitans is sutured to the upper eyelid or bulbar conjunctiva, incorporating buttons or Silastic tubing to prevent tissue necrosis from the sutures.	• *Pocket:* an incision is made along the margins of the gland into the palpebral conjunctiva. A pocket is formed, and the gland is returned to its normal position. The incision is then sutured together over the gland. • *Pursestring:* the third eyelid is exposed and stabilized. A pursestring suture is placed over both ends of the gland. The gland is returned to normal position with a cotton-tipped applicator, and the pursestring suture is pulled tight and knotted.
NOTES	• *Client Education:* painful, blind eyes will not benefit from the above-mentioned surgeries and should be enucleated	• *Complications:* sutures may pull through with excess tension • *Client education:* suture removal varies between 10 days and 4 weeks	• *Client Education:* removal of the gland is no longer recommended because of later complications

ORTHOPEDIC

Table 12-13 Orthopedic Surgery

Procedure	Orthopedic Surgery
DEFINITION	• See particular surgery
INDICATIONS	• See particular surgery
PREPARATION — INSTRUMENTS	• Orthopedic pack • Pin set • Screw set • Implant set • Periosteal elevator set
PREPARATION — PATIENT	• Lateral recumbency • Scrub midhock to ventral midline with the leg suspended by gauze
PREPARATION — SURGICAL TECHNIQUE	• See particular surgery
COMPLICATIONS — PROCEDURAL	• Failure of intended surgery • Infection (e.g., osteomyelitis) • Malunion or non-union from inadequate immobilization
COMPLICATIONS — PATIENT	• Gait alterations
FOLLOW-UP — PATIENT CARE	• ± Bandage • Physical therapy (See Skill Box 6-8) • Analgesia postoperatively • Standard postoperative care • Confine and restrict activity until suture/staple removal or as directed by DVM
FOLLOW-UP — CLIENT EDUCATION	• Recheck/Suture removal in _____ days • Medication: _____ • Lab results in _____ days

Table 12-14 Orthopedic Surgery (Continued)

Procedure	Cranial Cruciate Ligament Rupture	Femoral Head Ostectomy (FHO)	Fracture Repair
DEFINITION	• To stabilize the joint by ↓ or eliminating abnormal forces exerted on the stifle joint because of ligament loss, and thereby to prevent further injury and return the leg to normal function	• Removal of the femoral head and part of the neck	• To provide stability so fracture healing may occur with the least amount of disruption to the natural healing process
INDICATIONS	• Progressive lameness and degenerative joint disease	• Cats and small dogs with hip dysplasia or hip injury	• Any type of break in a bone, typically a long bone
SURGICAL TECHNIQUE	• *Fibular Head Transposition:* extracapsular technique using cranial advancement of the fibular head to fix the stifle in external rotation • *"Over-the-Top" Fascia Strip:* intracapsular technique using a strip of fascia passed through the bone tunnels to mimic the cranial cruciate ligament • *"Over-the-Top" Patellar Tendon Graft:* intra-articular technique using a patellar tendon graft to replace the cranial cruciate ligament • *Retinacular Imbrication:* extracapsular technique using sutures placed both laterally and medially to stabilize the stifle short-term and allow fibrous tissue to form for long term stabilization • *Tibial Plateau Leveling Osteotomy (TPLO):* repositioning of the tibial plateau through osteotomy to allow surrounding muscles to provide stifle stability	• A craniolateral incision is made. The hip joint is dissected down and the hip is luxated to allow ↑ visibility. The femoral head and a portion of the neck are removed, and the end of the bone is smoothed over. Tendons and muscles are returned to original location and sutured. Routine closure of the tissue in layers is performed.	• *Cerclage wire:* wire placed around the bone fracture for stabilization • *Tension band wiring:* wire and intramedullary pins placed to fix and apply compression to the tension side of a fracture • *Interlocking Nail and Intramedullary Pin Fixation:* pins and locking nails placed down the intramedullary canal of long bones • *Stack-Pinning:* multiple intramedullary pins placed for internal fixation • *Screw Fixation:* screws placed along fracture sites for stabilization
NOTES	• *Client Education:* a 4–5-month recovery period is typically necessary, but the patient should follow DVM's postoperative instructions for optimal recovery	• *Patient Care:* anti-inflammatory drugs are typically used • *Client Education:* vigorous activity is started immediately after surgery for short periods and return to complete activity typically takes 6–12 months	• *Patient Preparation:* ± traction on the affected bone

Table 12-15 Orthopedic Surgery (Continued)

Procedure	Patellar Luxation	Triple Pelvic Osteotomy (TPO)	Total Hip Replacement
DEFINITION	• To stabilize the patella in the trochlea and allow movement of the limb without luxation	• Rotation of the acetabulum portion of the pelvis to help prevent degenerative joint disease in hip dysplasia	• Replacement of the femoral head and acetabular cup with artificial prostheses
INDICATIONS	• Patella that luxates spontaneously or with palpation	• Young dogs (5–18) months with hip dysplasia and no signs of degenerative joint disease	• Dogs >9 months old with a disabling condition of the hip
SURGICAL TECHNIQUE	• *Trochleoplasty:* to deepen the trochlear groove by removal of the current cartilage • *Chondroplasty:* to deepen the trochlear groove by forming a flap of cartilage, removing underlying bone, and replacing the flap • *Wedge recession:* to deepen the trochlear groove by cutting a wedge of cartilage out and replacing it further recessed into the groove • *Tibial tuberosity translocation:* transplantation of the attachment of the patellar ligament to a more lateral position, using wires for stabilization	• Three incisions are made into the wing of the ilium, pubis, and ischium around the acetabulum. The acetabulum is then free to be rotated to provide more dorsal coverage of the femoral head. Bone plates, wires, or screws are then placed to secure the acetabulum in its new position. Routine closure of the tissue in layers is then performed.	• A craniolateral incision is made. The femoral head and a portion of the neck is removed and replaced with the prosthetic. The location of the original acetabular cup is widened, and the prosthetic acetabular cup is cemented to the medial pelvic wall. The femoral head is then reduced into the acetabular cup, and the joint is closed tightly. Then routine closure of the tissue in layers is performed.
NOTES	• *Patient care:* at least 3 weeks of restricted activity	• *Complications:* infection and loosening of bone plates	• *Patient Preparation:* IV antibiotics are started the day before the procedure, and the surgery site is clipped to check for skin infections • *Complicatons:* infection of implants

REPRODUCTIVE TRACT SURGERY

Table 12-16 Reproductive Tract Surgery		
Procedure	**Reproductive Tract Surgery**	
PREPARATION	DEFINITION	• See particular surgery
	INDICATIONS	• See particular surgery
	INSTRUMENTS	• General surgical pack
	PATIENT	• See particular surgery
COMPLICATIONS	SURGICAL TECHNIQUE	• See particular surgery
	PROCEDURAL	• Adhesions of uterine stump, bladder, or scrotal skin • Failure to remove all gonadal tissue completely (e.g., ovarian remnant syndrome) • Hemorrhage • Peritonitis/sepsis • Inadvertent damage to vital urinary structures (e.g., ureters)
	PATIENT	• Vomiting • Inappetance
FOLLOW-UP	PATIENT CARE	• Standard postoperative care • Confine and restrict activity until suture/staple removal (typically 5–7 days) or as directed by DVM
	CLIENT EDUCATION	• Recheck/Suture removal in _____ days • Medication: • Lab results in _____ days

Table 12-17 Reproductive Tract Surgery (Continued)

Procedure	Ceasarean Section (C-section, Hysterotomy)	Orchiectomy (Alter, Neuter, Castration)	Ovariohysterectomy (Spay, OVH, OHE)
DEFINITION	• Removal of all fetuses from the uterus through the abdomen	• The removal of the testes	• The removal of the uterus and both ovaries
INDICATIONS	• Dystocia, uterine inertia, prolonged gestation, fetal death, trauma, or toxemia	• Sterilization, reduction of aggressiveness, wandering, and marking behavior, cancer, traumatic injury, infections, and prostate gland problems	• Sterilization, uterine infections, cancer, uterine torsion, congenital abnormalities, ovarian-induced hormone imbalances, elimination of estrus, and extensive injury
PATIENT PREPARATION	• Dorsal recumbency • Prepare xiphoid to pubis • **Prepare as much of the surgical site as possible before induction of anesthesia to limit depression of neonates** • **Caution:** Avoid narcotic premedications that might compromise fetal condition via placental blood flow	• Verify the patient is a male, has not previously been neutered, and has 2 palpable testicles *Canine:* • Dorsal recumbency • Prepare the prepuce to the area surrounding and including the scrotum *Feline:* • Ventral recumbency • Prepare the area surrounding and including the scrotum	• Verify the patient is a female and has not previously been spayed • Dorsal recumbency • Manually express the bladder • Prepare entire ventral abdomen

Table 12-17 Reproductive Tract Surgery (Continued)

Procedure	Ceasarean Section (C-section, Hysterotomy)	Orchiectomy (Alter, Neuter, Castration)	Ovariohysterectomy (Spay, OVH, OHE)
SURGICAL TECHNIQUE	• A ventral midline incision is made and the horns of the uterus are exteriorized. The incision is packed with saline moistened gauze or laparotomy pads to avoid abdominal contamination. An incision is made into the uterus and one by one each fetus is milked down to the incision and gently pulled out. The fetal membranes are removed to allow breathing and the umbilical cord is clamped 2-3 cm from the abdomen. Once all the fetuses have been removed, the uterine horns are checked for any remaining fetuses or placentas. The uterine incision is closed, moistened with saline, covered with omentum and returned to the abdominal cavity. Routine closure of the tissue in layers is performed.	*Canine:* • An incision is made just cranial to the scrotum, and one testicle is exposed through the fascia. The entire spermatic cord may be ligated to remove the testicle (closed), or the outer tunic may be incised to reveal the spermatic vessels and cord. These structures are then ligated or knotted onto themselves (open). Gentle traction is placed on the scrotum to allow the remaining tunic tissue to retract into the scrotum. The procedure is repeated for the second testicle. *Feline:* • An incision is made into the scrotum over each testicle in a caudoventral position, and the open or closed technique may then be applied.	• A ventral midline incision is made, and the left uterine horn is located. The suspensory ligament is stretched or broken, and the ovary is ligated and detached. The right uterine horn is located, and the broad ligament is broken and the ovary is ligated and detached. Then the uterus is ligated at the stump, and the combined uterus and ovaries are removed. Routine closure of the tissue in layers is performed.
NOTES	• *Surgical:* intense monitoring (especially circulatory) once the neonates are delivered to prevent shock in the dam • *Patient Care:* bloody vaginal discharge is to be expected for 3–7 days, but copious amount of clotted or foul-smelling vaginal discharge should be reported to the DVM • *Patient Care:* avoid post-op analgesics that will be passed into the milk (See Skill Box 12-3) • *Client Education:* once an animal has had a C-section, they are more likely to need one with the next litter and multiple C-sections cause scarring at the incision line and may complicate surgery	• *Patient Care:* monitor for scrotal hematoma • *Client Education:* insemination is still possible for several weeks after neuter • *Client Education:* behavioral changes after neutering may take several months to show; and may not show at all in an older dog	• *Patient Care:* Monitor for extreme listlessness, persistent bleeding, urinary incontinence, and skin problems • *Client Education:* healthy animals should be spayed around 6 months of age, when their bodies are best able to tolerate the anesthesia and before the first estrus cycle to prevent a more complicated surgery and to ↓ the risk of mammary tumors • *Client Education:* ↓ caloric intake; the activity of a spayed animal ↓ and so should their caloric intake

Skill Box 12-3 / Postoperative Care of Neonates and the Dam

Neonate Care:

1. Remove fetal membranes and verify that the umbilical cord is temporarily clamped

2. Assess the condition: whether a heartbeat can be palpated, clear the mouth and nose of fluid and mucus by gentle suction or cotton swabs

3. Stimulate respiration

   a. Rub the neonate briskly with a towel

   b. Grasp the neonate firmly in both hands and gently swing it from over head to between your legs

      - **Caution: strong force may cause brain damage**

   c. Administer doxapram (1–2 gtt sublingually or 0.1 mL IV in the umbilical vein) or naloxone (0.01 mg/kg IM or IV)

   d. Place an acupuncture needle or a small-gauge needle ($\leq$ 25g) between the upper lip and the nose to a depth of 2–4 mm while firmly holding the head extended and elevated above the heart

   - **If the above methods do not produce a neonate that is breathing and crying, emergency resuscitation must take place**

4. Once the neonates are stable, place them in a warm, confined location (e.g., incubator, box with towels, or circulating hot water pad)

5. Verify the neonates are free of congenital abnormalities and are nursing appropriately before discharge

   - **Caution: Neonates are often small enough to fall between the bars on a cage door**

Dam Care:

1. Mammary glands should be cleaned of surgical preparation solutions, blood, or fetal fluids

2. Dam should be allowed to recover from anesthesia alone and then returned to her litter once there is not risk of injury to the neonates

3. Monitor for the first few hours after surgery for relapses into shock because of uterine hemorrhage

4. Discharge dam and litter once she is able to stand and shows appropriate mothering instinct

THORACIC SURGERY

Table 12-18 Thoracic Surgery

Procedure	Thoracic Surgery
DEFINITION	• See particular surgery
INDICATIONS	• See particular surgery
INSTRUMENTS	• Electrocautery • Hemostat pack • Retractor pack • Suction tips and tubing pack • Thoracic pack
PATIENT	• See particular surgery
SURGICAL TECHNIQUE	• Ventilation support and circulation monitoring required throughout surgery
PROCEDURAL	• Hemorrhage (e.g., hemothorax) • Pleuritis/sepsis • Pneumothorax • Ventricular arrhythmias
PATIENT	• Pain • Difficulty breathing
PATIENT CARE	• Monitor radiographs for signs of pleural effusion • Monitor for pain and discomfort • Analgesia postoperatively • Standard postoperative care • Confine and restrict activity until suture/staple removal or as directed by DVM
CLIENT EDUCATION	• Recheck/Suture removal in _____ days • Medication: • Pain medication: • Lab results in _____ days

PREPARATION — COMPLICATIONS — FOLLOW-UP

Table 12-19 Thoracic Surgery (Continued)

Procedure	Diaphragmatic Hernia	Sternotomy, Median	Thoracotomy, Intercostal
DEFINITION	• Variably sized hole in the diaphragm allowing passage of the abdominal contents into the thoracic cavity	• To gain access to the thoracic cavity except the structures in the dorsal mediastinum (e.g., esophagus and bronchial hilus)	• To gain access to one third of the left or right side of the thorax and expose selected thoracic organs via an intercostal approach
INDICATIONS	• Herniation of liver, spleen, GIT, or omentum into the thoracic cavity	• Cardiac and respiratory diseases, neoplasia, correction of cardiovascular defects, and to obtain biopsy specimens	• Cardiac and respiratory diseases, neoplasia, correction of cardiovascular defects, and to obtain biopsy specimens
PATIENT PREPARATION	• Dorsal recumbency • Prepare bottom half of sternum to 2–3 inches below umbilicus	• Dorsal recumbency • Prepare entire thorax	• Lateral recumbency • Prepare lateral thorax
SURGICAL TECHNIQUE	• A ventral midline abdominal incision is made. Any herniated structures are examined for extended strangulation/obstructive damage and then placed back into the abdominal cavity. The abdominal cavity contents, lungs, and pleural space are examined for any further damage. The diaphragm is examined for any other tears and then the defect(s) is sutured closed. A chest tube is placed and maintained for 8–12 hours to ensure control of the pleural space. Air can also be aspirated as the last suture is tied, but does not allow pleural space maintenance if needed. Routine closure is performed on the abdominal wall.	• An incision is made over the midline on the sternum. The sternum is cut with an oscillating saw or sternal splitter. Retractors are placed, and the exploratory is performed. Before closure, a chest tube is placed. The thoracic wall is sutured closed in many layers. A pleural vacuum is created through the chest tube, and a light bandage is placed over the tube entrance.	• An incision is made based on the location in the thorax desired. The correct intercostal space is chosen, and an incision is made from the costovertebral junction to the sternum, and then the muscles are dissected through to the thoracic cavity. The pleura is punctured, and the thoracic organs are accessed. Before closure, a temporary or permanent chest tube is placed. The thoracic wall is sutured closed in many layers. A pleural vacuum is created through the chest tube and a light bandage is placed over the tube entrance.
NOTES	• *Surgery:* IPPV is crucial to allow the surgeon to work while avoiding injury to pulmonary tissue • *Patient Care:* monitor pain, heart rate, CRT, MM color, pulse strength and character, respiratory rate, blood pressure (BP), blood gases, and pulse oximetry	• *Instruments:* Oscillating saw or sternal splitter • *Patient Care:* monitor pain, heart rate, CRT, MM color, pulse strength and character, respiratory rate, BP, blood gases, and pulse oximetry	• *Patient Care:* monitor pain, heart rate, CRT, MM color, pulse strength and character, respiratory rate, BP, blood gases, and pulse oximetry

UROGENITAL TRACT SURGERY

Table 12-20 Urogenital Tract Surgery	
Procedure	**Urogenital Tract Surgery**
PREPARATION	
DEFINITION	• See particular surgery
INDICATIONS	• See particular surgery
INSTRUMENTS	• Abdominal pack • Curettes pack • General surgical pack • Saline bowl • Saline, warmed • Suction tips and tubing pack • Syringe, 60-mL catheter tip • Urethral catheter(s)
PATIENT	• See particular surgery
SURGICAL TECHNIQUE	• See particular surgery
COMPLICATIONS	
PROCEDURAL	• Urinary leakage or obstruction • Hemorrhage
PATIENT	• Stranguria
FOLLOW-UP	
PATIENT CARE	• Hematuria for 12–36 hours up to 5–7 days is normal • Remove catheter 1–2 days postoperatively • Monitor ease and amount of urine production • Standard postoperative care • Confine and restrict activity until suture/staple removal
CLIENT EDUCATION	• Recheck/Suture removal in ____ days • Medication: ____ • Lab results in ____ days • Diet: ____ • Repeat urinalysis or radiographs in ____ days/weeks

Table 12-21 Urogenital Tract Surgery (Continued)

Procedure	Cystotomy	Urethrostomy, Perineal
DEFINITION	• An incision made into the urinary bladder	• The creation of a new urethral orifice
INDICATIONS	• Cystic or urethral calculi, neoplasia, and urethral reimplantation	• Recurrent cystic calculi, trauma, and urethral stricture
PATIENT PREPARATION	• Dorsal recumbency • Place and secure a urinary catheter and empty urinary bladder • Prepare from umbilicus to ventral abdomen	• Ventral recumbency with rear legs draped over end of table and tail secured cranially • Place and secure a urinary catheter and empty urinary bladder • Prepare the entire perineal area, including the base of the tail
SURGICAL TECHNIQUE	A caudal midline abdominal incision is made. The caudal abdomen is examined for additional abnormalities. The bladder is isolated, exteriorized, packed with saline-moistened gauze sponges, and stay sutures are placed. A ventral cystotomy incision is made into the bladder, and all calculi or tumor are removed. The bladder is flushed by retrograde propulsion via the urinary catheter, and any grit is removed via curettes or suction. The bladder wall is securely closed and distended with saline to check for leakage. Routine closure is performed on the abdominal wall.	An elliptical incision is made around the scrotum, starting halfway between the anus and scrotum. If the patient is not neutered, it is done so in the normal fashion. The area is dissected down to the urethra, and an incision is made into the dorsal midline of the urethra and enlarged to 3 cm. The urethra mucosa and skin are sutured together to make a single edge around the elliptical incision, leaving a new urethral orifice. The penis is then removed caudal to the urethral incision and sutured. The urinary catheter is removed, and a new one is placed in the new urethral orifice and sutured into place.
NOTES	• *Patient Care:* calculi must be sent out for analysis and appropriate medical management started	• *Complications:* urethral stricture, rectal prolapse, urocystitis, infection, and fecal and urinary incontinence • *Client Education:* use shredded paper litter until suture removal

Table 12-22 Urogenital Tract Surgery (Continued)

Procedure	Urethrostomy, Scrotal	Urethrostomy, Prescrotal
DEFINITION	• The creation of a new urethral orifice	• An incision made into the urethra
INDICATIONS	• Recurrent cystic calculi, trauma, and urethral stricture	• Urethral calculi
PATIENT PREPARATION	• Dorsal recumbency with rear legs abducted and secured caudally • Place and secure a urinary catheter and empty urinary bladder • Prepare the prepuce to the area surrounding and including the scrotum	• Dorsal recumbency • Prepare from umbilicus to ventral abdomen
SURGICAL TECHNIQUE	An elliptical incision is made over the base of the scrotum. If the patient is not neutered, this is done in the normal fashion. The area is dissected down to the urethra and an incision is made into the ventral midline of the urethra and enlarged to 2.5–4 cm. The urethra mucosa and skin are sutured together to make a single edge around the elliptical incision, leaving a new urethral orifice.	An incision is made from just caudal to the prepuce and cranial to the scrotum. The area is dissected down to the urethra, and the urethra is incised. All calculi are removed, and a catheter is placed in the incision into the proximal urethra to identify further calculi or obstruction. The catheter is also advanced distally to dislodge any calculi in the penile urethra. The urethral incision may be left open to heal by secondary intention or sutured closed.
NOTES	• *Complications:* urocystitis and urethral stricture • *Patient Care:* apply petroleum jelly around incision to ↓ urine scald until ↓ inflammation	• *Complications:* urethral stricture • *Patient Care:* monitor renal function, electrolyte concentrations, and hydration status

Appendix

Listed below are the common conversions used in veterinary medicine. In cases in which the conversion is not useful, a "-" has been listed.

Prefix	Symbol	Power	Base 10
Kilo	k	10^3	1,000
Hecto	h	10^2	100
Deca	da	10^1	10
Unity		1	1
Deci	d	10^{-1}	0.1
Centi	c	10^{-2}	0.01
Milli	m	10^{-3}	0.001
Micro	μ or r	10^{-6}	0.000001
Nano	n	10^{-9}	0.000000001
Pico	p	10^{-12}	0.000000000001

Weights

	Kilogram (kg)	Gram (g)	Milligram (mg)	Microgram (mcg or µg)	Pound (lb.)	Ounce (oz)	Grain (gr)
1 kilogram	1 kg	1,000 g	1×10^6 mg	1×10^9 µg	2.2 lb.	36 oz	-
1 gram	0.001 kg	1 g	1,000 mg	1×10^6 µg	-	-	15 gr
1 milligram	1×10^{-6} kg	0.001 g	1 mg	1,000 µg	-	-	-
1 microgram	1×10^{-9} kg	1×10^{-6} g	0.001 mg	1 µg	-	-	-
1 pound	0.454 kg	454 g	-	-	1 lb.	16 oz	-
1 ounce	0.028 kg	28.4 g	-	-	0.0625 lb.	1 oz	-
1 grain	-	0.065 g	65 mg	-	-	-	1 gr

Liquid Measure

	Liter (L)	Milliliter (mL)/Cubic centimeter (cc)	Gallon (gal.)	Quart (qt)	Pint (pt)	Cup (c.)	Tablespoon (Tb)	Teaspoon (t)	Ounce (oz)	Drop (gtt)	Dram
1 liter	1 L	1,000 mL	1/4 gal.	1 qt	2 pts.	4 c.	-	-	34 oz	-	250 dram
1 milliliter	.001 L	1 mL	-	-	-	-	-	1/5 t	-	12 gtt	1/4 dram
1 gallon	3.84 L	3,840 mL	1 gal.	4 qts.	8 pts.	16 c.	-	-	128 oz	-	-
1 quart	.960 L	960 mL	1/4 gal.	1 qt	2 pts.	4 c.	-	-	32 oz	-	250 dram
1 pint	1/2 L	480 mL	1/8 gal.	1/2 qt	1 pt	2 c.	32 Tbsp	-	16 oz	-	120 dram
1 cup	1/4 L	240 mL	1/16 gal.	1/4 qt	1/2 pt	1 c.	16 Tbsp	48 tsp	8 oz	-	60 dram
1 tablespoon	-	15 mL	-	-	-	-	1 Tbsp	3 tsp	1/2 oz	180 gtt	4 dram
1 teaspoon	-	5 mL	-	-	-	-	1/3 Tbsp	1 tsp	1/6 oz	60 gtt	1 dram
1 ounce	-	30 mL	-	-	-	-	2 Tbsp	6 tsp	1 oz	360 gtt	8 dram
1 dram	-	4 mL	-	-	-	-	1/3 Tbsp	1 tsp	1/8 oz	60 gtt	1 dram
1 drop	-	-	-	-	-	-	-	-	-	1 gtt	-

Length

	Meter (m)	Centimeter (cm)	Millimeter (mm)	Yard (yd)	Feet (ft)	Inch (in)
1 meter	1 m	100 cm	1,000 cm	1.0936 yd	3.2808 ft	39.37 in
1 centimeter	0.01 m	1 cm	10 mm	0.0109 yd	0.03281 ft	0.3937 in
1 millimeter	0.001 m	0.1 cm	1 mm	0.0011 yd	0.00328 ft	0.03937 in
1 yard	0.9144 m	91.44 cm	914.40 mm	1 yd	3 ft	36 in
1 foot	0.3048 m	30.48 cm	304.8 mm	0.333 yd	1 ft	12 in
1 inch	0.0254 m	2.54 cm	25.4 mm	0.0278 yd	0.0833 ft	1 in

Kilograms to Body Surface Area (m²):

Common equations used to calculate body surface area:

Canine: $\dfrac{10.1 \times (\text{weight in grams})^{2/3}}{10,000}$

Feline: $\dfrac{10 \times (\text{weight in grams})^{2/3}}{10,000}$

Canine and Feline: $\dfrac{(\text{weight in kg})^{2/3}}{10}$

Canine						Feline			
Kg	m²	Kg	m²	Kg	m²	Kg	m²	Kg	m²
0.5	0.06	14	0.58	28	0.92	0.5	0.063	5.5	0.311
1	0.10	15	0.60	29	0.94	1	0.1	6	0.330
2	0.15	16	0.63	30	0.96	1.5	0.131	6.5	0.348
3	0.20	17	0.66	35	1.07	2	0.159	7	0.366
4	0.25	18	0.69	40	1.17	2.5	0.184	7.5	0.383
5	0.29	19	0.71	45	1.26	3	0.208	8	0.400
6	0.33	20	0.74	50	1.36	3.5	0.231	8.5	0.416
7	0.36	21	0.76	55	1.47	4	0.252	9	0.432
8	0.40	22	0.78	60	1.55	4.5	0.273	9.5	0.449
9	0.43	23	0.81	65	1.64	5	0.292	10	0.464
10	0.46	24	0.83	70	1.72				
11	0.49	25	0.85	75	1.80				
12	0.52	26	0.88	80	1.88				
13	0.55	27	0.90	85	1.96				

Temperature Conversion:

Celsius to Fahrenheit $(°C \times 1.8) + 32 = °F$

Fahrenheit to Celsius $(°F - 32) \times 0.555 = °C$

Celsius	Fahrenheit
0	32.0
4.0	39.2
25.0	77.0
32.0	89.6
37.0	98.6
38.6	101.5
39.1	102.5
39.4	103

Glossary

ABG (arterial blood gases) Gases found in the blood; clinically useful oxygen and carbon dioxide

Absorber Filters out carbon dioxide particles from the patient's exhaled gases

ACh (acetylcholine) A chemical neurotransmitter substance; thought to play an important role in nerve impulse transmissions

Acini Smallest division of a gland; a group of secretory cells surrounding a cavity

ADH Antidiuretic hormone

Adrenergic The nerve fibers that release epinephrine when stimulated

Akinesia A loss of motor response (movement) caused by paralysis of nerves

Allodynia A condition in which a normal painless stimulus is now perceived as painful

Alopecia Absence or loss of hair

Amyloidosis A metabolic disorder marked by deposition of amyloid in organs and tissue

Analgesia A temporary loss of pain

Anechoic To not produce any or only a few echoes

Anesthetic An agent that produces loss of feeling or sensation

Aphakic Absence of the crystalline lens of the eye

Apnea The cessation of respiration

Apneustic breathing Breathing in which there is inspiratory hold or pause before exhalation; often seen in dissociative anesthesia

Aqueous flare Increased turbidity of aqueous humor

Arthralgia Pain in the joint

Arthrodesis Surgical immobilization of a joint

Artificial colloid Intravenous solution containing protein or starch molecules

Ascites Accumulation of serous fluid in the peritoneal cavity

Ataxia Defective muscular coordination

Atelectasis Collapsed or airless condition of the lung

Auscultate To examine by listening to the sounds produced within the body

Azotemia Presence of nitrogenous bodies

Biot's respiration Sequence of uniformly deep breaths, apnea, and then deep breaths again

Blepharospasm Twitching of the spasmodic contraction of the orbicularis oculi muscle

Breathing tubes Corrugated tubing connecting the endotracheal tube of the patient to the anesthetic machine

Bronchial sounds Produced by air movement in the trachea and larger bronchi; louder on expiration

Buphthalmos	Condition of infantile glaucoma resulting in uniform enlargement of the eye, particularly the cornea
Cachexia	A state of ill health, malnutrition, and wasting
Cataract	Opacity of the lens of the eye and/or its capsule
Catelepsy	A state in which there is malleable rigidity of the limbs and the patient is generally unresponsive to aural, visual, or minor painful stimuli
Caudate	Possessing a tail
Cellularity	Quality of the cell (e.g., component size and shape)
CVP (central venous pressure)	Pressure within the superior vena cava; represents the pressure of the blood returning to the right atrium
Chelate	To chemically grasp a toxic substance, making it nonactive
Chemosis	Edema of the conjunctiva around the cornea
Chest wall coupage	Striking the chest to loosen bronchial secretion and thus facilitate drainage
Cholinergic	Nerve fibers that release acetylcholine when stimulated
Chyle	The milklike, alkaline contents of the lacteals and lymphatic vessels of the intestines, consisting of the products of digestion and principally absorbed fats
Colobomas	Lesion or defect of the eye, usually a fissure or cleft of the iris, ciliary body, or choroid
Colostrum	Mammary fluid produced by the animal a few days before and after birthing; containing proteins, calories, antibodies, and lymphocytes
Comedones	Discolored dried sebum plugging an excretory duct of the skin
Convex	Curved evenly; resembling the segment of a sphere
CPAP (continuous positive airway pressure)	Used to manage or prevent alveolar collapse or atelectasis
Crepitus	Having or making a crackling sound
CRTZ (chemoreceptor trigger zone)	The area of the brain which stimulates vomiting when certain toxins enter the bloodstream
Crystalloid	Isotonic or electrolyte solution typically used as a replacement or maintenance solution
Cycloplegic	Medication that results in paralysis of the ciliary muscle in the eye
Danger level	The point at which the level of a specific chemistry in the blood is reaching a critical (dangerous) point
Dead Space, anatomic	The volume of air from the nose and the mouth to the alveoli
Dead Space, physiologic	The anatomic dead space and the volume of air in any nonfunctioning alveoli, and the volume of air in excess of the amount needed to convert oxygen content of capillary blood to that of arterial blood
Decubital	Bedsores

Definitive host	An animal harboring a sexually mature parasite
Dehiscence	Rupture of a wound
Descemetocele	Protrusion of a fine membrane between the endothelial layer of the cornea and the substantia propria
Desquamative cells	Shedding epidermal cells
Diatheses	Constitutional predisposition to certain disease conditions
Dissociative anesthesia	The state in which that patient is disconnected from its environment; interruption of information flow from the unconscious to the conscious parts of the brain
Dyschezia	Painful or difficult bowel movement
Dyscoria	Abnormal form or shape of the pupil
Dysphonia	Difficulty in speaking
Echogenicity	Strength or amplitude of returning echoes
Echoic	To produce echoes
Eczema, miliary	Acute or chronic cutaneous inflammatory condition with erythema, papules, vesicles, pustules, scales, crusts, or scabs alone or in combination
EDTA (ethylenedi-aminetetraacetic acid)	An anticoagulant
Embryonated	Having an embyro
Endophthalmitis	Inflammation of the inside of the eye that may or may not be limited to a particular chamber
Epidural anesthesia	The deposition of local anesthesia within the epidural space
Epiphora	Abnormal overflow of tears down the cheek caused by excess secretion of tears or obstruction of the lacrimal duct
Erythema	A form of macula showing diffused redness over the skin
Evisceration	Surgical removal of intraocular contents
Exenteration	Removal of the eye and all orbital tissues
Extrinsic	No forming part of or belonging to a thing
Facultative	Having the ability to live under certain circumstances
Fetid	Rank or foul in odor
Fibroblasts	Any cell or corpuscle from which connective tissue is developed
Field block	The creation of "walls" of anesthesia encircling the surgical field by means of injection of a local anesthetic
Fistula	An abnormal passage from one cavity to another
Floccose	A growth made up of short and densely but irregularly interwoven filaments
Flocculent	Culture containing whitish shreds of mucus
Flowmeter	Controls the rate at which a particular gas is delivered to the patient
Fontanelle	Unossified space of tissue lying between the cranial bones of a fetus; also known as the soft spot

FSH (follicle-stimulating hormone)	Promotes growth and maturation of ovarian follicles in females and spermatogenosis in males
Furunculosis	A condition resulting from boils
Genal	Pertaining to the cheek
General anesthesia	A controllable and reversible loss of consciousness induced by intoxication of the CNS
GnRH (gonadotropin-releasing hormone)	Stimulates the release of LH or FSH or the activity similar to the hormones
Hematemesis	Blood in the vomitus
Hematochezia	Blood in the feces
Hemoptosis	Expectoration of blood arising from the oral cavity, larynx, trachea, bronchi, or lungs
HPA	Hypothalamic-pituitary-adrenal axis
Hyperalgesia	Increased sensitivity to pain
Hypercapnia	Excessively high level of carbon dioxide in the blood
Hyperechoic	To produce more echoes than the surrounding tissue
Hyperesthesia	Increased sensitivity to sensory stimuli (touch, sight, sound)
Hyperosmolar	Increased osmolarity of the blood
Hypertonic	Having a higher osmotic pressure than a compared solution; >300 mOsm/L
Hypnosis	Artificially induced sleep or a trance resembling sleep from which the patient can be aroused by stimuli
Hypoechoic	To produce less echoes than the surrounding tissue
Hypoperfusion	Abnormally low amount of tissue blood flow resulting in decreased oxygen and nutrients to the body as well as failure to remove wastes
Hypotonic	Solution having a lower osmotic pressure than a compared solution; <300 mOsm/L
Hypotony	Defective muscular tension or tone
Hypovolemia	Abnormally low blood volume
Idiopathic	Conditions without clear pathogenesis, or disease without recognizable cause, as of spontaneous origin
Immunization/vaccination	Process of administering a vaccine to produce a protective immune response from the host
Infarctions	Area of tissue in an organ or part that undergoes necrosis after cessation of blood supply
Intermediate host	Animal used during the immature stages of the parasite's life cycle to continue their development
Intrinsic	Originating or due to causes within a body organ or part
Intussusception	Invagination; the slipping of one part of the intestines into another part
IPPV (intermittent partial pressure ventilation)	The manual method of placing air into a patient's lungs

Iridodonesis	Tremulousness of iris, seen in an aphakic eye or one with subluxated lens
Ischemic	Local and temporary deficiency of blood supply caused by obstruction of circulation to a part
Isoechoic	To produce similar echoes as the surrounding tissue
Isothenuric	Condition of urine being of a uniform specific gravity and osmolarity despite fluctuations in fluid uptake
Isotonic solution	Exerting an equivalent osmotic pressure to the compared solution; = 300 mOsm/L
Karyo-	Referring to a cell's nucleus
Left shift	Increased number of immature neutrophils in the blood
LH (luteinizing hormone)	Stimulates ovulation in females and testosterone in males
Local anesthesia	An injection of an anesthetic agent into the tissues that are to be incised or manipulated
Lochia	Clear, odorless, serosanguineous normal postpartum discharge
Luxation	Displacement of organs or articular surfaces
Lymphadenopathy	Disease of the lymph nodes
Maintenance solution	Solution that contains less sodium and more potassium than replacement solutions
Manometer	Monitors pressure within the breathing system
Melena	Black, tarry feces caused by action of intestinal secretions on free blood
Menace response	A rapid eye closure, with or without head withdrawal, in response to a threatening or unexpected image suddenly appearing in the near field vision
Meniscus	Concavoconvex lens
Metabolic acidosis	Condition in which there is an excess of hydrogen ions resulting in a decrease in the body pH
Micturition	The act of voiding urine from the body
Mixed echogenicity	For one structure to produce more than one echogenicity
Myasthenia gravis	A disease characterized by muscle weakness and progressive fatigue
Myoclonus	Repetitive, rhythmic twitching or clonic spasm of a muscle or group of muscles
Mydriasis	Abnormal dilation of the pupil
Myxedema	Condition resulting from hypofunction of the thyroid gland
Narcosis	A drug-induced stupor or sedation in which the patient is oblivious to pain, with or without hypnosis
Neonate	Newborn up to 6 weeks of age
Nephrogram	Radiograph showing the opacification of the functional parenchyma of the kidneys
Nerve block	Injection of an anesthetic agent close to the major nerves whose conductivity is to be cut off
Neurolept-analgesia	State characterized by lack of apprehension and anxiety (neurolepsis) and loss of pain perception (analgesia)

Nictitans	Third eyelid; nictitating membrane
NMB (new methylene blue)	Stain used in microbiology
Nocturia	Excessive urination at night
Nystagmus	Constant, involuntary, cyclical movement of the eyeball
Oliguria	Diminished amount of urine formation
Oncosphere	Embyronic phase of a tapeworm in which it has hooks
Oocyst	Encysted form of a fertilized gamete occurring in certain sporozoa
Operculum	Any covering
Osmolality	Determination of a particle's ability to attract water based on a relative number of solute particles in 1 kg of the solution
Oxygen flush Valve	Delivers oxygen to the anesthetic system at 35–75 L/min
PABA	Trade name for para-aminobenzoic acid
Pallor	Lack of color, paleness
Palpate	To examine the consistency of body areas by touch, using your fingers with light pressure
Papule	Red elevated area on the skin, solid and circumscribed
Paradoxical respiration	When the affected side of a pneumothorax bulges out during expiration and caves in during inspiration
Paratenic host	Animal serving as a transport for an immature parasite; no development takes place
Paresis	Partial or incomplete paralysis
PEEP (positive end-expiratory pressure)	A respiration method used to hold alveoli open during expiration
Penn-HIP	Additional method to evaluate hip laxity and hip dysplasia when radiographs are inconclusive. The procedure uses the OFA VD view distraction and compression views. A distractor unit is used in one view, and this method requires special training and certification by the veterinarian. Acronym for (University of) Pennsylvania Hip Improvement Program.
Petechiae	Small, purplish hemorrhagic spots on the skin or mucous membranes
Pleomorphic	Having many shapes
Pollakuria	Abnormally frequent passage of urine
Polycythemia	An excess of RBCs
Postprandial	After a meal
Postprandial alkaline tide	↑ Secretion of alkaline ions by the kidney after a meal to compensate for acid ions secreted in the stomach to aid digestion, resulting in alkaline urine
Preprandial	Before a meal
Prepatent period	Period between the time of introduction of parasitic organisms into the body and their appearance in the blood or tissues until they reach reproductive maturity

Pressure relief valve (Pop-off valve)	Allows the release of excess pressure from the anesthetic system; the volume of gas in excess of the animal's minute consumption is vented from the system
Proglottids	Segment of a tapeworm; containing both male and female reproductive organs
Pronotal	Before or in front of the dorsal area
Pyelogram	A radiograph showing the opacification of pelvic recesses, renal pelves, and ureters
Pyknotic	Thickness
Radiopharmaceutical drug	A compound mixed with a radionuclide
Rales	Abnormal thoracic sounds caused by a secretion from or a thickening of bronchial walls; "crackling sounds"
Rebreathing bag	Used as a reservoir of gases in the anesthetic system to ventilate the patient as necessary
Redundant	More than necessary; an overflow
Regional anesthesia	Producing the loss of sensation in a portion of the body by interrupting sensory nerve conduction from that region of the body
Regulator	Reduce the variable pressure of the gas within the cylinder to a constant pressure of approximately 50 psi
Replacement solution	Solutions that are typically more similar to extracellular fluid
Retrograde	Moving backward
Rhonchi	Abnormal sounds of the thorax typically indicating an airway obstruction; "musical sounds"
Scavenger system	Removes waste gas to an outside environment or filtering system
Second-gas effect	The uptake of one gas is sped up by the uptake of another
Sedation	A mild depression of the CNS during which the patient is awake, calm, and sometimes drowsy
Septate	Having a dividing wall
Slough	Dead matter or necrosed tissue separated from living tissue
Specific gravity	Weight of a substance compared with an equal volume of water
Sporangia	The supporting stalk for a spore sac of certain fungi
Sporulated	Production of spores
Stenosis	Constriction or narrowing of a passage or orifice
Stertor	Snoring or laborious breathing caused by obstruction of air passages in the head
Stridor	Harsh sound during respiration, high pitched and resembling the blowing of wind, caused by obstruction of air passages; wheezing sound made on inspiration typically indicating a laryngeal obstruction
Supernatant	Clear liquid remaining at the top after a precipitate settles
Suppurative	Producing or associated with generation of pus
Symblepharon	Adhesions between conjunctiva of lens and eyeball
Syncope	A transient loss of consciousness caused by inadequate blood flow to the brain

Synechia	Adhesions of iris to lens and cornea
Tenesmus	Spasmodic contraction of anal or vesical sphincter with pain and persistent desire to empty bowel or bladder, with involuntary ineffectual straining efforts
Tetany	A nervous affection characterized by intermittent tonic spasms that are usually paroxysmal and involve extremities
Thrombus	Blood clot that obstructs a blood vessel or a cavity of the heart
Tonicity	State of normal tension
Topical anesthesia	Application of a local anesthetic agent to the surface of the skin or mucous membranes
Tortuous	Having many twists and turns
Toxic change	Prominent purplish cytoplasmic granules, cytoplasmic vacuolation, cytoplasmic basophilia, or Döhle bodies of a cell
Tranquilization	State of relaxation and calmness without drowsiness
Transducer	The probe that sends and receives the sound wave signal of an ultrasound machine
Trismus	Tonic contraction of the muscles of mastication
Trocarization	Insertion of a large-bore needle to relieve distension
Trophozoite	Sporozoan nourished by its host during its growth stage
Turgor	Resistance of skin to be changed from its normal position on the body
Unidirectional valves	Prevent exhaled gas from being rebreathed before it passes through the absorbent cannister in an anesthetic system
Uremic	Toxic condition associated with renal insufficiency produced by the retention in the blood of nitrogenous substances normally excreted by the kidneys
Urticaria	Eruption of itchy wheals (hives)
USG (urine specific gravity)	Clinically relates to the concentration of the urine
Vaccine	Biologic product that stimulates the immune system to produce antibodies.
Vaporizer	Delivers specified concentrations of anesthetic gas to the patient
Vesicular sounds	Sounds produced by the small bronchi, bronchioles, and alveoli; typically louder on inspiration; sounds like "rustling leaves"
Volvulus	A twisting of the bowel on itself, causing obstruction
VPC (ventricular premature contractions)	An impulse originating in the ventricles instead of the SA node
Xerostomia	Dryness of the mouth

Bibliography

Abbott Laboratories Insert for Dextrose and Sodium Chloride Injection, USP, 1989.

Abrams K. Cataracts. (On-line). Available: http://users.ids.net/peteyes/cataract.htm, 1996.

Abrams K. Glaucoma.(On-line). Available: http://users.ids.net/peteyes/glaucoma.htm, 1996.

Accuvet. Advantages of Laser Surgery. (On-line). Available: http://petlasers.com/site/content/avl_laservet.asp, 2000.

Allen DG, Pringle JK, Smith DA, et al. *Handbook of Veterinary Drugs* (2nd ed.). Philadelphia, PA: Lippincott, Williams and Wilkins, 1998.

American Association of Feline Practitioners/ Academy of Feline Medicine. Panel report on feline senior health care. *Compendium on Continuing Education for the Practicing Veterinarian* 1999;21:531-539.

Anderson WD, Anderson BG. *Atlas of Canine Anatomy*. Philadelphia, PA: Lea & Febiger, 1994.

Bach E. *Bach Flower Essences for the Family*. London: Wigmore Publications Ltd., 1996.

Baldwin K. Step-by-step placing an intraosseous catheter in the canine trochanteric fossa. *Veterinary Technician*, 1999;20:656-659.

Barbe P, Addison's Disease (Hypoadrenocorticism) (On-line) http://www.mirage-samoyeds.com/Addison.htm, 2000.

Barger AM, Grindem CB. Analyzing the results of a complete blood cell count. *Veterinary Medicine* 2000;95:535-545.

Battaglia-Lawrence A. Shock: Recognition, treatment and monitoring. *Veterinary Technician*, 1997;18:167-178.

Battaglia-Lawrence A. Step-by-step placing a peripheral intravenous catheter. *Veterinary Technician*, 1998;19:86-88.

Baxter Inserts for Dextrose Injection, USP, Lactated Ringer's Injection, USP, and Sodium Chloride Injection, USP.

Bergerson WO. Golden opportunities: technical, economic, and professional aspects of urinalysis. *Veterinary Technician* 1998;19:574-583.

Birchard SJ, Sherding RG. *Saunders Manual of Small Animal Practice*. Philadelphia, PA: W. B. Saunders Company, 1994.

Bistner SJ, Ford R, Raffe M. *Kirk and Bistner's Handbook of Veterinary Procedures and Emergency Treatment*, 7th ed. Philadelphia, PA: W.B. Saunders Company, 2000.

Bolette DP. Worming their way in: identifying cestodes, trematodes, and acanthocephala. *Veterinary Technician* 1998;19:510-517.

Bolton G. *Handbook of Canine Electrocardiography*. Philadelphia, PA: W.B. Saunders Company, 1975.

Boon JA. *Manual of Veterinary Echocardiography*, Philadelphia, PA: Lippincott, Williams & Wilkins, 1998.

Borjab JM, Ellison GW, Slocum B. *Current Techniques in Small Animal Surgery*. Philadelphia, PA: Lippincott Williams & Wilkins, 1998.

Boyd B. Internet Vets (On-line) http://www.internetvets.com, 1999-2000.

Brooks WC. *Pet Health Care Library: What is a Cataract?* (On-line). Available: http://www.vin.com/members/searchdb/misc/m05000/m01291.htm, Veterinary Information Network, 2000.

Brooks W. *Pet Health Care Library: Radiotherapy.* (On-line). Available: http://www.vin.com/members/searchdb/misc/m05000.htm, Mar Vista Animal Medical Center, 2001.

Burkholder WJ. Age-related changes to nutritional requirements and digestive function in adult dogs and cats. *JAVMA* 1999;215:625-629.

Burris P. It's the Little Things... *Cryptosporidium. Veterinary Technician* 2000;21:192-201.

Cappuccino JG, Sherman N. *Microbiology, A Laboratory Manual,* 4th Ed. Menlo Park, CA: The Benjamin/Cummings Publishing Company, Inc., 1996.

Cartee RE. and contributors. *Practical Veterinary Ultrasound,* Philadelphia, PA: Williams & Wilkins, 1995.

Carter GR, Chengappa MM, Roberts AW. *Essentials of Veterinary Microbiology,* 5th Ed. Baltimore, MD: Williams and Wilkins, 1995.

Chandler ML, Guilford WG, Payne-James J. Use of peripheral parenteral nutritional support in dogs and cats. *JAVMA* 2000;216:669-673.

Chew DJ, DiBartola SP. *Interpretation of Canine and Feline Urinalysis.* Wilmington, DE: The Gloyd Group, Inc., 1998.

Cook CS, Mughannam AJ, Szymanski CM. *Cataract Surgery: The Current State of the Art.* (On-line). Available: http://www.veterinaryvision.com/dvm_forum/dvm-cataracts/htm, Veterinary Vision, 1998.

Cook CS, Mughannam AJ, Szymanski CM. *Glaucoma* (On-line). Available: http://www.veterinaryvision.com/dvm_forum/dvm-glaucoma/htm, Veterinary Vision, 1998.

Cordell D, Duke A, Mack JD, et al. Delivering Compassionate Care: A Roundtable Discussion Part II. Good Medicine is Only the Beginning. *Veterinary Technician* 2000;21:284-288.

Cornick-Seahorn J, Marks SL. Emergency! Treating Patients in Shock. *Veterinary Technician.,* 1998;19:355-369.

Corwin RM, Nahm J. *Veterinary Parasitology.* (On-line). Available: www.parasitology.org, University of Missouri-Columbia, 1997.

Cowell RL, Tyler RD, Meinkoth JH. *Diagnostic Cytology and Hematology of the Dog and Cat,* 2nd Ed. St. Louis, Mosby-Year Book, Inc., 1999.

Crawford P, Connor K. A breath of a chance: Pleural effusions in small animals. Part I. *Veterinary Technician* 2000;21:455-461.

Crowe Jr. DT, Devey J. Peel-away long venous catheter technique minimizes placement steps. *DVM Newsmagazine* 2000:15-35.

Douglas SW, Williamson HD. *Principles of Veterinary Radiography,* 2nd Ed. London, England: Bailliere Tindall, 1972.

Eigner DR. CFA Health Committee Feline Vaccine Guidelines. (On-line). Available: www.cfainc.org/health/vaccination-guidelines.html, 1998.

Emily P, Penman S. *Handbook of Small Animal Dentistry.* Oxford: Pergamon Press, 1990.

Ettinger SJ, Feldman EC. *Textbook of Veterinary Internal Medicine.* Philadelphia, PA: W. B. Saunders, 1995.

Ettinger SJ, Feldman EC. *Textbook of Veterinary Internal Medicine,* 4th Ed. Philadelphia, PA: W. B. Saunders, 1995.

Ettinger SJ, Feldman EC. *Textbook of Veterinary Internal Medicine,* 5th Ed. Philadelphia, PA: W. B. Saunders, 2000.

Ettinger SJ, Feldman EC. *Textbook of Veterinary Internal Medicine,* 5th Ed., Vol. 2. Philadelphia, PA: W. B. Saunders, 2000.

Evans HE, deLahunta A. *Miller's Guide to the Dissection of the Dog.* Philadelphia, PA: W.B. Saunders Company, 1971.

Evans HE, Christensen GC. *Miller's Anatomy of the Dog,* Philadelphia, PA: W.B. Saunders Company, 1979.

Feldman EC, Nelson RW. *Canine and Feline Endocrinology and Reproduction,* 2nd Ed. Philadelphia, PA: W.B. Saunders, 1996.

Feline Leukemia Virus. *Veterinary Technician,* 1997;18:680-682.

Fenner WR. *Quick Reference of Veterinary Medicine.* Philadelphia, PA: Lippincott Williams & Wilkins, 2000.

Firth AM, Haldane SL. Development of a scale to evaluate postoperative pain in dogs. *JAVMA* 1999;214:651-659.

Foreyt WJ. *Veterinary Parasitology Reference Manual.* Pullman: Washington State University, 1994.

Fossum TW. *Proceedings from Veterinary Post Graduate Institute Seminar on Soft-Tissue Surgery.* Texas A & M, 1997.

Frost P. *The Veterinary Clinics of North America–Dentistry* Vol 16, no. 5. Philadelphia, PA: W. B. Saunders Company, 1986.

Gaynor JS. Is postoperative pain management important in dogs and cats? *Veterinary Medicine* 1999;94:254-257.

Gilbert SG. *Pictorial Anatomy of the Cat,* 9th Ed. Seattle, WA: University of Washington Press, 1991.

Glaze K. Treating a broken heart: Congenital heart disease—Part I. *Veterinary Technician* 1998;19:169-179.

Glaze K. Treating a broken heart: Congenital heart disease—Part II. *Veterinary Technician* 1998;19:339-347.

Goodwin C. Canine cilia disorders. *Veterinary Technician* 1998;19:115-124.

Gourley IM, Vasseur PB. *General Small Animal Surgery,* Philadelphia, PA: J. B. Lippincott Company, 1985.

Graff SL. *A Handbook of Routine Urinalysis.* Philadelphia, PA: J.B. Lippincott Company, 1983.

Greene CE. *Infectious Disease of the Dog and Cat,* 2nd Ed. Philadelphia, PA: W.B. Saunders, 1998.

Greiner EC, McIntosh A. Comparison of the efficacy of three fecal flotation media. *Veterinary Technician* 1997;18:283-287.

Griffith D. *Herbal Medicine.* (On-line). Available: http://www.vin.com/members/searchdb/rounds/lc990523.htm, Veterinary Information Network, 1999.

Griffith D, Limehouse J. *Holistic Medicine.* (On-line). Available: http://www.vin.com/members/searchdb/rounds/lc970706.htm, Veterinary Information Network, 1997.

Harari J. *Surgical Complications and Wound Healing in the Small Animal Practice.* Philadelphia, PA: W.B. Saunders Company, 1993.

Harvey CE, Emily PP. *Small Animal Dentistry.* St. Louis: Mosby, 1993.

Harvey CE. *The Veterinary Clinics of North America—Feline Dentistry,* Vol 22. Philadelphia, PA: W. B. Saunders Company, 1992.

Hawkins BJ, Down in the Mouth: Examining the Feline Oral Cavity, Veterinary Technician, 1997; Vol. 18:671-678.

Hawkins J. *Waltham Applied Dentistry.* Veterinary Learning Systems Co., Inc., 1993.

Heath D. Lifeline to recovery: Intravenous catheterization techniques. *Veterinary Technician,* 1998;19:614.

Heath D. Step-by-step placing an over-the-needle catheter in the cephalic vein. *Veterinary Technician,* 1998;19:617

Heins AL. A new approach to treatment of periodontal disease. *Veterinary Technician* 1997;18:372-378.

Hendrix CM. *Diagnostic Veterinary Parasitology.* St. Louis: Mosby-Year Book, Inc., 1998.

Hickman A. Parenteral Nutrition. Paper presented at Spring Conference, Kansas State University (Spring 1997).

Holloway C, Buffington T. A clinical problem: obesity and related health risks. *Veterinary Technician* 2000;21:281-283.

Holloway C, Buffington T. Basic guidelines for dogs and cats. *Veterinary Technician* 1999;20:499-505.

Holmstrom SE, Frost P, Gammon RL. *Veterinary Dental Techniques for the Small Animal Practitioner.* Philadelphia, PA: W. B. Saunders Company, 1998.

Holmstrom SE. *Veterinary Dentistry for the Technician & Office Staff.* Philadelphia, PA: W. B. Saunders Company, 2000.

Hoskins JD. Pediatric Health Care and Management, *The Veterinary Clinics of North America Small Animal Practice* 1999;29: 837-852.

Hoskins JD. *Veterinary Pediatrics: Dogs and Cats from Birth to Six Months.* Philadelphia, PA: W.B. Saunders, 1995.

IGI-EVCSO Pharmaceuticals (On-line) http://www.evscopharm.com (no dates noted).

Ikram M, Hill E. *Microbiology for Veterinary Technicians.* St. Louis, MO: Mosby-Year Book, Inc., 1991.

Introduction to Sonography (On-line). Available: http://www.webvet.cornell.edu/cvm/imaging/notes_US.html

Ivens VR, Mark DL, Levine ND. *Principal Parasites of Domestic Animals in the United States, Biological and Diagnostic Information.* Urbana, IL: University of Illinois, 1981.

Jensen MM, Wright DN, Robison RA. *Microbiology for the Health Sciences.* 4th Ed. Upper Saddle River: Prentice Hall, 1997.

Jewett L. *Test Directory.* Phoenix Central Laboratory, Everett, WA 98024 Updated in April 2000.

Joseph D. Step-by-step placement of jugular catheters in small animals. *Veterinary Technician* 2000;21:587-590.

Kealy JK. *Diagnostic Radiology of the Dog and Cat.* Philadelphia, PA: W.B. Saunders Company, 1979.

Kesel ML. *Veterinary Dentistry for the Small Animal Technician.* Ames, IA: Iowa State University Press, 2000.

King L, Hammond R. *Manual of Canine and Feline Emergency and Critical Care.* Shurdington, Cheltenham: British Small Animal Veterinary Association, 1999.

King L, Hammond R. *Manual of Canine and Feline Emergency and Critical Care*, Chapter 2: Fluid Therapy. Dez Hughes, British Small Animal Veterinary Association, 1999.

Kirk RW. *Kirk's Current Veterinary Therapy X.* Philadelphia, PA: W. B. Saunders, 1989.

Kirk RW. *Kirk's Current Veterinary Therapy XI.* Philadelphia, PA: W. B. Saunders, 1992.

Kirk RW. *Kirk's Current Veterinary Therapy XII.* Philadelphia, PA: W. B. Saunders, 1995.

Kleine LJ, Warren FG. *Small Animal Radiology.* St. Louis, MO: The C.V. Mosby Co., 1983.

Laflamme DP, Kealy RD,. Schmidt DA. Estimation of body fat by conditioning score. *J Vet Intern Med* 1994;154:59-65.

LaFlamme D. Sweet success: Managing diabetes mellitus. *Veterinary Technician* 2001;22:24-25.

Lappin MR. Feline toxolasmosis. *Veterinary Technician* 1997;18:298-299.

Lavin LM. The imaging chain: Links to high-quality radiography. *Veterinary Technician,* 2001;22:230-241.

Lavin LM. *Radiography in Veterinary Technology.* Philadelphia, PA: W. B. Saunders Company, 1994.

Lemke KA., Dawson SD. Local and regional anesthesia. *The Veterinary Clinics of North America Small Animal Practice* 2000;30:839-857.

Little S. CFA Health Committee Establishing Vaccination Protocols for Catteries. (On-line). Available: www.cfainc.org/health/vaccination-protocol-catteries.html

Lumb WV, Jones EW. *Lumb & Jones' Veterinary Anesthesia.* Philadelphia, PA: Lippincott Williams & Wilkins, 1996.

Macintire DK. Pediatric intensive care. *The Veterinary Clinics of North America Small Animal Practice* 1999;29:971-988.

Mama K. New options for managing chronic pain in small animals. *Veterinary Medicine* 1999;94:352-357.

MarVista Animal Medical Center (On-line) http://www.marvistavet.com/html/pharmacy_center.html, 1997-2002.

Mathews KA. Pain assessment and general approach to management. *The Veterinary Clinics of North America Small Animal Practice* 2000;30:729-755.

Matteson V. Block that pain, local anesthesia in dogs and cats. *Veterinary Technician* 2000;21:332-339.

Mauldin G. Practical Clinical Nutrition. Paper presented at a lecture at Buffalo Academy, 2000.

McClure RC, Dallman MJ, Garrett PD. *Cat Anatomy,* Philadelphia, PA: Lea & Febiger, 1973.

McCormick TS. *The Essentials of Microbiology.* Piscataway, NJ: Research and Education Association, 1995.

McCurnin DM. *Clinical Textbook for Veterinary Technicians.* Philadelphia, PA: W.B. Saunders Company, 1994.

McCurnin DM. *Clinical Textbook for Veterinary Technicians,* 4th Ed. Philadelphia, PA: W. B. Saunders Company, 1994.

McCurnin DM., Bassert JM. *Clinical Textbook for Veterinary Technicians,* 5th Ed. Philadelphia, PA: W. B. Saunders Company, 2002.

McKelvey D, Hollingshead KW. *Small Animal Anesthesia.* St. Louis, MO: Mosby-Year Book, Inc., 1994.

McMichael M, Dhupa N. Pediatric critical care medicine: Physiologic considerations. *Compendium,* 2000;22:206.

Measurement of central venous pressure. *Small Animal Diagnostic and Therapeutic Techniques.* (On-line). Available: www.vetmed.wsu.edu/courses_samDX/cvp.htm, 2002

Meleo K. *Radiation Therapy: Machines, Fractions, and Doses.* (On-line). Available: http://www.vin.com/members/searchdb/rounds/lc000319.htm, Veterinary Information Network, 2000.

Mihatov L. So what is *Giardia* anyway? *Veterinary Technician* 2000;21:188-190.

Muir W III, Hubbell JAE. *Handbook of Veterinary Anesthesia.* St. Louis: Mosby-Year Book, Inc., 1995.

Muir WW III, Hubbell JAE, *Handbook of Veterinary Anesthesia,* 2nd Ed. St. Louis, MO: Mosby, 1995.

Mullane PA. Practical neonatal care: Tube feeding. *Veterinary Technician* 1998;19:532-535.

Novartis Canada, (On-line) http://www.ah.ca.novartis.com/product/index.html, 2001.

Novotny B. Nutritional assessment. *Hill's HealthCare Connection* 1996;95:139-149.

O'Brien TR. *Radiographic Diagnosis of Abdominal Disorders in the Dog and Cat.* Davis, CA: Covell Park Veterinary Company, 1981.

Ogilvie GK, Moore AS. *Managing the Veterinary Cancer Patient.* Trenton, NJ: Veterinary Learning Systems Co., Inc., 1995.

Olsen JL, Ablon L, Giangrasso A. *Medical Dosage Calculations,* 6th Ed. Menlo Park, CA: Addison-Wesley Nursing, 1995.

Osborne CA, Stevens JB. *Handbook of Canine and Feline Urinalysis.* St. Louis, MO: Ralston Purina Company, 1981.

Osborne CA, Stevens JB. *Urinalysis: A Clinical Guide to Compassionate Patient Care.* Trenton, NJ: Veterinary Learning Systems Co., Inc., 1999.

Osborne JN, Sharp NJH. Putting "wobblers" back on track—Part II. *Veterinary Technician* 1998;19:519-527.

"Otoscopy in Veterinary Practice", (On-line). Available: http://www.ksvea.com/small _otoscopy.html

Owens JM, Biery DN. *Radiographic Interpretation for the Small Animal Clinician,* 2nd Ed. Philadelphia: Lippincott Williams & Wilkins, 1999.

Owens JM. Radiographic Interpretation for the Small Animal Clinician, Ralston Purina, 1982.

Pascoe PJ. Perioperative pain management. *The Veterinary Clinics of North America Small Animal Practice* 2000;30:917-932.

Pfizer Inserts for Bordetella Bronchiseptica Vaccine.

Pitcairn RH, Pitcairn SH. *Dr. Pitcairn's Complete Guide to Natural Health for Dogs and Cats.* Emmaus, NJ: Rodale Press, Inc, 1995.

Placement of a jugular catheter. *Small Animal Diagnostic and Therapeutic Techniques* (On-line). Available: www.vetmed.wsu.edu/courses_samDX/jugcath.htm

Plumb DC. *Veterinary Drug Handbook*, 3rd Ed. Ames, IA: Iowa State University Press, 1999.

Plunkett SJ. *Emergency Procedures for the Small Animal Veterinarian*, Philadelphia, PA: W.B. Saunders Company, 1993.

Poundstone M. Emergency medicine: CPR techniques. *Veterinary Technician* 1992;13:357–362

Pratt PW. *Laboratory Procedures for Veterinary Technicians*. St. Louis, MO: Mosby-Year Book, Inc., 1997.

Pratt PW. *Lab Procedures for Veterinary Technicians*, 3rd Ed. St. Louis, MO: Mosby, 1997.

Prince J. Endoscopy (On-line) http://www.peteducation.com/vet_proc/endoscoopy.htm, 1997-2001.

Hancock R, Rashmir-Raven A. Principles and techniques of the Robert-Jones bandage. *Veterinary Technician* 2000;21:463-465.

Randall A. The (hook)worms crawl in: *Ancylostoma* infection in humans. *Veterinary Technician* 1999;20:189-197.

Rebar AH. *Handbook of Veterinary Cytology*. St. Louis, MO: Ralston Purina Company, 1980.

Reding J. Bordetelia Bronchiseptica: Is your cattery at risk? (On-line). http://www.fanciers.com/other-faqs/bordetalla.html, 1996

Richards JR, et al. Caring for the senior cat, American Association of Feline Practitioners/Academy of Feline Medicine Update Vol 2. *Veterinary Technician* 1999;20:368-372.

Richards JR, et al. "Caring for the senior cat, American Association of Feline Practitioners/Academy of Feline Medicine Update Vol 3. *Veterinary Technician* 1999;20:438-441.

Rivera MJ. Homeopathy: Like cures like. *Veterinary Technician* 2000;21:681-684.

Rivera MJ. A pointed approach: The fundamentals of veterinary acupuncture. *Veterinary Technician* 2000;21:32-40.

Rivera MJ, Rivera PL. Veterinary chiropractic. *Veterinary Technician* 2000;21:301-304.

Root C. Contrast radiography for veterinary technologists. 1985 Annual Veterinary Technology Convention.

Royer N. Step by step, performing cystocentesis. *Veterinary Technician* 1997;18:298-299.

Sandman KM., Harari J. Canine cranial cruciate ligament repair techniques: Is one best? *Veterinary Medicine* 2001;96:850-855.

Schebitz H, Wilkens H. *Atlas of Radiographic Anatomy of the Dog and Cat*, 3rd Ed. Philadelphia, PA: W.B. Saunders Co., 1978.

Schoen AM, Wynn SG. *Complementary and Alternative Veterinary Medicine*. St. Louis, MO: Mosby, 1998.

Severin GA. *Severin's Veterinary Ophthalmology Notes*, 3rd Ed. Fort Collins, CO: Veterinary Ophthalmology Notes, 1996.

Shaffran N. Blood gas analysis. *Veterinary Technician* 1998;19:95-103.

Shaffran N. Pain in critically ill small animals: Ethical aspects. *Veterinary Technician* 1998;19:349-353.

Shipp AD, Fahrenkrug P. *Practitioners' Guide to Veterinary Dentistry*, 1st Ed. Glendale, CA: Griffin Printing, Inc., 1992.

Skarda RT. Anesthesia case of the month. *JAVMA*, 1999;214:37-39.

Slater DH. *Textbook of Small Animal Surgery*, Vol 1., Philadelphia, PA: W.B. Saunders Company, 1985.

Slatter D. *Fundamentals of Veterinary Ophthalmology*, 2nd Ed. Philadelphia, PA: W. B. Saunders Company, 1990.

Slatter D. *Textbook of Small Animal Surgery*, 2nd Ed, Vol. 2.. Philadelphia, PA: W. B. Saunders, 1993.

Spellane-Newman M. Laser surgery: The cutting edge. *Veterinary Technician* 2001;22: 412-416.

Stafford D. The great mimic: Canine Addison's disease. *Veterinary Technician* 1999;20: 490-497.

Stedman TL. *Stedman's Concise Medical Dictionary*, 3rd Ed. Baltimore, MD: Williams & Wilkins, 1997.

Stein D. *Natural Healing for Dogs & Cats*. Freedom, IA: The Crossing Press, 1993.

Strombeck DR. *Home-Prepared Dog & Cat Diets: The Healthful Alternative*. Ames, IA: Iowa State University Press, 1999.

Swaim SF, Henderson RA Jr. *Small Animal Wound Management*, 2nd Ed. Philadelphia, PA: Williams & Wilkins, 1997.

Tabers CW. *Taber's Cyclopedic Medical Dictionary*. Philadelphia, PA: F. A. Davis Company, 1989.

Thrall DE. *Textbook of Veterinary Diagnostic Radiology*. Philadelphia, PA: W.B. Saunders, 1986.

Ticer JW. *Radiographic Technique in Veterinary Practice*. Philadelphia, PA: W. B. Saunders, 1984.

Tighe MM, Brown M. *Mosby's Comprehensive Review for Veterinary Technicians*, Baltimore, MD: Mosby, 1998.

Tilley LP. *Essentials of Canine and Feline Electrocardiography Interpretation and Treatment*, 3rd Ed. Philadelphia, PA: Lippincott Williams and Wilkins, 1992.

Tilley LP, Smith FWK Jr. *The 5-Minute Veterinary Consult, Canine and Feline*, 2nd Ed. Philadelphia, PA: Lippincott, Williams and Wilkins, 2000.

Tracy DL. *Mosby's Fundamentals of Veterinary Technology Small Animal Surgical Nursing*. St. Louis, MO: Mosby, 1994.

Volhard W, Brown K. *The Holistic Guide for a Healthy Dog*. New York: Howell Book House, 1995.

Wagner AE. Is butorphanol analgesic in dogs and cats? *Veterinary Medicine* 1999;94:346-351.

Wanamaker BP, Pettes CL. *Applied Pharmacology for the Veterinary Technician*. Philadelphia, PA: W. B. Saunders, 1996.

Williams JF, Zajac A. *Diagnosis of Gastrointestinal Parasitism in Dogs and Cats*. St. Louis, MO: Ralston Purina Company, 1980.

Williams LT, Bagley RS. Pot-bellied dogs? Diagnosing and managing canine hyperadrenocorticism. *Veterinary Technician* 1998;19:47-56.

Wilson S. Feeding tube care. *Internal Medicine and Endoscopy*, Photocopy.

Wingfield WE, Bowen RA. *Enteral Feeding Calculations*. (On-line). Available: http:/www.cvmbs.colostate.edu/clinsci/wing/enteral.html, Colorado State University, 1998.

Wingfield SG, Wingfield WE. Triage in trauma: Nursing implications and initial assessment. *Veterinary Technician, 1997;18*:183-190.

Wingfield WE. *Enteral Nutritional Support in Critically Ill Dogs and Cats: Making the Right Decisions*. Colorado State University, Fort Collins, 1998.

Wischnitzer S. *Atlas and Dissection Guide for Comparative Anatomy*, 5th Ed. New York: W.H. Freeman and Company, 1993.

Wortinger A. Learning and teaching from pet food labels. *Veterinary Technician* 1999;19:586-590.

Wortinger A. Managing inflammatory bowel disease. *Veterinary Technician* 1998;19:689-695.

Wortinger A. Nutritional support for hospitalized pets. *Veterinary Technician* 1999;20:316-323.

Wynn SG. *Herb Doses for Small Animal Patients*. (On-line). Available: http://www.vin.com/members/searchdb/misc/m05000/m00923.htm, Veterinary Information Network, 2000.

Zigler M. *Glaucoma of the Veterinary Patient*. (On-line). Available: http://www.eyevet.ca, Eyevet Consulting Services, 2001.

Zigler M. *Prolapsed Gland of the Third Eyelid*. (On-line). Available: http://www.eyevet.ca, Eyevet Consulting Services, 2001.

Zsombor-Murray E, Freeman LM. Peripheral parenteral nutrition. *Compendium on Continuing Education for the Practicing Veterinarian* 1999;21:512-523.

Index

Page numbers in *italics* denote figures.